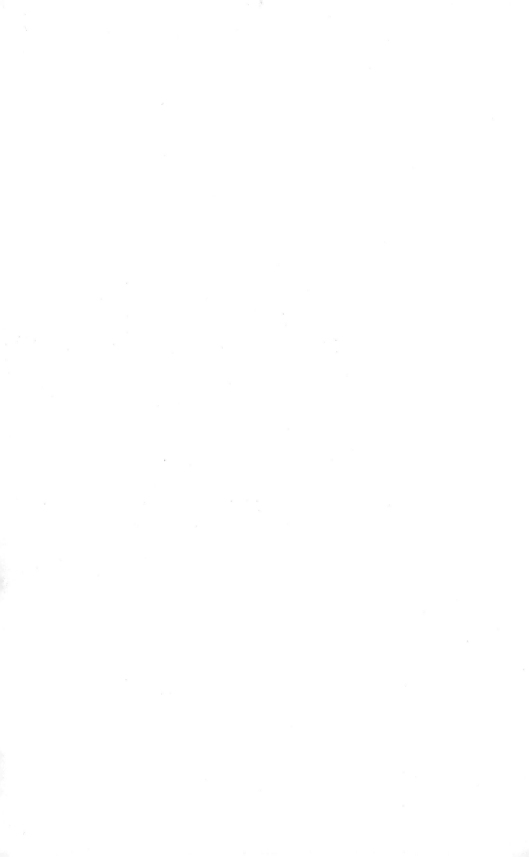

THE DENTAL CLINICS OF NORTH AMERICA

Dental Therapeutics Update

PAUL A. MOORE, DMD, PhD, MPH,
ELLIOT V. HERSH, DMD, MS, PhD, GUEST EDITORS

VOLUME 46 • NUMBER 4 • OCTOBER 2002

W.B. SAUNDERS COMPANY
A Division of Elsevier Science
PHILADELPHIA   LONDON   TORONTO   MONTREAL   SYDNEY   TOKYO

W.B. SAUNDERS COMPANY
A Division of Elsevier Science

The Curtis Center • Independence Square West • Philadelphia, Pennsylvania 19106

http://www.wbsaunders.com

THE DENTAL CLINICS OF NORTH AMERICA
October 2002
Editor: John Vassallo

Volume 46, Number 4
ISSN 0011-8532

Reprints: For copies of 100 or more, of articles in this publication, please contact the commercial Reprints Department, Elsevier Science Inc., 360 Park Avenue South, New York, New York, 10010-1710. Tel. (212) 633–3813 Fax: (212) 633–3820 email: reprints@elsevier.com.

The ideas and opinions expressed in *The Dental Clinics of North America* do not necessarily reflect those of the Publisher. The Publisher does not assume any responsibility for any injury and/or damage to persons or property arising out of or related to any use of the material contained in this periodical. The reader is advised to check the appropriate medical literature and the product information currently provided by the manufacturer of each drug to be administered to verify the dosage, the method and duration of administration, or contraindications. It is the responsibility of the treating physician or other health care professional, relying on independent experience and knowledge of the patient, to determine drug dosages and the best treatment for the patient. Mention of any product in this issue should not be construed as endorsement by the contributors, editors, or the Publisher of the product or manufacturers' claims.

The Dental Clinics of North America (ISSN 0011-8532) is published quarterly by W.B. Saunders Company. Corporate and Editorial Offices: The Curtis Center, Independence Square West, Philadelphia, PA 19106-3399. Accounting and circulation offices: 6277 Sea Harbor Drive, Orlando, FL 32887-4800. Periodicals postage paid at Orlando, FL 32862, and additional mailing offices. Subscription prices are $135.00 per year (US individuals), $187.00 per year (US institutions), $160.00 per year (Canadian individuals), $234.00 per year (Canadian institutions), $68.00 per year (US students/residents), $182.00 per year (foreign individuals), and $234.00 per year (foreign institutions) and $93.00 (Canadian and foreign students/residents). Foreign air speed delivery is included in all *Clinics* subscription prices. All prices are subject to change without notice. POSTMASTER: Send address changes to *The Dental Clinics of North America*, W.B. Saunders Company, Periodicals Fulfillment, Orlando, FL 32887–4800. **Customer Service: 1-800-654-2452 (US). From outside of the US, call 1-407-345-4000.**

The Dental Clinics of North America is covered in *Index Medicus, Current Contents/Clinical Medicine, ISI/BIOMED and Clinahl.*

Printed in the United States of America.

GUEST EDITORS

PAUL A. MOORE, DMD, PhD, MPH, Professor, Pharmacology and Dental Public Health; Director, Oral Health Science Institute, Department of Dental Public Health, University of Pittsburgh School of Dental Medicine, Pittsburgh, Pennsylvania

ELLIOT V. HERSH, DMD, MS, PhD, Associate Professor, Oral Surgery and Pharmacology; Associate Dean for Clinical Research, University of Pennsylvania School of Dental Medicine, Philadelphia, Pennsylvania

CONTRIBUTORS

GEORGE ABDELSHEHID, BS, Pre-doctoral Fellow, Harvard School of Dental Medicine, Boston, Massachusetts

GEORGE ACS, DMD, MPH, Chairman, Department of Dentistry, Children's National Medical Center; Associate Professor, Pediatrics, George Washington University School of Medicine, Washington, District of Columbia

DANIEL BECKER, DDS, Professor, Allied Health Technology, Sinclair College; Director, Dental Anesthesia Education, General Practice Residency, Miami Valley Hospital, Dayton, Ohio

MICHAEL T. BRENNAN, DDS, MHS, Director, Oral Medicine Residency, Department of Oral Medicine, Carolinas Medical Center, Charlotte, North Carolina

SCOTT S. DEROSSI, DMD, Assistant Professor, Department of Oral Medicine, University of Pennsylvania School of Dental Medicine, Philadelphia, Pennsylvania

RAYMOND A. DIONNE, DDS, PhD, Clinical Director, Pain and Neurosensory Mechanisms Branch, National Institute of Dental and Craniofacial Research, National Institutes of Health, Bethesda, Maryland

RICHARD L. FINDER, DMD, MS, Clinical Associate Professor, Physiology and Pharmacology, University of Pittsburgh School of Dental Medicine; Private Anesthesia Practice, Ambulatory Anesthesia Associates, Pittsburgh, Pennsylvania

PHILIP C. FOX, DDS, Visiting Scientist, Department of Oral Medicine, Carolinas Medical Center, Charlotte, North Carolina

J. MAX GOODSON, DDS, PhD, Senior Staff, Department of Periodontology, The Forsyth Institute, Boston, Massachusetts

JAMES GUGGENHEIMER, DDS, Professor, Department of Oral Medicine and Pathology; Professor, Department of Otolaryngology, University of Pittsburgh School of Dental Medicine, Pittsburgh, Pennsylvania

WENDY S. GULDEN, DDS, MS, Assistant Professor, Department of Restorative Sciences—Endodontics, University of Minnesota School of Dentistry, Minneapolis, Minnesota

DANIEL A. HAAS, DDS, PhD, FRCD(C), Associate Dean, Clinical Sciences, Faculty of Dentistry; Professor and Head, Anesthesia, Faculty of Dentistry; Professor, Department of Pharmacology, Faculty of Medicine; Active Staff, Sunnybrook and Women's College Health Sciences Center, University of Toronto, Toronto, Ontario, Canada

J. MEL HAWKINS, DDS, BScD(An), FADSA, DADBA, Director, Intravenous Sedation, Continuing Education Program, Faculty of Dentistry, University of Toronto; Private Practice, Toronto, Ontario, Canada

MARC W. HEFT, DMD, PhD, Director, Claude D. Pepper Center for Research on Oral Health in Aging; Associate Chairman, Professor, Department of Oral and Maxillofacial Surgery and Diagnostic Sciences, University of Florida, Gainesville, Florida

ELLIOT V. HERSH, DMD, MS, PhD, Associate Professor, Oral Surgery and Pharmacology; Associate Dean for Clinical Research, University of Pennsylvania School of Dental Medicine, Philadelphia, Pennsylvania

DOUGLASS L. JACKSON, DMD, MS, PhD, Associate Professor, Department of Oral Medicine, University of Washington School of Dentistry, Seattle, Washington

BARTON S. JOHNSON, DDS, MS, Associate Professor, Departments of Restorative Dentistry and Hospital Dentistry, University of Washington School of Dentistry, Seattle, Washington

ASMA A. KHAN, BDS, PhD, Clinical Research Fellow, Department of Oral and Craniofacial Biological Sciences, Dental School, University of Maryland, Baltimore, Maryland; National Institutes of Dental and Craniofacial Research, National Institutes of Health, Bethesda, Maryland

PETER B. LOCKHART, DDS, Chairman, Department of Oral Medicine, Carolinas Medical Center, Charlotte, North Carolina

ANGELO J. MARIOTTI, DDS, PhD, Chairman, Associate Professor, Department of Periodontics, The Ohio State University College of Dentistry, Columbus, Ohio

NINA MARKOVIC, PhD, Assistant Professor, Department of Dental Public Health, Department of Epidemiology, Graduate School of Public Health, University of Pittsburgh School of Dental Medicine, Pittsburgh, Pennsylvania

JOHN G. MEECHAN, BSc, BDS, FDSRCPS, PhD, Senior Lecturer, Department of Oral and Maxillofacial Surgery, University of Newcastle upon Tyne, Newcastle upon Tyne, United Kingdom

PAUL A. MOORE, DMD, PhD, MPH, Professor, Pharmacology and Dental Public Health; Director, Oral Health Science Institute, Department of Dental Public Health, University of Pittsburgh School of Dental Medicine, Pittsburgh, Pennsylvania

LENNY W. NAFTALIN, DDS, Chief Resident, Section of Anesthesiology, University of California at Los Angeles School of Dentistry, Los Angeles, California

RICHARD NIEDERMAN, DMD, Senior Scientist, Department of Cytokine Biology; Director, Center for Evidence-Based Dentistry, The Forsyth Institute, Boston, Massachusetts

JAMES C. PHERO, DMD, Professor, Clinical Anesthesia, Pediatrics, and Surgery; Faculty, University of Cincinnati Physicians Pain Center, Anesthesia Department, College of Medicine, University of Cincinnati, Cincinnati, Ohio

ERIK SCHEIFELE, DMD, Assistant Professor, Division of Pediatric Dentistry, Temple University School of Dentistry, Philadelphia, Pennsylvania

ROBIN A. SEYMOUR, BDS, PhD, Professor, Department of Restorative Dentistry, The Dental School, Newcastle upon Tyne, United Kingdom

GALIB SHARIFF, DDS, Resident, Oral Medicine, Department of Oral Medicine, Carolinas Medical Center, Charlotte, North Carolina

DEBORAH STUDENPAVLOVICH, DMD, Professor and Director, Predoctoral Pediatric Dentistry, Department of Pediatric Dentistry, University of Pittsburgh School of Dental Medicine, Pittsburgh, Pennsylvania

JAMES Q. SWIFT, DDS, Director, Oral and Maxillofacial Surgery; Associate Professor, Department of Diagnostic and Surgical Sciences, University of Minnesota School of Dentistry, Minneapolis, Minnesota

ANUPAMA RAO TATE, DMD, Director, Satellite Facilities, Department of Dentistry, Children's National Medical Center; Assistant Professor, Pediatrics, George Washington University School of Medicine, Washington, District of Columbia

MICHAEL D. WEBB, DDS, Associate Professor, Director, Graduate Program, Pediatric Dentistry, Baylor College of Medicine; Chief, Clinical Department of Dentistry, Attending Pediatric Dentist/Dental Anesthesiologist, Children's Medical Center of Dallas; Attending Pediatric Dentists/Dental Anesthesiologist, Texas Scottish Rite Hospital for Children, Dallas, Texas

JOHN M. WHITWORTH, BChD, PhD, Senior Lecturer, Department of Restorative Dentistry, The Dental School, Newcastle upon Tyne, United Kingdom

JOHN A. YAGIELA, DDS, PhD, Professor and Chair, Division of Diagnostic and Surgical Sciences, University of California at Los Angeles School of Dentistry, Los Angeles, California

CONTENTS

Preface   xv
Paul A. Moore and Elliot V. Hersh

Section I: Antimicrobial Agents

Antibiotic Therapy—Managing Odontogenic Infections   623
James Q. Swift and Wendy S. Gulden

>   Several pharmaceuticals have been developed in the past 10 years
>   that have made a significant impact on the health of the human race.
>   There have been few advances, however, that have proved more ef-
>   ficacious than the pharmacotherapies we have had available for
>   many decades for the treatment of odontogenic infections. Many
>   new antibiotics/antimicrobials have been developed, but none have
>   been determined to be of significant benefit to replace or supplant the
>   use of penicillins for the management of orofacial infections caused
>   by pathogens in and around the oral cavity. Judicious use of antibio-
>   tics in conjunction with surgical therapy is the most appropriate
>   method to treat odontogenic infections. Using the antibiotic "du
>   jour," many times promoted by pharmaceutical representatives, re-
>   sults in costly and unnecessary complexity of care. A return to the
>   basics is indicated for the antibiotic management of odontogenic
>   infections.

**Antibiotic Prophylaxis for Endocarditis, Prosthetic Joints,
and Surgery**   635
Robin A. Seymour and John M. Whitworth

>   Antibiotics are prescribed in dentistry for two main reasons: to
>   treat infections and to prevent infections. It is the latter that can
>   be regarded as prophylactic use of these drugs. For the perspective
>   of this article, we consider the main indications (or controversies)
>   relating to prophylactic use of antibiotics in dentistry, notably the
>   prevention of infective endocarditis, infections in patients with
>   hip and joint prostheses, and the prevention of infection following
>   various dental surgical procedures.

Antibiotics and Oral Contraceptives   653

Scott S. DeRossi and Elliot V. Hersh

> Oral contraceptives and antibiotics are among the most widely
> used prescription medications in the United States. The proposed
> interaction between oral contraceptives and antibiotics has long
> been a major source of controversy and discussion. Considering
> the relatively high usage of both antibiotics and oral contracep-
> tives, there is little scientific evidence to support this interaction.
> However, sporadic case reports of oral contraceptive failure during
> concomitant antibiotic therapy do appear in the literature. This ar-
> ticle challenges the scientific basis of the alleged interaction and
> summarizes the results of key clinical studies.

**Periodontal Therapy Using Local Delivery of
Antimicrobial Agents**   665

Richard Niederman, George Abdelshehid,
and J. Max Goodson

> Anitmicrobial agents, systemic and/or local, are thought by some
> to be effective agents for treating periodontal infections. Here the
> authors determine the costs and benefits of local delivery agents
> for treating periodontal disease. Applying this cost-benefit analysis
> to patient care, however, will depend upon a clinician's expertise
> and a patient's value system.

Section II: Analgesic and Anti-Inflammatory Agents

**The COX-2 Inhibitors: New Analgesic
and Anti-Inflammatory Drugs**   679

Asma A. Khan and Raymond A. Dionne

> Selective cyclooxygenase-2 (COX-2) inhibitors are a new class of
> nonsteroidal anti-inflammatory drugs (NSAIDs) designed to
> achieve the therapeutic effects of traditional NSAIDs without the de-
> leterious side effects associated with their use. This article reviews
> the therapeutic use of the selective COX-2 inhibitors celecoxib and
> rofecoxib in the management of acute and chronic orofacial
> pain, with emphasis on the potential safety associated with their use.

Rational Use of Analgesic Combinations   691

James C. Phero and Daniel Becker

> The rational use of analgesic combinations offers significant benefit
> to patient's suffering from acute and chronic pain. This article dis-
> cusses the current oral analgesic options commonly available to the
> practitioner and offers prescribing recommendations.

Dental Postoperative Pain Management in Children 707
Anupama Rao Tate and George Acs

Misconceptions have existed about the need for pain management in pediatric patients. We now understand that children feel pain and respond to pain medication in much the same way as adults. With this new understanding, practitioners must recognize all the factors that affect the feeling of pain. Pain can be variable and each patient brings a unique set of characteristics to be evaluated. The first objective should be to assess the patient's previous treatment history, medical condition, extent of treatment needed, and age. An effective pain management protocol begins with preoperative pain and anxiety control, with the use of agents such as nitrous oxide and local anesthetics. Postoperative pain medication should be given at the correct dosage and time intervals for the appropriate duration. With our commitment to pain management in children, these protocols should easily translate into improved clinical practice.

Section III: Local Anesthetic Agents

Local Anesthesia: Advances in Agents and Techniques 719
J. Mel Hawkins and Paul A. Moore

The improvements in agents and techniques for local anesthesia are possibly the most important advances in dental science to have occurred in the past 100 years. The agents currently available in dentistry have most of the characteristics of an ideal local anesthetic. Today's anesthetics can be administered with minimal irritation and little concern for stimulating allergic reactions. A variety of agents are available that provide rapid onset of surgical anesthesia with adequate duration. This article provides a brief review of the local anesthetic agents, formulations, and techniques used in dentistry with special emphasis on newly introduced agents and procedures.

Vasoconstrictors: Indications and Precautions 733
Lenny W. Naftalin and John A. Yagiela

Vasoconstrictors are useful additives to local anesthetic solutions. They can enhance the duration and quality of the anesthetic block while also decreasing surgical blood loss. Precautions must be taken, however, when using vasoconstrictors with certain patients, especially those with cardiovascular disease. Several drug interactions must also be considered before administration of a local anesthetic with a vasoconstrictor, and special care must be taken when injecting such preparations in patients on nonspecific β-adrenergic blockers, tricyclic antidepressants, catechol-O-methytransferase inhibitors, cocaine, and certain general anesthetics. Lastly, in the patient with true sulfite allergy, local anesthetics without a vasoconstrictor should be used.

Adverse Drug Reactions to Local Anesthesia   747
Richard L. Finder and Paul A. Moore

A dentist's ability to safely administer regional anesthesia is essential for dental practice. Local anesthetic solutions used in the United States for dental anesthesia are formulated with several components. The contents of a standard local anesthetic cartridge may include an amide or ester local anesthetic drug, an adrenergic vasoconstrictor, and an antioxidant. In susceptible patients, any of these components may induce systemic, dose-dependent adverse reactions. Although extremely rare, allergic reactions may also occur. Signs and symptoms of the various adverse reactions associated with local anesthetics are quite distinctive, permitting rapid diagnosis and treatment. Serious reactions are extremely infrequent and, when treated properly, unlikely to result in significant morbidity or mortality.

Effective Topical Anesthetic Agents and Techniques   759
John G. Meechan

One technique used to reduce the discomfort of intraoral injection is to apply a topical anesthetic prior to needle penetration. This article describes the published evidenced concerning the pharmacologic benefits of topical anesthesia in the mouth. A number of different factors such as variations in materials, injection site, and duration of topical anesthetic application are important in relation to efficacy.

Section IV: Sedatives and Anxiolytic Agents

Conscious Sedation for Dentistry: Risk Management and Patient Selection   767
Douglass L. Jackson and Barton S. Johnson

The goal of this article is to review the many aspects of risk management that need to be considered when using N_2O/O_2 inhalational sedation and enteral sedation in adults and children. Understanding the regulations and guidelines that need to be followed when delivering conscious sedation greatly increases the margin of safety. This article reviews the definitions and guidelines for delivering conscious sedation, establishes the criteria for selecting appropriate patients, and discusses the many aspects of clinical preparedness.

Inhalational and Enteral Conscious Sedation for the Adult Dental Patient   781
Douglass L. Jackson and Barton S. Johnson

There are clearly many safe and effective sedatives available to the dental practitioner for reducing patient fear and improving their level of comfort. Careful consideration needs to be given to the objectives of the sedation when deciding which pharmacologic agents to use because they all possess slightly different clinical characteristics and various degrees of risk. Patient selection is also critical when making decisions about sedation because the patient's expectations and general health status factor into keeping the procedure safe.

Sedation for Pediatric Dental Patients 803
Michael D. Webb and Paul A. Moore

There are few areas of dental therapeutics as controversial as the pharmacologic management of fearful and uncooperative pediatric dental patients. A pediatric dentist is faced with one of the most difficult tasks in our profession: maximizing comfort and cooperation while minimizing risks and costs of dental care for the unmanageable child. Pharmacosedation provides the means for children to avoid psychologically traumatic experiences that might inhibit regular oral health care when they become adults. By controlling disruptive behaviors, the pediatric dentist is able to provide quality dental care in an environment that is pleasant for the child, the parent, and the practitioner.

Emergency Drugs 815
Daniel A. Haas

It can be assumed that there is universal agreement that dentists require emergency drugs to be readily available. Where there are differences in opinion is the specific drugs that should comprise an emergency kit. This article provides one opinion. Oxygen, epinephrine, nitroglycerin, injectable diphenhydramine or chlorpheniramine, albuterol, and aspirin should be readily available in a dental office. Other drugs, such as glucagon, atropine, ephedrine, hydrocortisone, morphine or nitrous oxide, naloxone, midazolam or lorazepam, and flumazenil also should be considered.

Section V: Agents to Treat Oral Pathology

Practitioner's Guide to Fluoride 831
Erik Scheifele, Deborah Studen-Pavlovich,
and Nina Markovic

The current health care trend is to provide evidence-based recommendations and treatment. Many literature reviews have shown fluoride's effectiveness against caries. The current use of fluoride in the prevention of dental caries is based on community, professional, and individual strategies. Personalized fluoride regimens should include a risk analysis and a review of the patient's current fluoride exposure. The future of fluoride may be found in its slow release and retention in the oral cavity through various modalities. Because of the many uncertainties still associated with fluoride, further research is needed.

Treatment of Xerostomia: A Systematic Review of Therapeutic Trials   847

Michael T. Brennan, Galib Shariff, Peter B. Lockhart, and Philip C. Fox

The purpose of the present article is to systematically assess the level of evidence available in therapeutic clinical trials for the management of xerostomia. Specifically, the authors examine and rate the quality of randomized controlled trials in peer-reviewed journals, using established objective criteria. The goal is to determine the strength of the clinical trial evidence for proposed xerostomia therapies.

Oral Manifestations of Drug Therapy   857

James Guggenheimer

A variety of oral abnormalities may result from side effects of medications that are being taken for medical conditions. The increased availability and use of prescription, over-the-counter, and herbal medications make this a more likely occurrence. Dental practitioners need to be prepared for this and recognize when an oral anomaly may be a manifestation of drug therapy so that the patient can receive appropriate treatment and/or preventive interventions.

Geriatric Pharmacology   869

Marc W. Heft and Angelo J. Mariotti

With the dramatic demographic change that has resulted in the "graying of the population" has come a compelling interest in the health and health concerns of older adults. The increasing incidence and prevalence of systemic diseases, especially chronic diseases, among older adults, and the concomitant increase in medication use, have provided impetus for the subspecialty of geriatric pharmacology. This article reviews the physiologic changes, nonphysiologic aspects, and pharmacologic changes associated with aging and their implications for dental practice.

Cumulative Index 2002   887

FORTHCOMING ISSUES

January 2003

Minority Oral Health
Racquel Z. LeGeros, PhD, and
Norman S. Braveman, PhD, *Guest Editors*

April 2003

Nutrition and Oral Health
Laura Romito, DDS, MS, *Guest Editor*

July 2003

Update on Infectious Diseases and Dentistry
Michael Glick, DMD, *Guest Editor*

RECENT ISSUES

July 2002

Dental Informatics
Titus Schleyer, DMD, PhD, *Guest Editor*

April 2002

Restorative Dentistry
Franklin García-Godoy, DDS, MS, *Guest Editor*

January 2002

Evidence Based Dentistry
Gary R. Goldstein, DDS, *Guest Editor*

THE DENTAL
CLINICS OF
NORTH
AMERICA

Dent Clin N Am 46 (2002) xv–xviii

Preface

Dental therapeutics update

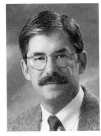
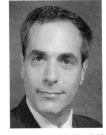

Paul A. Moore, DMD, PhD, MPH   Elliot V. Hersh, DMD, MS, PhD
Guest Editors

Dental pharmacotherapeutics is advancing rapidly. It is a field that requires constant updates in the knowledge of new drugs, drug interactions, and useful therapeutic trends. The goal of this issue of the *Dental Clinics of North America* is to provide an update of therapeutic agents of interest to general practitioners of dentistry. These agents include antimicrobial agents, analgesic and anti-inflammatory drugs, local anesthetic formulations, and sedative and anxiolytic agents. In addition, drugs of special importance for managing unique patient populations such as geriatric patients, pediatric patients, and dry mouth patients are presented. Other topics of importance include supplemental fluoride requirements, oral manifestations of drug therapy, and emergency drugs. Because of the wide variety of therapy used in dentistry, this issue limits therapeutic information to agents useful for the general practitioner. The concise presentations that have been included focus on therapies that are maximally effective and safe.

Patient demographics for the 21st century

Expected changes in the nation's demographics, patient populations, and drug consumption make this review and update of drug therapy particularly timely. The number and proportion of elderly dental patients in the United States will continue to grow. Compared with geriatric patients a decade ago, the prevalence of edentulism and tooth loss has decreased; subsequently, the need for restorative dentistry and periodontal therapy is expected to increase [1,2].

Complex medical and drug histories have become routine for many dental practitioners. Elderly patients tend to have more chronic health problems, and they usually take more medications. The risks associated with new drugs and the implications of multiple drug therapy challenge our understanding of clinical pharmacology and adverse drug reactions.

General practitioners need clear and concise information to keep abreast of the plethora of drug advances. Continual learning is a lifelong enterprise for anyone in a health-related profession; information transfer regarding current drug therapy is particularly demanding because of the rapid changes in drug administration that have occurred in the last few decades. For example, of the 20 drugs most frequently prescribed in 1997, only 10 existed in 1987 [3]. In addition, as many as 30 new drugs are introduced to the market by the pharmaceutical industry each year in the United States [4]. The knowledge of safe and effective drug therapy learned during dental school rapidly becomes irrelevant, and the demand for obtaining reliable new information is a constant challenge for practicing dentists. The authors of this issue of the *Dental Clinics of North America* recognize that one of the most effective means of optimizing therapy is to rapidly and clearly inform practitioners of the existence of these potential complications and recommend alternative therapeutic strategies.

Patients who have chronic diseases, have multiple physician prescribers, and take many different types of drugs will require a thorough patient evaluation. Many obstacles exist to obtaining an accurate medical and drug history. Patients cannot always remember the names and the doses of the drugs they are taking, and many forget to include over-the-counter (OTC) drugs in their histories. Older patients may have limited recall abilities. Not only is it important to know which drugs are being taken by a patient, but the dose and duration of use should be noted. Patients taking higher doses of drugs for longer periods may be at higher risk for a drug interaction. Consulting with prescribing physicians, the patient's pharmacist, and family members may be required in some circumstances.

All drugs taken (including prescription medications, OTC drugs, drugs of abuse, and herbal remedies) as well as compliance with drug regimens should be documented in the patient's dental record. The dental practitioner should have a working knowledge of how these drugs act and any potential drug interactions. Selecting dental therapeutic agents with proven records of clinical efficacy and minimal risks is also recommended. Caution is particularly necessary when treating the high-risk patient. Because of the abundance of newly marketed drugs and drug combinations, the dental practitioner should be suspicious of possible unreported drug interactions until experience is gained with new drug entities.

Various electronic and printed resources are available as resources to the dentist. The *Physician's Desk Reference* provides complete product information for currently marketed drugs and quick drug references such as Lexicomp's *Drug Information Handbook for Dentistry*, Mosby's *Dental Drug*

Reference, the *ADA Guide to Dental Therapeutics*, and The Medical Letter's *Handbook of Adverse Drug Interactions* are extremely useful guides [5–9]. Additionally, the Internet has many websites that permit a practitioner to rapidly source drug information. A valuable review of electronic drug databases useful for a dental practitioner has recently been published [10].

Dental pharmacotherapeutics

Many of the characteristics of drug therapy in dentistry are unique and limit the likelihood of serious drug interactions (see following list). Drug therapy in dentistry is typically administered either as a single dose or for only a short duration. Many of the adverse drug reactions and drug interactions that are associated with changes in the rate of drug metabolism and excretion require repeated dosing before blood concentrations are altered significantly. Most of the drugs used in dental therapy have large margins of safety, which limits the likelihood of many drug interactions. In addition, much of dental therapy is elective and can be postponed if the medical status of a patient is in question or increases the risk of an adverse drug interaction. Finally, there are a limited number of drugs routinely used in dental therapeutics: antibiotics, local anesthetics and vasoconstrictors, analgesics, and sedatives and anxiolytic agents. Consequently, many dental practitioners have a thorough knowledge of the indications, contraindications, and precautions of the drugs they routinely use. Dental practitioners are able to focus their drug information needs toward the clinical significant drug interactions of only a few drugs and drug classes.

Unique characteristics of dental therapeutics
- There are a limited number of agents in a practitioner's armamentarium.
- Either single-dose regimens or therapies with short durations are most common.
- Most dental drug therapies have large margins of safety.
- There is limited use of intravenously administered drugs.
- Elective dental procedures may be scheduled to avoid concomitant medical treatment.
- Research using the third molar extraction model provides robust data sources regarding use of analgesics, local anesthetics, and pharmacosedation.

As the population becomes older and drug consumption subsequently increases, adverse drug interactions will continue to be a major concern in dental practice. The number of elderly patients in the United States will increase for at least the next few decades. Because older patients tend to have more chronic health problems and tend to take more medications, complex medical and drug histories have become routine requirements for many dental practitioners. The risks associated with new drug therapies and the implications of multiple drug therapy challenge our understanding of clinical pharmacology and adverse drug interactions. Fortunately, when used within acceptable dosage guidelines, drugs routinely used in dental practice are relatively safe, and few significant adverse drug reactions or drug interactions are encountered.

The drug therapies described in this issue of the *Dental Clinics of North America* fall into the realm of basic dental therapeutics. Local anesthetic agents are administered for regional anesthesia during one setting and within accepted dose recommendations. Sedative and anxiolytic agents are administered orally immediately before (or possibly the day before) dental treatment. Intravenous drug use and dental therapies lasting beyond a few weeks are not considered common dental therapies and are not included in establishing the significance of drug interactions that are most important for general practitioners.

References

[1] Burt BA, Eklund SA. Dentistry, dental practice, and the community. 4th edition. Philadelphia: WB Saunders Co; 1992.
[2] Marcus SE, Drury TF, Brown LJ, Zion GR. Tooth retention and tooth loss in the permanent dentition of adults: United States, 1988–1991. J Dent Res 1996;75:684–95.
[3] The top 200 drugs. American Druggist 1997;Feb:30–7.
[4] New drugs approved by the FDA in 1997. Pharmacists Letter 1998;2:14.
[5] Physcian's desk reference. 55th edition. Montvale (NJ): Medical Economics; 2001.
[6] Wynn RL, Meiller TF, Crossley HL. Drug information handbook for dentistry. 7th edition. Hudson (OH): Lexicomp; 2001.
[7] Gage TW, Pickett FA. Dental drug reference. 4th edition. St. Louis: Mosby, Inc; 1999.
[8] Rizack MA. The Medical Letter handbook of adverse drug interactions. New Rochelle (NY): Medical Letter, Inc; 1998.
[9] Ciancio SG, editor. ADA guide to dental therapeutics. 2nd edition. Chicago: ADA Publishing; 2000.
[10] Wynn RL. Internet Web sites for drug information. Gen Dent 1998;46:12–8.

Paul A. Moore, DMD, PhD, MPH
Professor, Pharmacology and Dental Public Health
Department of Dental Public Health
University of Pittsburgh
School of Dental Medicine
552 Salk Hall, 3501 Terrace Street
Pittsburgh, PA 15261, USA

Elliot V. Hersh, DMD, MS, PhD
Associate Professor of Oral Surgery and Pharmacology
Department of Oral Surgery and Pharmacology
University of Pennsylvania School of Dental Medicine
4001 Spruce Street, Philadelphia, PA 19104-6003, USA

THE DENTAL
CLINICS OF
NORTH
AMERICA

Dent Clin N Am 46 (2002) 623–633

Antibiotic therapy—managing odontogenic infections

James Q. Swift, DDS[a],*, Wendy S. Gulden, DDS, MS[b]

[a]*Oral and Maxillofacial Surgery, Department of Diagnostic and Surgical Sciences,
University of Minnesota School of Dentistry, 515 Delaware Street Southeast,
7-174C Moos T, Minneapolis, MN 55455, USA*
[b]*Department of Restorative Sciences—Endodontics, University of Minnesota
School of Dentistry, Minneapolis, MN 55455, USA*

Several pharmaceuticals have been developed in the past 10 years that have made a significant impact on the health of the human race. There have been few advances, however, that have proved more efficacious than the pharmacotherapies we have had available for many decades for the treatment of odontogenic infections. Many new antibiotics/antimicrobials have been developed, but none have been determined to be of significant benefit to replace or supplant the use of penicillins for the management of orofacial infections caused by pathogens in and around the oral cavity. Judicious use of antibiotics in conjunction with surgical therapy is the most appropriate method to treat odontogenic infections. Using the antibiotic "du jour," many times promoted by pharmaceutical representatives, results in costly and unnecessary complexity of care. A return to the basics is indicated for the antibiotic management of odontogenic infections.

Chemotherapy is defined as the use of synthetic, semi-synthetic, and naturally occurring chemicals that selectively inhibit specific organisms causing disease. The term antibiotic means "against life" (*anti* = against and *bio-sis* = life).

The decision to use an antimicrobial/antibiotic agent in managing an odontogenic infection is based on several factors. The clinician must first diagnose the cause of the infection and determine the appropriate dental treatment that may include multiple modalities, including initiation of endodontic therapy and pulpectomy, odontectomy, or surgical or mechanical disruption of the infectious environment. The determination as to whether

---

* Corresponding author.
E-mail address: swift001@umn.edu (J.Q. Swift).

conjunctive antibiotic therapy is indicated is based on several factors, including host defense mechanisms, severity of the infection, magnitude of the extension of the infection, and expected pathogen. Because of the lack of circulation within dental pulp, the normal host defenses (inflammation and immunity) are compromised and the root canal system becomes a unique environment to harbor a limited group of bacteria.

Most odontogenic infections are polymicrobial and are composed of at least two predominating bacteria [1]. Most bacteria comprising the oral flora are nonpathogenic and have not been shown to proliferate and grow in host tissue [1]. When the dental pulp is overwhelmed from the bacterial attack, a local acute inflammatory response is seen, followed by nonspecific and specific immunologic reactions with the presence of lymphocytes, plasma cells, and macrophages. Eventually polymorphonuclear lymphocytes (PMNs) are chemotactically attracted to the area of damaged tissue. An abscess, a fibro-collagenous layer of tissue, may form around an accumulation of PMNs in the region of infection, isolating it from surrounding tissue. Because the host may be unable to resorb the abscess and resolve the infection, root canal treatment, extraction, or other surgical therapy is needed to remove the cause. Recent studies demonstrate that a localized abscess may be an inflammatory/immunologic phenomenon and in some patients represents a non-bacterial cause for the periapical localized clinical symptoms [2,3]. The effectiveness of an oral antibiotic as primary and sole treatment for an infection of odontogenic etiology is highly questionable because of the lack of effective circulation in a necrotic pulp system and an abscess. This concept reinforces the idea that surgery of some kind is the primary treatment of an infection of odontogenic source, and that antibiotic therapy is adjunctive care. Observations reveal that many clinicians, however, do treat odontogenic infections primarily with antibiotics, especially when there is a question as to the etiology of the symptoms of a potential infective process. Endorsement of a philosophy of care that antibiotic administration is low risk and potential high yield cannot be substantiated, especially with the current concern regarding bacteria that have developed resistance to current antibiotic therapy. Antibiotics should not be prescribed as a substitute for proper dental treatment.

Mechanism of action

Antibiotics have various effects on bacteria based on their pharmacologic action. The most commonly used antibiotics in dentistry (penicillins, cephalosporins, and vancomycin) work by attacking the cellular processes necessary for the bacterial cell wall synthesis while having no effect on host cells. Other commonly used antibiotics in dentistry exert their effect by inhibiting translation needed for bacterial protein synthesis (erythromycins, tetracyclines, aminoglycosides, and chloramphenicol). Metronidazole, indicated in dentistry for anaerobic bacterial infections, is a direct-acting agent that binds and degrades DNA in bacteria. Still other antibiotics (amphotericin B, polymixins) act by inhibiting cell membrane function. Further development in determining the difference between host and bacterial protein synthesis may lead to the development of alternative sensitive and specific antibiotic therapeutics.

The emergence of resistant bacteria is growing. The microbial ecosystem is engaged in trying to remain opportunistic and by mutating and adapting, resistant strains develop. Specific enzymes can destroy the antibiotic once it has entered the bacteria, permeability into the cell wall can become difficult, and an alteration of certain targets that the drug attaches to become apparent. Mutations in any of these functions can result in loss of sensitivity and specificity to any of the previously mentioned antibiotics.

New synthetic antibiotics for potential use in dental-related infections are the quinolones (cinoxacin, nalidixic acid, and methenamine) and the fluoroquinolones (ciprofloxacin, norfloxacin, and ofloxacin). These agents should be considered when culture results have revealed that these antibiotics are warranted. They have a broader spectrum of action and inhibit bacterial DNA replication (fluoroquinolones inhibit DNA gyrase that inhibits the uncoiling of DNA for replication). The limited indication and the high cost of these drugs is a serious consideration before prescribing. They are rarely used in the management of odontogenic infections.

Bacteria have two major advantages that allow them to survive and prosper in the host system. They replicate quickly and can produce multiple mutations spontaneously. Once a mutation is present, all bacteria offspring generally acquire the new trait. Genetic transfer is another process that bacteria possess. Genetic transfer allows families of bacteria to share desirable traits with a wide range of microbial species. It has recently been found that antibiotic-resistant genes can be passed among every species of bacteria.

Indications for the use of antibiotics

Clinical effectiveness in treating an infection is based on correct diagnosis. Once the source of the infection has been established, dental procedures should be used immediately to disrupt the microorganisms involved. Antibiotic therapy should be used as an adjunct to dental treatment and never used alone as the first line of care. Antibiotics are indicated when systemic signs of involvement are evident. Pain alone or localized swellings do not require antibiotic treatment. Fevers greater than 100° F, malaise, lymphadenopathy, or trismus are clinical signs that possible spread of the infection has occurred. A rapidly spreading infection or persistent infections are other indications for which one may prescribe an antibiotic. Clinicians should consider consulting a specialist if the swelling spreads to extraoral spaces or obstructs breathing or swallowing. The choice of an antibiotic should be based on knowledge of the usual causative microbe. The empiric approach usually results in favorable outcomes [4,5]. Penicillin is the first choice in managing odontogenic infections because it is susceptible to gram-positive aerobes and intraoral anaerobes, organisms found in alveolar abscesses, periodontal abscesses, and necrotic pulps. Patients with compromised host defense systems may indicate antibiotic therapy in conjunction with their dental treatment. Organ transplant patients and patients with poorly controlled diabetes are two examples that point toward the use of antibiotic therapy.

Indications for culturing

Although culturing is rarely required in managing odontogenic infections, at times it is necessary to resolve a progressive infection. Culturing methods have improved over the years; however, one should keep in mind that a bias may occur during the isolation and culturing of bacteria. Many anaerobic microbes are killed quickly when exposed to oxygen. Needle aspiration techniques and transfer under inert gas should be used when culturing for aerobic and anaerobic bacteria in the oral cavity. The antibiotic is then chosen to treat the predominant microbe found in the culture if empiric therapy has failed. The following are indications for culturing an odontogenic infection.

1. The patient is not responding to the first antibiotic prescribed after 48 hours and appropriate dental treatment has been completed.
2. The infection is progressing to other facial spaces.
3. The patient is immunocompromised or has a history of bacterial endocarditis and is not responding to the antibiotic therapy.

Antibiotic treatment should begin immediately even when a culture is taken because of the rapid spread of oral infections.

Antibiotics of choice

Penicillin is still the gold standard in treating dental infections. Penicillin has contributed to a dramatic decrease in mortality in serious odontogenic infections such as Ludwig's angina and diffuse orofacial cellulitis [6]. Aerobic and anaerobic microorganisms are susceptible to penicillin [7]. Pen VK is the obvious choice over Pen G because of the greater oral absorption by Pen VK. Pen VK is bactericidal and active against replicating bacteria often encountered in odontogenic infections [8]. The side effect encountered most often in penicillin is hypersensitivity, which is found in roughly 3–5% of the population. Certain bacteria can develop resistance to the penicillins because of the B-lactamase enzymes that inactivate the penicillin. A combination antibiotic consisting of a penicillin and clavulanic acid, a B-lactamase inhibitor, or the use of clindamycin, an antibiotic specific for infections caused by staphylococci, streptococci, pneumococci, and other bacterial species may be necessary in an infection not responding to penicillin alone. Cephalexin, cephradine, or cephadroxil, all first generation cephalosporins, provide a slightly broader antibiotic spectrum, especially when gram-positive organisms are suspected to be the cause of the infection being treated. Cephalosporins beyond the first generation are not indicated in most odontogenic infections.

If an antibiotic is warranted, providing adequate blood levels is essential. A loading dose of 2000 mg Pen VK approximately 1 hour before beginning surgical therapy followed by 500 mg every 6 hours for 5–7 days is optimal. If the infectious signs and symptoms continue beyond 5–7 days, additional antibiotic therapy may be indicated. If within 48 hours the patient is not responding to penicillin, one could consider adding metronidazole. It is prescribed in a 500-mg dose every 8 hours for the duration of the antibiotic therapy. Metronidazole is active only against obligate anaerobic bacteria by penetrating all bacterial cells and inhibiting DNA replication. It should not be used in pregnant patients or patients with a history of seizures, and if combined with ethyl alcohol can produce nausea and vomiting. Another alternative to treat an infection that is not responding to penicillin is clindamycin. It may be used as a first-line antibiotic if the infection is deemed to be more mature and potentially has spread to bone. Indiscriminate use should be avoided (see later discussion). A loading dose of 600 mg may be administered approximately 1 hour before surgical therapy begins, followed with 300 mg every 6 hours for the duration of the infection (5–7 days).

Appropriate diagnosis and surgical therapy coupled with the empiric use of antibiotics and sound clinical judgment in assessing improvement is the standard of care in the management of odontogenic infections

Antibiotic preparations for odontogenic infections for adults

Pen VK 500 mg every 6 hours, tablets: 125 mg, 250 mg, and 500 mg
Amoxicillin 500 mg every 8 hours, tablets: 250 mg
Metronidazole 500 mg every 8 hours, tablets: 250 mg and 500 mg
Clindamycin 150–300 mg every 6 hours, capsules: 75 mg and 150 mg

Myths

There are many myths that pervade the clinical practice of dentists regarding the diagnosis and management of odontogenic infections. These behaviors have been observed repeatedly in the course of clinical practice. To dispel the continued improper use of antibiotics in the dental environment, these myths are exposed in this discussion.

Myth #1: antibiotics are not harmful

The unwarranted administration of antibiotics is not without risk. The risks for pseudomembranous colitis and allergic reaction must be taken into consideration before prescribing.

Many antibiotics can disturb the normal microbial flora of the gastrointestinal tract, which may cause severe diarrhea and potentially fatal pseudomembranous colitis. These reactions occur more frequently when using oral administration of antibiotics versus parenteral administration, based on variation of hepatic circulation of the drug associated with the two mechanisms of administration. Various degrees of allergic responses have been reported with the use of common antibiotics used for odontogenic infections. Dermatologic reactions such as rash or hives represent milder reactions, whereas life-threatening anaphylactoid reactions have occurred. It has been estimated that 100–300 fatal allergic reactions to penicillin occur annually in the United States [9,10]. For an allergic reaction to have occurred, previous exposure to the drug is necessary. This may have occurred by the patient receiving the antibiotic in beef, milk, or poultry products where the uncontrolled use leaves a residue of the antibiotic in food products [11]. It has been estimated when given amoxicillin that 1 in every 10 patients develops a rash, 1 in every 10,000 develops anaphylactic reactions, and 1 in every 100,000 dies from an allergic reaction [12–14]. Two types of allergic reactions can arise. An acute allergic response or an anaphylactic reaction occurs within 30 minutes of receiving the drug and the reactions include bronchoconstriction, urticaria, angioedema, and shock. Treatment of this type of reaction involves the administration of epinephrine, antihistamine, and possible corticosteroids. Delayed allergic responses take longer than 2 hours to develop and demonstrate mild skin rashes, glossitis, and local inflammatory reactions. Therefore, antibiotic therapy should not be prescribed unless justification for the need is warranted. The improper use of antibiotics can cause the patient serious adverse effects. It is the clinician's responsibility to determine the benefit:risk ratio before administrating the antibiotic.

Myth #2: doses and duration of antibiotic treatment should be nonspecific and variable for most odontogenic infections

Inappropriate dosing of an antibiotic can result in inadequate concentration of the drug at the site of the infection. This practice can promote recurrence of infections and development of resistant bacterial strains. As vulnerable microorganisms die, the number of surviving microbes increases, making each successive bacterial generation better equipped to resist future antibiotic challenges. This selection process accelerates when the drugs are administered in doses small enough to allow stronger bacteria to survive the antibiotic assault. Eventually, strains of bacteria are created that can resist antibiotic therapy. In an average size patient with an odontogenic infection serious enough to warrant antibiotic therapy, there is little indication for the use of doses of penicillin as low as 250 mg. Five hundred mg of penicillin is the lowest dose that should be prescribed for an adult. Inadequate duration of the therapy or overdosing of the antibiotic can also result in damaging the host response and producing toxic effects. A rule of thumb when prescribing is that the antibiotic should last for 3 days after the patient's symptoms have resolved. Treatment of most odontogenic infections requires an average of 5–7 days of therapy; however, treatment of severe infections or immunocompromised patients' therapy may be of longer duration.

Patient compliance is another complication in effective treatment. The drug may be too expensive or not covered by a third party payer and the prescription remains unfilled. Dosing frequency may be complicated. The compliance issue most often observed is missed doses after clinical symptoms have subsided. Another challenge to compliance is the untoward or unexpected side effects that can occur when taking antibiotics. In all these cases, mutated microbes can flourish and cause serious consequences.

*Myth #3: antibiotics are always indicated when treating
dental pain (odontalgia)*

Irreversible pulpitis is a result of severe inflammation of the pulp system. A large quantity of inflammatory mediators and neuropeptides are present, which results in vascular permeability and elevated capillary pressure. Because of the hard tissue in which the pulp is encased and its low-compliance environment, the pulp is unable to neutralize these mediators. Pain is often caused by the release of these mediators that lower pain thresholds and causes spontaneous firing of sensory nerves. Pain of irreversible pulpitis may be sharp, dull, localized, or diffuse, and may last minutes to days. Chemomechanical removal of the pulpal tissue is the treatment of choice. An old but often popular idea was the use of intracanal medicaments to help alleviate the patient's pain complaint. This concept can be dismissed as it is ineffectual. Cleaning and shaping of the root canal with the use of sodium hypochlorite, a dry cotton pellet, and temporization of the access is the desired treatment [15]. Odontectomy may be indicated if the tooth is deemed to be nonrestorable. Appropriate analgesics may be indicated but antibiotics are not. The patient's condition should improve rapidly once the source of the infection is eliminated. If the problem persists, consultation with a specialist may be warranted.

Myth #4: clindamycin is a first line drug for infections

Clindamycin is an antimicrobial reserved for anaerobic, later stage odontogenic infections. It exhibits bacteriostatic activity, thereby inhibiting protein synthesis. Clindamycin should be considered only as the first line of choice if the patient has had an allergic reaction to penicillin or if it can be determined that an osteomyelitis caused by anaerobic microbes is present [7]. It is an excellent choice for treating serious intraosseous infections. Clindamycin has less antigenic potential than penicillin, but has a slightly higher incidence of gastrointestinal adverse effects caused by the overgrowth of *Clostridium difficile* [16]. Recent studies show that colitis is a possible adverse effect of most antibiotics, especially broad-spectrum penicillins and cephalosporins. This condition is often observed in recently hospitalized elderly patients who have had previous abdominal complaints and received high doses of an antibiotic.

*Myth #5: if a periapical radiolucency, sinus tract, fistula,
or localized abscess is present, antibiotics are always indicated*

A periapical radiolucency, sinus tract, or fistula indicates a necrotic pulp. A vital pulp cannot exist with any of these objective signs. Because there is not significant vascularization to necrotic canals or abscesses, the effectiveness of antibiotic therapy is highly questionable. Therapeutic concentrations of an antibiotic at the site of the infectious process cannot be obtained. A localized abscess (swelling) begins from the necrotic debris in the root canal and diffuses into the surrounding bone at the apex of the tooth, resulting in a swelling or sinus tract formation.

Controlled clinical trials using penicillin, placebo, and neither medication in patients presenting with pulpal necrosis and periapical pain or localized swelling showed no differences between groups in the course of recovery or symptoms after debridement of the root canal system [17].

Local dental treatment is most important in resolving the infection. Root canal treatment or extraction if the tooth is not restorable accomplishes the removal of the irritants and drainage of the swelling. Incision and drainage is indicated if there is no drainage obtained from the tooth or tooth socket. Drainage helps in decreasing discomfort the patient is experiencing by releasing blood and serous fluids that contain bacteria and their byproducts. Intraoral drainage removes these local irritants and improves circulation.

Myth #6: antibiotics must be given for several days before implementation of surgical treatment

The polymicrobial environment of odontogenic infections persists until the source of the irritation is removed. Dental treatment establishes a favorable environment to the host to alleviate the disease. The key to successful resolution of the infection is initial drainage of the infection coupled with either thorough chemo-mechanical debridement of the root canal system or extraction of the tooth or as an emergency measure until such time that definitive dental therapy can be implemented. The vast majority of localized odontogenic infections can be successfully treated by appropriate dental treatment alone. Medically compromised patients who present with dental pain, sinus tracts, radiolucencies, apical periodontitis, or localized intraoral swellings do not routinely require antibiotics [17]. It is appropriate however to administer oral antibiotics approximately 1 hour before surgical therapy is initiated as the surgical therapy disrupts vascular supply to the infected area. Some antibiotic is delivered to the areas approximating the infection where tissues are minimally affected by the infection. Any time differential greater than 1 hour between administration of oral antibiotic and surgical therapy is not warranted. If the antibiotic is administered parenterally, tissue levels adjacent to the infection are established in much less than 1 hour.

Myth #7: indurated soft tissues means drainage is not indicated

The clinician need not wait until a swelling become soft or fluctuant before incising and draining. Diffuse fluctuant or indurated soft tissues are a more severe manifestation of the localized abscess. Surgical therapy (root canal treatment or extraction) is indicated primarily if the etiology is a necrotic tooth. If adequate drainage is not accomplished, soft tissue incision and drainage may be indicated. If soft tissue swellings (cellulitis) are left untreated, infection can spread to adjacent facial spaces resulting in serious consequences such as airway compromise, sepsis, blindness, mediastinal involvement, and death. Fluctuant swellings usually emit purulence immediately when incised, whereas a more indurated swelling results in small quantities of blood and serous fluid. Draining both types of swellings releases pressure from the area and facilitates good recovery by providing oxygen to an anaerobic environment, increasing blood circulation, and thereby optimizing host defense mechanisms. A culture and sensitivity should be obtained when draining an infection, not to guide the initial antibiotic selection, but to be available should the empiric antibiotic therapy used fail.

Myth #8: overprescription of antibiotic therapy does not occur in dentistry

Overuse and improper use of prescription drugs by dentists has been well documented. The national Centers for Disease Control and Prevention estimate that approximately one third of all outpatient antibiotic prescriptions are unnecessary. Nearly $23 billion worldwide has been spent on antibiotics in the last year [11]. Approximately 10% of antibiotics are now rendered ineffective [11]. The patient who demands to leave the appointment with a prescription in hand may drive the misuse of antibiotics. The reality is that appropriate dental treatment, analgesic therapy, and education of the patient will alleviate the patient's symptoms and build trust in the doctor–patient relationship.

A step-by-step approach for diagnosing and treating odontogenic infections

1. Listen to the chief complaint of the patient. This is the symptom that the patient is experiencing and describes in his or her own words.
2. Take a comprehensive health history. Review systemic diseases, past surgeries, injuries, and medications the patient is taking. Review any allergic responses a patient may have experienced.
3. Obtain a thorough dental history of existing problems: When did the problem begin, is it getting worse or better, and what medications is the patient taking for it?
4. Extraoral and intraoral examination for the presence and extent of pathosis. Percussion, palpation, and pulp vitality testing are indicated to diagnose pulpal and periodontal disease.
5. Radiographic examination is an adjunct in determining dental disease. Most pathologic states in pulpal tissue are not visible on a radiograph. Only when the cortical plate has been resorbed does the dental radiograph become helpful in identifying disease.
6. Treatment planning is discussed with the patient once the nature of the pathosis has been identified. Determine the difficulty of the case and whether handling it is within your comfort level or if the case should be referred. The clinician should calculate a prognosis for each case

including a contingency prognosis if problems are encountered after treatment has begun.

7. Designing the appropriate dental treatment should be rendered: emergency and definitive treatment.

8. Case selection completed and referral to a specialist if found that the patient's needs are beyond the capacity of the clinician's capabilities.

9. Appropriate analgesics and postoperative instructions given.

10. Selection of an antibiotic if warranted:

   a) Choose the narrowest spectrum antibiotic possible to prevent disturbing the host's normal microbial flora.

   b) Prescribe the medication with the appropriate dose and duration.

   c) Educate the patient about the importance of taking the medication for the proper length of the time.

   c) Provide adequate analgesic therapy along with antibiotic therapy if the patient is also experiencing pain.

   e) Closely monitor the patient and follow up in 48 hours to make sure the dental treatment and antibiotic therapies have reduced the patient's symptoms. If there has not been a reduction in symptoms, consider adding another antibiotic, culturing the infection, or referring the patient to a specialist.

New developments

Advances in science and molecular developments in studying bacterial function may help researchers "customize" future antibiotics to kill certain bacteria. New technologic advancements, such as radiographic crystallography, that help in studying the enzymes that promote drug resistance are advances that help control antibiotic resistance in humans. Genetics is yet another promising avenue for exploring bacterial functions.

References

[1] Montgomery EH. Antibiotics used in dentistry. In: Neidle EA, Kroeger DC, Yagiela JA, editors. Pharmacology and therapeutics for dentistry. St. Louis (MO): Mosby; 1985. p. 548–87.

[2] Torabinejad M. Mediators of acute and chronic periradicular lesions. Oral Surg Oral Med Oral Pathol 1994;78:511.

[3] Kettering JD, Torabinejad M, Jones SL. Specificity of antibodies present in human periapical lesions. J Endodon 1991;17:213.

[4] Yamamoto K, Fukushima H, Tsuchiya H, Sagawa H. Antimicrobial susceptibilities of *Eubacterium, peptostreptococcus* and *Bacteroides* isolated from root canals of teeth with periapical pathosis. J Endodon 1989;15:112.

[5] Baker PT, Evans RT, Siots J, Genco RJ. Antibiotic susceptibility of anaerobic bacteria from the human oral cavity. J Dent Res 1985;64:1233.

[6] Owens BM, Schuman NJ. Ludwig's angina: historical perspective. J TN Dent Assoc 1993; 73(1):19–21.

[7] Sabiston CB, Gold WA. Anaerobic bacteria in oral infections. Oral Surg Oral Med Oral Pathol 1974;38:187–92.

[8] Smith CM, Reynard AM. Antibiotic chemotherapy. The penicillins, vancomycin, and bacitracin. In: Smith CM, Reynard AM, editors. Textbook of pharmacology. Philadelphia: WB Saunders; 1992. p. 817–28.

[9] Rudolph AH, Price EV. Penicillin reactions among patients in venereal disease clinics. A national survey. JAMA 1973;223:499–501.

[10] Turck M. Alternatives to penicillin. Drug Ther 1976;6:8–19.

[11] Slavkin H. Emerging and re-emerging infectious diseases: a biological evolutionary drama. J Am Dent Assoc 1997;1:108–13.

[12] Bigby M, Jick H, Arndt K. Drug-induced cutaneous reactions. A report from the Boston collaborative drug surveillance program on 15,438 consecutive inpatients, 1975 to 1082. JAMA 1986;256:3358–63.

[13] Saxon A, Beall GN, Rohr AS, et al. Immediate hypersensitivity reactions to beta-lactam antibiotics. Ann Intern Med 1987;107:204–5.

[14] Doern GV, Ferraro MJ, Bruggemann AB, et al. Emergence of high rates of antimicrobial resistance among virdans group streptococci in the United States. Antimicrob Agents Chemother 1996;40:891–4.

[15] Hasselgren G, Reit C. Emergency pulpotomy; Pain relieving effect with and without the use of sedative dressings. JOE 1989;15:254.

[16] Condon RE, Anderson MJ. Diarrhea and colitis in clindamycin treated patients. Arch Surg 1978;113:794–7.

[17] Fouad A, Rivera E, Walton R. Penicillin as a supplement in resolving the localized acute apical abscess. Oral Surg Oral Med Oral Pathol 1996;81(5):590–5.

[7] Sabiston CB, Gold WA. Anaerobic bacteria in oral infections. Oral Surg Oral Med Oral Pathol 1974;38:187–92.

[8] Smith CM, Reynard AM. Antibiotic chemotherapy. The penicillins, vancomycin, and bacitracin. In: Smith CM, Reynard AM, editors. Textbook of pharmacology. Philadelphia: WB Saunders; 1992. p. 817–28.

[9] Rudolph AH, Price EV. Penicillin reactions among patients in venereal disease clinics. A national survey. JAMA 1973;223:499–501.

[10] Turck M. Alternatives to penicillin. Drug Ther 1976;6:8–19.

[11] Slavkin H. Emerging and re-emerging infectious diseases: a biological evolutionary drama. J Am Dent Assoc 1997;1:108–13.

[12] Bigby M, Jick H, Arndt K. Drug-induced cutaneous reactions. A report from the Boston collaborative drug surveillance program on 15,438 consecutive inpatients, 1975 to 1082. JAMA 1986;256:3358–63.

[13] Saxon A, Beall GN, Rohr AS, et al. Immediate hypersensitivity reactions to beta-lactam antibiotics. Ann Intern Med 1987;107:204–5.

[14] Doern GV, Ferraro MJ, Bruggemann AB, et al. Emergence of high rates of antimicrobial resistance among virdans group streptococci in the United States. Antimicrob Agents Chemother 1996;40:891–4.

[15] Hasselgren G, Reit C. Emergency pulpotomy; Pain relieving effect with and without the use of sedative dressings. JOE 1989;15:254.

[16] Condon RE, Anderson MJ. Diarrhea and colitis in clindamycin treated patients. Arch Surg 1978;113:794–7.

[17] Fouad A, Rivera E, Walton R. Penicillin as a supplement in resolving the localized acute apical abscess. Oral Surg Oral Med Oral Pathol 1996;81(5):590–5.

THE DENTAL
CLINICS OF
NORTH
AMERICA

Dent Clin N Am 46 (2002) 635–651

Antibiotic prophylaxis for endocarditis, prosthetic joints, and surgery

Robin A. Seymour, BDS, PhD*,
John M. Whitworth, BChD, PhD

*Department of Restorative Dentistry, The Dental School, Framlington Place,
Newcastle upon Tyne, England, NE2 4BW, United Kingdom*

Antibiotics are prescribed in dentistry for two main reasons: to treat infections and to prevent infections. It is the latter that can be regarded as prophylactic use of these drugs. For the perspective of this article, we consider the main indications (or controversies) relating to prophylactic use of antibiotics in dentistry, notably the prevention of infective endocarditis, infections in patients with hip and joint prostheses, and the prevention of infection following various dental surgical procedures.

Antibiotic prophylaxis to prevent infective endocarditis

Infective endocarditis (IE) is a microbial infection involving the cardiac valves. The condition is uncommon, with a prevalence of 15–30 cases per 1 million per year [1]. The prevalence of IE has remained consistent even after the introduction of antibiotic prophylaxis in the 1940s [2].

Dental procedures, especially those that result in a bacteremia, are frequently blamed for IE and hence result in the need for antibiotic prophylaxis to cover such procedures in at-risk patients. This has been the clinical doctrine and teaching for the past 60 years. Evidence from the United States [3] and studies from the Netherlands [1,4] have presented further data that challenge the practice of antibiotic prophylaxis to prevent IE. Thus there exist several controversial areas surrounding the association between dentistry and IE. These can be broadly classified as follows:

1. Is infective endocarditis caused by a dental procedure-induced bacteremia or from spontaneous bacteremia?

---

* Corresponding author.
E-mail address: r.a.seymour@ncl.ac.uk (R.A. Seymour).

0011-8532/02/$ - see front matter © 2002, Elsevier Science (USA). All rights reserved.
PII: S 0 0 1 1 - 8 5 3 2 (0 2) 0 0 0 3 3 - 2

2. Which patients are at risk for infective endocarditis?
3. Which procedures require antibiotic coverage?
4. Are the risks of providing such coverage greater than the risks for contracting infective endocarditis?
5. Are the antibiotic regimens effective?

A major pitfall in trying to address these questions is the lack of a randomized controlled clinical trial to evaluate the efficacy of antibiotic coverage. Such a study would require at least 6000 at-risk patients and raise considerable ethical issues.

Is infective endocarditis caused by a dental procedure-induced bacteremia or from spontaneous bacteremia?

Poor oral health, especially periodontal status, is an important risk factor for infective endocarditis. Gingival inflammation correlates positively with the prevalence and magnitude of bacteremia [5]. Bleeding per se, however, is a poor indicator of odontogenic bacteremia.

Certain periodontal procedures are associated with bacteremia, although the magnitude varies. The prevalence of such bacteremia and the associated procedures is shown in Table 1. Also, by contrast, is the prevalence of bacteremia arising after various oral hygiene practices and after chewing. In many instances their magnitudes are comparable with the listed procedures. It has been suggested that oral hygiene practices and chewing are responsible for so-called "random" or "spontaneous" cases of bacteremia. Such bacteremia, either from periodontal procedures or oral hygiene practices, is of low-grade intensity ($1 \leftrightarrow 10^1$–$2 \leftrightarrow 10^2$ cfu ml^{-1} of blood) and of short duration [6].

Table 1
Prevalence of bacteremia arising after various types of dental procedures and oral activity

Procedure	Prevalence of bacteremia
Extractions (single)	51%
Extractions (multiple)	68–100%
Endodontics (intracanal instrumentation)	0–31%
Endodontics (extracanal instrumentation)	0–54%
Periodontal surgery (flap procedure)	36–88%
Periodontal surgery (gingivectomy)	83%
Scaling and root planing	8–80%
Periodontal prophylaxis	0–40%
Toothbrushing	0–26%
Dental flossing	20–58%
Interproximal cleaning with toothpicks	20–40%
Irrigation devices	7–50%
Chewing	17–51%

Dental treatment is often regarded as the cause of infective endocarditis. In many instances, the occurrence of endocarditis does not relate to the so-called "dental-induced" bacteremia. It may well transpire that random or spontaneous bacteremia may be more causative in infective endocarditis than dental surgeons carrying out treatment.

Further evidence to support this hypothesis comes from an analysis of cases of infective endocarditis in which dental treatment has been implicated as the cause. Oral Streptococci cause approximately 50% of all infective endocarditis cases [7]. Similarly, only 15% of patients in whom infective endocarditis has been diagnosed reported medical or dental treatment within the previous 3 months [8]. It has been estimated that 4% or less of all infective endocarditis cases are related to dental-induced bacteremia [2,5]. Whether such bacteremias arise from dental treatment or were spontaneous is not discernible. It is suggested that if spontaneous, random bacteremias cause 96% of all cases of infective endocarditis, than these bacteremias as opposed to those arising from dental treatment also may have caused the remaining 4% [9].

Three major studies have investigated the link between dental procedures and infective endocarditis [1,3,4]. Of these 3 studies, one was a case study [1], and the remaining two were of case-control design [3,4]. The conclusion from the Dutch studies [1,3] suggest that strict adherence to generally accepted recommendations for prophylaxis might do little to decrease the total number of patients with endocarditis in the community. The Strom [4] study is more far-reaching in their findings. They found that dental treatment was no more frequent among patients with IE than control subjects (adjusted odds ratio 0.8), and that among patients with known cardiac lesions (the target of antibiotic coverage) dental treatment was significantly less common than among control subjects. Few participants received chemoprophylaxis. The authors concluded that the lack of a link between dental treatment and IE, together with the rare occurrence of this disease, does not justify the routine use of antibiotic prophylaxis.

Two of the studies [3,4] were of case-control design, and this may weaken their conclusions. Although such studies can demonstrate a risk, the addition of control subjects allows the risk to be quantified. Case control studies, however, are not first rate in hierarchies of evidence that reflect the degree to which different study designs are susceptible to bias, or how certain it is that the observed effects are attributable to the intervention and are not the results of other factors.

Other criticisms of the cited studies have been aired. For example, a letter published in the Lancet raises three points [10]. The first was that although the number of cases of endocarditis prevented was negligible in population terms, the effect on individual patients could not be ignored. Second, concern was expressed at the small numbers of cases eventually entered into the trial, and the even smaller number who received adequate prophylaxis. Finally, doubt was expressed over the feasibility of maintaining a sufficiently large trial to settle this question and comment was made that it might be fruitless anyway. For these reasons, the authors did not see any good reason to waive current antibiotic prophylaxis practice for at-risk patients undergoing a high-risk dental procedure.

Yet this is the dilemma. Few are prepared to say that dental treatment and the resulting bacteremia do not cause IE, or even advocate for less prophylaxis to demonstrate that some cases of endocarditis follow dental treatment. So it might be impossible to devise a trial in which some individuals would be denied antibiotic coverage. In the meantime, clinicians and their patients will find it difficult to abandon such coverage while circumstantial evidence exists, on an individual level, that it confers some benefit (or more precisely, may reduce a theoretic risk). It might be difficult to change clinical practice, even if an unequivocal randomized controlled trial was done. Until such a trial can be completed, current regimens are likely to remain in place, even if subjected to review and modification.

Which patients are at risk from infective endocarditis?

The most detailed list of patients at risk for IE has been published by the American Heart Association (AHA) [11] (Table 2). They categorize their patients as high, moderate, and negligible risk based on their cardiac history. The negligible risk patients are at no greater risk than the rest of the general population. Differentiating between high and moderate risk does seem somewhat arbitrary, as these patients require antibiotic coverage for most procedures. The main problem relates to mitral valve prolapse (MVP), which is a common condition that affects approximately 5% of the adult population [12]. It is only those patients who have valvular prolapse with regurgitation or thickened leaflets, however, who are at risk for IE. MVP can only be diagnosed by angiography or from echocardiograms. In most cases neither the dental surgeon nor the patient is aware of any disorder of their mitral valves and will receive treatment without antibiotic coverage.

Guidelines on identifying patients at risk for IE vary from country to country. The consensus view is that antibiotic coverage is often overprescribed for many seemingly innocuous cardiac conditions.

Which procedures require coverage?

Again, the AHA is prescriptive in identifying those procedures that require coverage [11] (see box below). From the periodontal perspective, these include all types of periodontal surgery, the placement of implants, scaling and root planing, probing periodontal pockets, subgingival placement of antibiotic fibers or strips, and prophylactic cleaning of the teeth when bleeding is anticipated. There may be concern among dental surgeons over procedures such as probing periodontal pockets, placement of

Table 2
American Heart Association guideline for antibiotic prophylaxis

Cardiac conditions associated with endocarditis
  High risk category
    Prosthetic heart valves, including bioprosthetic and homograft valves
    Previous bacterial endocarditis
    Complex cyanolic congenital heart disease (eg, single ventricle states, transposition of the
      great arteries, tetralogy of Fallot)
    Surgically-constructed systemic pulmonary shunts or conduits
  Moderate risk category
    Most other congenital cardiac malformations
    Acquired valvular dysfunction (eg, rheumatic heart disease)
    Hypertrophic cardiomyopathy
    Mitral valve prolapse with valvular regurgitation or thickened leaflets
  Negligible risk category (no greater risk than the general population)
    Isolated secundum atrial septal defect
    Surgical repair of atrial septal defect, ventricular septal defect, or patent ductus arteriosis
      (without residue beyond 6 m)
    Previous coronary artery bypass graft surgery
    Mitral valve prolapse without valvular regurgitation
    Physiologic, functional, or innocent heart murmurs
    Previous Kawasaki disease without valvular dysfunction
    Previous rheumatic fever without valvular dysfunction
    Cardiac pacemakers and implanted defibrillators

Antibiotic regimes

Situation	Regimen
Standard general prophylaxis	Adults: amoxicillin 2 g, children: amoxicillin 50 mg/kg, oral 1 h before procedure
Unable to take oral medications	Adults: ampicillin 2 g IV or IM Children: ampicillin 50 mg/kg IM or IV, within 30 min before procedure
Allergic to penicillin	Adults: clindamycin 600 mg Children: clindamycin 20 mg/kg 1 h before procedure or Adults: azithromycin or clarithromycin 500 mg Children: azithromycin or clarithromycin 15 mg/kg orally 1 h before procedure
Allergic to penicillin and unable to take oral medication	Adults: clindamycin 600 mg IV or IM Children: 20 mg/kg IV within 30 min before procedure

subgingival antibiotic fibers, and prophylactic cleaning of the teeth. Although bacteremias arising from such procedures have not been quantified, they are likely to be similar in magnitude to the bacteremia arising from tooth-brushing or other oral hygiene practices. This issue brings into question whether such procedures require coverage, whereas those that the patient can generate on their own do not. Although the AHA guidelines for certain periodontal procedures may be an overstatement, they do need to be adhered to until evidence becomes available that refutes them.

Dental procedures for which antibiotic prophylaxis is recommended to prevent infective endocarditis (AHA recommendations)

Dental extractions
Periodontal procedures, including surgery, scaling, root planing, probing periodontal pockets, and recall maintenance
Dental implant placement and reimplantation of avulsed teeth
Endodontic (root canal) instrumentation or surgery beyond the apex
Subgingival placement of antibiotic fibers or strips
Initial placement of orthodontic bands, but not brackets
Intraligamentary local anesthetic injections
Prophylactic cleaning of teeth or implants in which bleeding is anticipated
Incision and drainage or other procedures involving infected tissues

---

Are the risks for providing antibiotic coverage greater than the risk for contracting IE?

When antibiotics are given prophylactically to prevent IE, the dental surgeon needs to consider the risk and cost benefit of such treatment. The most significant adverse event associated with amoxicillin is hypersensitivity reactions. These can range from a troublesome rash to a life-threatening anaphylactic reaction. One to ten percent of patients report a penicillin allergy [13], although many of these are not confirmed if subjected to the appropriate test. More importantly, the chance of an allergic reaction following administration of the drug is in the range of 0.7–5% [14]. This prevalence does vary with the route of drug administration, with the intramuscular route causing a 5% prevalence and oral penicillin a 0.3% prevalence. High doses of oral amoxicillin, however, can cause an allergic reaction rate similar to that of intramuscular penicillin [15].

Data from the United States show that 400–800 deaths are caused each year by anaphylactic reactions to penicillin, although only a portion of these arise from penicillin prophylaxis to prevent IE. To put the risk–benefit ratio into perspective, it has been estimated that 1.36 people per 1 million population are likely to die from penicillin anaphylaxis to prevent IE, whereas only 0.26 deaths per 1 million population are caused by dental procedure-induced endocarditis [16]. Put another way, patients receiving penicillin (amoxicillin) prophylaxis to prevent IE are five times more likely to die from an anaphylactic reaction to the drug than to die from contracting endocarditis. It would thus seem from these statistics that the risk for providing antibiotic coverage to prevent IE is far greater than not providing coverage.

Are the antibiotic regimens effective?

One of the most telling statistics on the efficacy of antibiotic prophylaxis relates to the prevalence of the disease. The overall prevalence of IE is approximately 15 per 1 million patients per year. This figure has not changed with the advent of antibiotic prophylaxis. Thus, it could be inferred that the provision of such prophylaxis has had little impact on the occurrence of the disease. This would also question the value of providing such antibiotic coverage.

The efficacy of antibiotic prophylaxis to prevent IE has not been subjected to a randomized, placebo-controlled study. Evidence to date on efficacy has come from case-controlled studies, animal experiments, and antibiotic efficacy studies on bacteremia after tooth extractions. There is uncertainty as to whether prophylactic administration of penicillins has an impact on orally induced bacteremia. Parental penicillin has been shown to reduce bacteremia by 84–86% at 5 minutes and 95–97% at 30 minutes after a bacteremia induction. These figures compare with a reduction of 24–42% and 49–76% respectively, when no prophylaxis is used [17]. By contrast, otherworkers have shown that single doses of penicillin 2 g and amoxicillin 3 g fail to reduce bacteremia after dental extractions [18]. There is now a growing consensus that antibiotic prophylaxis may not prevent IE by a bactericidal blood activity but may do so by decreasing microbial adherence to damaged cardiac valves or by eliminating bacteria after their attachment to valves [19–21].

Although most attention has focused on antibiotic prophylaxis, there is evidence that antiseptic mouthwashes such as chlorhexidine and povidone-iodine used before certain dental procedures may reduce the prevalence of bacteremia [16,22]. The AHA recommends the use of local irrigation with chlorhexidine before any treatment that can result in a bacteremia. Whether such a procedure is sufficient to prevent IE in high or moderate risk patients has yet to be determined. One possible disadvantage is that regular use of chlorhexidine may lead to the selection of resistant streptococci such as *Streptococcus sanguis* and other gram-negative bacteria. An endocarditis from such resistant organisms would have a higher mortality rate than one caused by viridans streptococci [23,24].

Antibiotic prophylaxis in patients with hip and joint prostheses

The provision of joint prostheses is a common orthopedic procedure. In the late 1950s and early 1960s, there was a high prevalence (15–25%) of postoperative infections associated with such surgery. Infections that occurred within 2 months of surgery were categorized as early, whereas those that occurred after this time were considered late infections. Early infections were related to the surgical procedure, whereas late infections were believed to be caused by hematogenous spread of bacteria from another site of infection elsewhere in the body. Antibiotic prophylaxis at the time of surgery reduced the prevalence of postoperative infection to approximately 1%. These findings suggest that most of the late infections were caused by wound contamination and not from hematogenous spread. Despite such evidence, many orthopedic surgeons insist that their patients receive antibiotic coverage before dental procedures that can induce bacteremia.

Microbiology of joint infections

Most joint infections (>66%) are caused by staphylococci and only 4.9% are related to viridans streptococci of possible oral origin [25]. Whether the S viridans infection arose directly from dental treatment or from other sources was not established. DNA fingerprinting techniques have not been used to confirm that isolates from infected joints are the same as those found in the mouth.

Is there evidence to suggest that dental-induced bacteremia causes joint infections?

There is little firm evidence to suggest that dental-induced bacteremia can cause hematogenous infection around a prosthetic joint [26]. By contrast, there are several studies that show the opposite. A review of 21 cases of prosthetic joint infections attributable to a dental procedure identified one patient in whom the same infecting organism was grown on culture from the mouth, blood, and prosthetic joint [27]. Whether the bacteremia arose from a dental procedure or occurred spontaneously was never ascertained. In a prospective 6-year study [28] on 1000 patients, only three developed joint infections. Of these 1000 patients, 224 had undergone an invasive dental procedure without antibiotic prophylaxis and there was no episode of late joint infections. Two further reviews of patients with joint infection [29,30] implicate skin and soft tissue infections as being the most likely primary cause. Four of 110 cases were reported to be attributable to S viridans [29]. All four patients had recent experience of an acute dental infection.

Guidelines from professional bodies

Despite the lack of evidence of an association between dental treatment and late joint infections, several professional bodies have produced guidelines on antibiotic prophylaxis before dental treatment. Most recent guidelines are those issued jointly by the American Dental Association (ADA) and the American Academy of Orthopaedic Surgeons (AAOS) [31]. They state that "antibiotic prophylaxis is not indicated for dental patients with pins, plates and screws, nor is it routinely indicated for most patients with total joint replacement." They do consider that certain immunocompromised patients undergoing high-risk procedures within 2 years of joint replacement or those patients with a previous history of joint infection might be considered for antibiotic prophylaxis. A similar view is adopted by the British Orthopaedic Association, but they also advocate antibiotic prophylaxis when dental treatment is complex, extensive, and of long duration (>45 minutes). It is encouraging to see that both professional bodies advocate the establishment and maintenance of good oral health in patients with joint prostheses. The British Society for Antimicrobial Chemotherapy (BSAC) takes a different view than those expressed by Orthopaedic Associations [32]. The BSAC does not recommend prophylactic use of antibiotics, and further states that exposing patients to the risk for adverse reactions to antibiotics when there is no evidence that such prophylaxis is of any benefit is unacceptable. With these differing views, it is not surprising that the dental profession is confused. There does, however, seem to be some agreement between the various professional bodies that the otherwise healthy patient with a joint prosthesis does not require antibiotic prophylaxis for most dental procedures. Some of the guidelines do need challenging, in particular those involving immunocompromised patients, patients with a joint prosthesis fitted within 2 years, and for procedures lasting >45 minutes.

Patients who would be categorized as at-risk include patients with insulin-dependent diabetes, patients with previous joint infection (first 2 years following joint placement), hemophiliacs, patients with a history of rheumatoid arthritis, and patients with either drug- or disease-induced immunosuppression. An overview of these factors has been presented previously [26]. Their conclusions were that the evidence implicating rheumatoid arthritis and hemophilia as predisposing factors for late infection around prosthetic joints is persuasive. Use of corticosteroid may also predispose a patient to late infection, but this may be because many patients who have rheumatoid arthritis take corticosteroids. Immunosuppression, diabetes mellitus, the type of prosthesis used, the use of bone grafting, and previous complications (infections) related to a prosthetic joint have been reported to be predisposing factors for late infection; however, the data do not currently support such contentions.

Antibiotic regimens and efficacy

As with infective endocarditis, the efficacy of antibiotic prophylaxis to prevent hematogenous infection in patients with joint prostheses has not been evaluated in a randomized controlled trial.

The ADA/AAOS [31] recommendation for cases in which prophylaxis is indicated includes single doses of cephalexin, cephradine, or amoxicillin 2 g orally 1 hour before the dental procedure. Patients allergic to penicillin are prescribed clindamycin 600 mg orally.

Various studies have investigated the risk–benefit ratio for providing antibiotic prophylaxis to patients with prosthetic joints [33–35]. It has been estimated that for every 100,000 patients with joint replacements, approximately 30 (0.03%) would acquire an infection that would necessitate joint replacement. This additional surgery would cost approximately

$900,000. Providing these same 100,000 patients with antibiotic prophylaxis would cost $1,500,000. The risk for providing the coverage, however, would be 40 cases of anaphylaxis and four deaths. These figures would be lower for cephalosporins, but even with this antibiotic, the number of deaths from anaphylactic reactions would be greater than deaths from joint infections [33].

Overview

The need for antibiotic prophylaxis for patients with joint prostheses remains a contentious issue and is certainly an area of conflict between orthopedic surgeons and the dental profession. There is certainly a lack of evidence-based information to support some of the recommendations listed in various published guidelines. The following seems to be a synopsis of the evidence to date:

1. Most joint infections are of staphylococcal origin and not related to dental-induced bacteremia;
2. If an oral commensal has been implicated in causing a joint infection, then it is much more likely to have arisen spontaneously from the patient's oral hygiene practice than from a dental procedure;
3. There is no evidence from randomized controlled studies to support the efficacy of antibiotic prophylaxis before dental procedures to prevent hematogenous joint infections;
4. The risk for providing antibiotic prophylaxis is considerably greater than the risk for a joint infection;
5. Patients with joint prostheses should maintain a high standard of oral health and be rendered dentally fit before joint surgery;
6. There is limited evidence to suggest that patients with rheumatoid arthritis may be more susceptible to dental-induced bacteremia and hence may require antibiotic coverage.

As with infective endocarditis, there is the specter of litigation that often clouds the issue of antibiotic prophylaxis. In this era of evidence-based dentistry, however, it would seem difficult to support the cause of antibiotic prophylaxis for patients with joint prostheses.

The prevention of infection following dental surgical procedures

There are numerous local surgical procedures and medical conditions that are routinely covered by systemic antimicrobials in an attempt to prevent postoperative complications. These can be considered as follows:

- Local wound infection that may not jeopardize the procedure (eg, impacted third molar removal);
- Local infection that may jeopardize the procedure (eg, installation of endosseous implants);

- Distant metastatic infection (eg, infection of an in-dwelling vascular stent);
- Fulminant sepsis (eg, the severely immunocompromised patient).

Local surgical procedures

Antibiotic prophylaxis can generally be justified for surgical procedures when it may safely and cost-effectively reduce the risk for:

1. Exposing a sterile body area to infection;
2. Acquiring an infection likely to cause major morbidity, including the implantation of prostheses [36].

Considered against these criteria, there are few clear indications to provide antibiotic coverage for dental and oral surgical procedures in fit and healthy individuals [37].

Impacted third molars

Surgical removal of impacted third molars is a high-volume procedure in dental practice. The operation carries a low postoperative infection rate on the order of 1–5% [38–41], though procedures involving bone removal carry a higher risk than simple extraction [42]. Such infections are rarely serious or life threatening in healthy, immunocompetent patients. Antibiotic prescribing to prevent these infections is widespread and highly controversial. There is some evidence that antibiotics may further reduce the incidence and severity of postoperative infection [41,43], but others have strongly suggested otherwise [44–48].

It is difficult to support the routine, empirical use of antibiotics to cover such procedures with a low risk for minor morbidity [37,41]. Wise local precautions may include the avoidance of surgery in the presence of acute infection, ensuring optimal plaque control in the preoperative period, and supporting postoperative plaque control with a chemical antiplaque agent.

Orthognathic surgery

Infection is a complication of orthognathic surgery in 1–15% of cases [49,50]. Depending on the nature of the procedure, the consequences of infection may be serious. Numerous studies have revealed lower postoperative infection rates following the use of antibiotics [49,51–53], whereas at least one has demonstrated no benefit [54]. Responsible prescribing demands that the risks and consequences of wound infection are carefully assessed for each patient and procedure, and that antimicrobial drugs are not prescribed without thought. Certainly for intraoral procedures, local plaque control measures should probably be emphasized more strongly.

Implant surgery

The installation of intraoral endosseous implants fits the stated criteria for antibiotic prophylaxis [36]. We know little about the effects of prophylactic antibiotics on implant infection and failure [55], however, and clear indications for their use before implant surgery have not been established [56]. Although the incidence of infection seems to be low, most surgeons have used a prophylactic regimen, including preoperative and long-term postoperative antibiotic therapy [57].

A prospective multi-center study of 2641 implants [56] concluded that significantly fewer failed before the completion of stage II surgery if preoperative antibiotics were used. A following report showed that infectious complications were reduced by almost 50% if patients used chlorhexidine mouthwash perioperatively [58]. The correlation between chlorhexidine use and implant survival was not presented. Conversely, a retrospective, single-center study of 1454 implants in 279 patients followed for 1–6 years showed no significant difference in outcome if antibiotics were not used, and concluded that there was no advantage to the patient from antibiotic prophylaxis in routine implant cases [59].

More clinical audit and research is needed to clarify the position, but the case for routine prophylaxis is by no means clear [57].

Medical conditions

Patients with a lowered local or general resistance to infection may be placed at special risk by invasive dental treatment. It is probable that the risks to these patients are higher than those in the categories considered earlier, and that their relative rarity does not raise the same public health issues.

Immunosuppression

Immune function may be impaired by a range of conditions and medical treatments including leukemias, lymphomas, anti-cancer chemotherapy, immunosuppressive drugs following organ transplantation, poorly controlled insulin-dependant diabetes, loss of splenic function, and HIV infection.

Odontogenic infections may potentially be life threatening, and preventive dental care should be pursued aggressively.

High-risk, invasive dental procedures such as deep scaling and tooth extraction should be avoided whenever possible, but if they become necessary, they should be treated with antibiotics in patients with hematological cancers, bone marrow suppression, and those patients taking anti-cancer chemotherapy [37,60,61]. These are not procedures to be undertaken lightly or without proper collaboration with hematologic, oncologic, and microbiologic specialists. The risk, for example, for opportunistic fungal infection promoted by broad-spectrum antibiotic treatment should not be underestimated.

Organ transplant patients are generally not covered for dental procedures after the immediate postoperative period.

The vast majority of diabetics are controlled well enough to ensure that they are at no major threat from bacteremia caused by dental treatment. Patients with unstable insulin-controlled diabetes may be debilitated and at some risk from invasive dental interventions. Although clear evidence is lacking, these vulnerable patients may benefit from antibiotic prophylaxis for high-risk procedures such as extractions [60].

Splenectomized patients are certainly vulnerable to some forms of infection, particularly from encapsulated microorganisms such as *Staphylococcus pneumoniae* and *Haemophilus* spp [62,63]. The importance of oral microorganisms is less clear. Antibiotic prophylaxis is generally not recommended for dental treatment in these patients [37,61], and the status of post-splenectomy sepsis in an age of routine *S pneumoniae* immunization is under review [62].

Most people with HIV infection are generally well and do not require antibiotic coverage for dental procedures [64,65]. Those with full-blown AIDS become increasingly vulnerable to infection, and it is wise to consider covering patients undergoing invasive procedures with a high risk for bacteremia, such as the removal of an abscessed tooth [60,61]. The balance of risks between fulminant sepsis without antibiotic coverage and the precipitation of another opportunistic infection if a broad-spectrum agent is used should again be carefully reviewed. The best course for these patients is to limit the need for treatment by implementing an effective preventive approach.

Locally reduced resistance to infection

Irradiated bone is poorly vascularized and liable to necrose following trauma or infection. Historically, it was recommended that patients were rendered edentulous before radiotherapy to the head and neck [66] to eliminate dental disease or treatment as a cause of osteoradionecrosis. Osteoradionecrosis is a significant risk after dental extraction [67], but the relative risks for infection and trauma are not known. Some clinicians have reported that extractions can be accomplished with minimal risk under antibiotic coverage, combined with careful technique and effective oral hygiene [68]. Others have observed that antibiotic coverage alone is not sufficient to prevent delayed healing and osteoradionecrosis [69]. There is some consensus that patients who have received radiotherapy to the head and neck should receive antibiotic coverage for dental extractions, that antibiotics should continue until healing is complete, and that complications can be further reduced by hyperbaric oxygen therapy to enhance angiogenesis and perfusion [69–71].

Infection of other in-dwelling devices

Bacteremia from dental treatment may theoretically present an infection risk to a range of in-dwelling devices including vascular grafts, catheters and shunts, neurosurgical shunts, cardiac pacemakers, and defibrillators.

Cardiac pacemakers and defibrillators have not been shown to be at special risk from dentally induced bacteremia, and antibiotic prophylaxis is not recommended [11,72].

By contrast, patients with vascular grafts involving the major vessels [37] and renal impairment, especially those with arteriovenous shunts for hemodialysis [73–76] should be considered for antibiotic prophylaxis before invasive dental procedures. A recent review [60] added extracranial shunts for the drainage of cerebrospinal fluid to this list.

For many of these special situations, there is no clear evidence base. Treatment planning is often complex, involving a variety of specialists and care providers. The prevention of serious dental disease cannot be overemphasized in all of the patient groups considered, and dentists should play an important role in multidisciplinary teams.

Summary

It would seem from a review of the evidence that the need for antibiotic prophylaxis in dentistry is overstated. In simple mathematic terms, the risk for providing coverage is greater than the outcomes that could arise if coverage is withheld. In addition, there is the increasing problem of the development of resistant strains and their impact on medicine and dentistry. Yet despite these observations, the profession continues to put their patients at this greater risk. Medico-legal issues do cloud judgments in this area and many dentists err on the side of caution. The profession does require clear, uniform guidelines that are evidence-based. At present, there is still significant debate as to who is at risk from dental-induced bacteremia and what procedures require chemoprophylaxis.

References

[1] Van der Meer JT, Thompson J, Valkenburg HA, Michel MF. Epidemiology of bacterial endocarditis in The Netherlands. II. Antecedent procedures and use of prophylaxis. Arch of Int Med 1992;152:1869–73.

[2] Bayliss R, Clark C, Oakley C, et al. The teeth and infective endocarditis. Br Heart J 1983;50:506–12.

[3] Strom BL, Abrutyn E, Berlin JA, Kinman JL, Feldman RS, Stolley PD, et al. Dental and cardiac risk factors for infective endocarditis. A population-based, case-control study. Ann Int Med 1998;729:761–9.

[4] Van der Meer JT, Van Wijik WM, Thompson J, Vandenbroucke JP, Vafkenburg HA, Michel MF. Efficacy of antibiotic prophylaxis for prevented native-valve endocarditis. Lancet 1992;339:135–9.

[5] Guntheroth WG. How important are dental procedures as a cause of infective endocarditis. Am J Cardiol 1984;54:797–801.

[6] Roberts GJ, Gardner P, Simmons NA. Optimum time for detection of dental bacteraemia in children. Int J Cardiol 1992;35:311–5.

[7] Kaye D. Prophylaxis for infective endocarditis: an update. Ann Intern Med 1986;104: 419–23.

[8] Cherubin CE, Neu HC. Infective endocarditis at the Presbyterian Hospital in New York City from 1938–1967. Am J Med 1971;51:83–96.

[9] Oakley CM. Controversies in the prophylaxis of infective endocarditis: a cardiological view. J Antimicrob Chemother 1987;20(Suppl A):99–104.

[10] Simmons NA, Ball AP, Cawson RA, et al. Antibiotic prophylaxis and infective endocarditis. Lancet 1992;339:1292–3.

[11] Dajani AS, Taubert KA, Wilson W, et al. Prevention of bacterial endocarditis. Recommendations of the American Heart Association. J Am Med Assoc 1997;277:1794–1801.

[12] Savage DD, Garrison RJ, Devereux RB, et al. Mitral valve prolapse in the general population. I. Epidemiological features; The Framingham study. Am Heart J 1983;106:571–6.

[13] Smith JW, Johnson JW, Cluff LE. Studies on the epidemiology of adverse drug reactions. II An evaluation of penicillin allergy. N Engl J Med 1966;274:998–1007.

[14] Parker CW. Allergic reactions in man. Pharmacol Rev 1982;34:85–104.

[15] Weiss ME, Adkinson NE. β-lactam allergy. In: Mandell GL, Douglas RG, Bennett JE, editors. Principles and practice of infectious diseases. 3rd edition. New York: Churchill Livingstone; 1990. p. 265.

[16] Tzukert AA, Leviner E, Benoliel R, Katz J. Analysis of the American Heart Association for the prevention of infective endocarditis. Oral Surg Oral Med Oral Pathol 1986;62:276–9.

[17] Baltch AL, Pressman HL, Schaffer C, et al. Bacteraemias in patients undergoing oral procedures: study following parenteral antimicrobial prophylaxis as recommended by the American Heart Association 1977. Arch Intern Med 1988;148:1084–8.

[18] Hall G, Hedstrom SA, Helmdahl A, Nord CE. Prophylactic administration of penicillins for endocarditis does not reduce the incidence of post extraction bacteremias. Clin Infect Dis 1993;17:188–94.

[19] Durack DT. Prevention of infective endocarditis. N Engl J Med 1995;332:38–44.

[20] Francioli O, Glauser MP. Successful prophylaxis of experimental streptococcal endocarditis with single doses of sublethal concentrations of penicillin. J Antimicrob Chemother 1985;15(Suppl A):297–302.

[21] Morellion P, Francioli P, Overholser D, et al. Mechanism of successful amoxicillin prophylaxis of experimental endocarditis due to streptococcus intermedins. J Infect Dis 1986;154:801–7.

[22] MacFarlane TW, Ferguson MM, Mulgrew CJ. Post-extraction bacteremia: role of antiseptics and antibiotics. Br Dent J 1984;156:179–81.

[23] Svinhufuud LB, Heimdahl A, Nord CE. Effect of topical administration of vancomycin versus chlorhexidine on α-hemolytic streptococci in oral cavity. Oral Surg Oral Med Oral Pathol 1988;66:304–9.

[24] Durack DT. Infective and noninfective endocarditis. In: Hurst JW, Schlant RC, Rackley CE, Sonneblick EH, Wenger NK, editors. The heart. 7th edition. New York: McGraw Hill; 1990. p. 1230–52.

[25] Inman RD, Gallegos KU, Brause BD, et al. Clinical and microbial features of prosthetic joint infection. Am J Med 1978;77:47–53.

[26] Deacon JM, Pagliaro AJ, Zelicof SB, et al. Prophylactic use of antibiotics for procedures after total joint replacement. J Bone Joint Surg 1996;78A(11):1755–71.

[27] Thyne GM, Ferguson JW. Antibiotic prophylaxis during dental treatment in patients with prosthetic joints. Br J Bone Joint Surg 1991;73(B):191–4.

[28] Ainscow DAP, Denham RA. The risk of haematogenous infections in total joint replacement. J Bone Joint Surg 1984;66(B):580–2.

[29] Ching DWT, Gould IM, Rennie JAN, Gibson PAH. Prevention of late haematogenous infection in major prosthetic joints. J Antimicrob Chemother 1989;23:676–80.

[30] Maderazo EG, Judson S, Pasternak H. Late infections of total joint prostheses. A review and recommendations for prevention. Clin Orthop 1988;229:131–42.

[31] Antibiotic prophylaxis for dental patients with total joint replacements [advisory statement]. J Am Dent Assoc 1997;128(7):1004–8.
[32] Simmons NA, Ball AP, Cawson RA, et al. Case against antibiotic prophylaxis for dental treatment of patients with joint prostheses. Lancet 1992;339:301.
[33] Jacobsen JJ, Schweitzer S, De Porter DJ, et al. Chemoprophylaxis of dental patients with prosthetic joints: a simulation model. J Dent Educ 1988;52:599–604.
[34] Norden CW. Prevention of bone and joint infections. Am J Med 1985;78:229–32.
[35] Tsevat J, Durand-Zaleski I, Pauker SG. Cost-effectiveness of antibiotic prophylaxis for dental procedures in patients with artificial joints. Am J Pub Health 1989;79:739–43.
[36] Paluzzi RG. Antimicrobial prophylaxis for surgery. Med Clin N Am 1993;77:427–41.
[37] Pallasch TJ, Slots J. Antibiotic prophylaxis and the medically compromised patient. Periodontology 2000 1996;10:107–38.
[38] Peterson L. Antibiotic prophylaxis against wound infections in oral and maxillofacial surgery. J Oral Maxillofac Surg 1990;48:617–20.
[39] Longman LP, Martin MV. The use of antibiotics in the prevention of post-operative infection: a re-appraisal. Br Dent J 1991;170:257–62.
[40] Loukota RA. The effect of peri-operative perioral skin preparation with povidone-iodine on the incidence of infection after third molar removal. Br J Oral Maxillofac Surg 1991;29:336–7.
[41] Piecuch JF, Arzadon J, Lieblich SE. Prophylactic antibiotics for third molar surgery: a supportive opinion. J Oral Maxillofac Surg 1995;53:53–60.
[42] MacGregor AJ. Aetiology of dry socket: a clinical investigation. Br J Oral Surg 1968;6: 49–58.
[43] Rood JP, Murgatroyd J. Metronidazole in the prevention of "dry socket". Br J Oral Surg 1979;17:62–70.
[44] Rud J. Removal of impacted lower third molars with acute pericoronitis and necrotising gingivitis. Br J Oral Surg 1970;7:153–60.
[45] Curran JB, Kenett S, Young AR. An assessment of the use of prophylactic antibiotics in third molar surgery. Int J Oral Surg 1974;3:1–6.
[46] Happonen RP, Backstrom AC, Ylipaavalniemi P. Prophylactic use of phenoxymethyl-penicillin and tinidazole in mandibular third molar surgery, a comparative placebo controlled trial. Br J Oral Maxillofac Surg 1990;28:12–5.
[47] Worrall SF. Antibiotic prescribing and third molar surgery. Br J Oral Maxillofac Surg 1998;36:74–6.
[48] Sekhar CH, Narayanan V, Baig MF. Role of antimicrobials in third molar surgery: prospective double blind, randomised, placebo-controlled clinical study. Br J Oral Maxillofac Surg 2001;39:134–7.
[49] Ruggles JE, Hann JR. Antibiotic prophylaxis in intraoral orthognathic surgery. J Oral Maxillofac Surg 1984;42:797–801.
[50] Cheynet F, Chossegros C, Richard O, Ferrara JJ, Blanc JL. Infectious complications of mandibular osteotomy. Rev Stomatol Chir Maxillofac 2001;102:26–33.
[51] Alfter G, Schwenzer N, Friess D, Mohrle E. Perioperative antibiotic prophylaxis with cefuroxime in oral-maxillofacial surgical procedures. J Craniomaxillofac Surg 1995;23:38–41.
[52] Bentley KC, Head TW, Aiello GA. Antibiotic prophylaxis in orthognathic surgery: a 1-day versus 5-day regimen. J Oral Maxillofac Surg 1999;57:226–30.
[53] Zijderveld SA, Smeele LE, Kostense PJ, Tuinzing DB. Preoperative antibiotic prophylaxis in orthognathic surgery: a randomised, double-blind, and placebo-controlled clinical study. J Oral Maxillofac Surg 1999;57:1403–6.
[54] Peterson LJ, Booth DF. Efficacy of antibiotic prophylaxis in intraoral orthognathic surgery. J Oral Surg 1976;34:1088–91.
[55] Esposito M, Hirsch J-M, Lekholm U, Thomsen P. Biological factors contributing to failures of osseointegrated oral implants (II). Etiopathogenesis. Eur J Oral Sci 1998;106:721–64.

[56] Dent CD, Olson JW, Farish SE, Bellome J, Casino AJ, Morris HF, et al. The influence of preoperative antibiotics on success of endosseous implants up to and including stage II surgery: a study of 2,641 implants. J Oral Maxillofac Surg 1997;55(Suppl 5):19–24.

[57] Larsen PE. Antibiotic prophylaxis for placement of dental implants. J Oral Maxillofac Surg 1993;51(Suppl 3):194–5.

[58] Lambert PM, Morris HF, Ochi S. The influence of 0.12% chlorhexidine digluconate rinses on the incidence of infectious complications and implant success. J Oral Maxillofac Surg 1997;55(Suppl 5):25–30.

[59] Gynther GW, Kondell PA, Moberg L-E, Heimdahl A. Dental implant installation without antibiotic prophylaxis. Oral Surg Oral Med Oral Pathol 1998;85:509–11.

[60] Tong DC, Rothwell BR. Antibiotic prophylaxis in dentistry: a review and practice recommendations. J Am Dent Assoc 2000;131:366–74.

[61] Scully C, Cawson RA. Immunodeficiencies. In: Scully C, Cawson RA, editors. Medical problems in dentistry. 4th edition. Oxford (UK): Wright; 1998. p. 408–37.

[62] Read RC, Finch RG. Prophylaxis after splenectomy. J Antimicrob Chemother 1994;33: 4–6.

[63] Holdsworth RJ, Irving AD, Cuschieri A. Post-splenectomy sepsis and its mortality rate: actual versus perceived risks. Br J Surg 1991;78:1031–8.

[64] Glick M, Abel SN, Muzyka BC, DeLorenzo M. Dental complications after treating patients with AIDS. J Am Dent Assoc 1994;125:296–301.

[65] Porter SR, Scully C, Luker J. Complications of dental surgery in persons with HIV disease. Oral Surg Oral Med Oral Pathol 1993;75:165–7.

[66] Daland EM. Radiation necrosis of the jaw. Radiology 1949;52:205–15.

[67] Murray CG, Herson J, Daly TE, Zimmerman S. Radiation necrosis of the mandible: a 10-year study. Part II. Dental factors; onset, duration and management of necrosis. Biology and physics. Int J Radiat Oncol 1980;6:549–53.

[68] Carl W, Schaaf NG, Sako K. Oral surgery and the patient who has had radiation therapy for head and neck cancer. Oral Surg Oral Med Oral Pathol 1973;36:651–7.

[69] Tong AC, Leung AC, Cheng JC, Sham J. Incidence of complicated healing and osteoradionecrosis following tooth extraction in patients receiving radiotherapy for treatment of nasopharyngeal carcinoma. Aust Dent J 1999;44:187–94.

[70] Scully C, Epstein JB. Oral health care for the cancer patient. Eur J Cancer 1996;32B: 281–92.

[71] Shaw MJ, Kumar NDK, Duggal D, Fiske J, Lewis DA, Kinsella T, Nisbet T. Oral management of patients following oncology treatment: literature review. Br J Oral Maxillofac Surg 2000;38:519–24.

[72] Arber N, Pras E, Copperman Y, Schapiro JM, Meiner V, Lossos IS, et al. Pacemaker endocarditis: report of 44 cases and review of the literature. Medicine (Baltimore) 1994;73:299–305.

[73] Bottomley WK, Cioffi RF, Martin AJ. Dental management of the patient treated by renal transplantation: preoperative and postoperative considerations. J Am Dent Assoc 1972; 85:1330–5.

[74] Manton SL, Midda M. Renal failure and the dental patient: a cautionary tale. Br Dent J 1986;160:388–90.

[75] Naylor GD, Hall EH, Terezhalmy GT. The patient with chronic renal failure who is undergoing dialysis of renal transplantation: another consideration for antimicrobial prophylaxis. Oral Surg Oral Med Oral Pathol 1988;65:116–21.

[76] De Rossi SS, Glick M. Dental considerations for the dental patient with renal disease receiving haemodialysis. J Am Dent Assoc 1996;127:211–9.

THE DENTAL
CLINICS OF
NORTH
AMERICA

Dent Clin N Am 46 (2002) 653–664

Antibiotics and oral contraceptives

Scott S. DeRossi, DMD[a],
Elliot V. Hersh, DMD, MS, PhD[b],*

[a]*Department of Oral Medicine, University of Pennsylvania School of Dental Medicine,
4001 Spruce Street, Philadelphia, PA 19104-6003, USA*
[b]*Department of Oral Surgery and Pharmacology, University of Pennsylvania School of
Dental Medicine, 4001 Spruce Street, Philadelphia, PA 19104-6003, USA*

Oral contraceptives and antibiotics are among the most widely used pre-scription medications in the United States. It is estimated that more than 11 million women in the United States use oral contraceptives, with up to 70 million women worldwide. Many more women of childbearing potential also periodically consume antibiotics. The proposed interaction between oral contraceptives and antibiotics has long been a major source of contro-versy and discussion in the literature [1]. Antibiotics are alleged to reduce blood concentrations and, therefore, the ultimate effectiveness of oral con-traceptive agents. The proposed mechanisms of these antibiotic-associated interactions include hepatic microsomal enzyme induction by the antibiotic of both the estrogen and progestin components of the oral contraceptive, interference with enterohepatic circulation of the oral contraceptive metab-olites, interference with oral contraceptive absorption from the gastrointes-tinal tract, alterations in plasma-protein binding of the oral contraceptive components, and increased excretion of the oral contraceptive. Considering the relatively high usage of both antibiotics and oral contraceptives, there is little scientific evidence to support this interaction. But sporadic case reports of oral contraceptive failure during concomitant antibiotic therapy do appear in the literature, and, to fully understand the rationale behind the proposed interaction, a discussion of the pharmacology of oral contracep-tives is necessary.

* Corresponding author.
E-mail address: evhersh@pobox.upenn.edu (E.V. Hersh).

The pharmacology of oral contraceptives

There are three types of oral contraceptives:

(1) The combined fixed-dose estrogen-progestin preparations (with high, medium, or low estrogen content)
(2) The combined sequential preparations with the doses of each steroid varied throughout the menstrual cycle
(3) The progestin-only preparations.

The goal of oral contraceptive therapy is to use a preparation that will minimize complications and side effects yet still prevent pregnancy.

Oral steroid contraceptives, or combination pills, are a mixture of semi-synthetic estrogens, usually ethinyl estradiol (EE) or mestranol, and semi-synthetic progesterones known as progestins (eg, norethindrone, levonorgestrel). In general, the estrogen component of oral contraceptives blocks ovulation by inhibiting the release of follicle-stimulating hormone (FSH) and leutinizing hormone (LH) via negative feedback on the pituitary gland and hypothalamus. The progestin component of oral contraceptives increases the viscosity of the cervical fluid, changes the endometrial lining to make it unsuitable for egg implantation, and provides some antiovulatory action [2,3].

To be effective, oral contraceptives must have adequate circulating concentrations of active hormone to prevent ovulation. In general, estrogens are present in very low concentrations (pg/ml) and sensitive and specific assays have only recently become available. Through these assays, it has become evident that even without any significant drug interactions, there is tremendous variation in plasma concentrations of active hormone among women. It is likely that women who have the lowest concentrations of estrogen are most likely to suffer interactions with other drugs.

Though it is the most effective form of reversible contraception, oral contraceptives, like any medication, are not 100% effective, and many women conceive while taking these preparations. When taken correctly, they reduce the chance of pregnancy to less than 1%. The reported failure rate among United States women is approximately 3% [4]. In the teenage population, the failure rate can be as high as 8%, often attributed to missed doses [5]. The most common causes of the pregnancies are thought to be missed pills, malabsorption, and drug interactions.

Oral contraceptives are not without side effects. The most critical side effect of the estrogen component is an increased risk of venous throboembolytic disease. The progestin component has been associated with increases in blood pressure, serum glucose, and serum lipid levels. An increased risk of myocardial infarction and stroke has been reported in oral contraceptive users who smoke and are greater than 35 years of age [6]. These significant adverse effects have led to the development of pills with reduced dosages of both estrogen and progestin components.

Interactions with rifampin

In the 1970s, reports began to appear regarding drug interactions between oral contraceptives and the antituberculosis drug rifampin. This was the first antibiotic implicated in reducing the effectiveness of oral contraceptives. Reimers and Jezek reported that 38 of 51 women (75%) taking rifampin and oral contraceptives concomitantly experienced breakthrough bleeding, an indicator of ovulation [7]. Two years later, another report of 88 women on oral contraceptive therapy associated concomitant rifampin use with 66 instances of breakthrough bleeding and five pregnancies [8]. Since then, other reports have followed associating increased risk of pregnancy with concomitant use of rifampin and oral contraceptives. Not surprisingly, over three-quarters of all alleged antibiotic–oral contraceptive interactions involve rifampin [9]. Clinical studies clearly demonstrate that rifampin significantly reduces blood levels of both the estrogen and progestin components of oral contraceptives [10–12] (Fig. 1). Though short-term exposure to rifampin or the related drug rifabutin may result in increased ethinyl estradiol and norethindrone clearance without reversing their contraceptive effect [12], long-term administration of these agents for tuberculosis therapy or prophylaxis is associated with both a diminution of hormonal blood levels and a reduction in contraceptive efficacy [7–11].

Rifampin is a potent inducer of the liver cytochrome p450 system and results in the increased metabolism and subsequent diminished blood levels of a number of drugs, including oral contraceptives [13]. Among antibiotics, only rifampin has been scientifically demonstrated to reduce blood levels and interfere with the effectiveness of oral contraceptives.

Interactions with other antibiotics

Anecdotal evidence implicating more commonly prescribed antibiotics with interference of oral contraceptive effectiveness began appearing in 1975. Dosseter reported three cases of pregnancy in patients taking oral contraceptives who were given ampicillin [14]. A few years later, another report was published describing a 20-year-old student who claimed to be totally compliant with her oral contraceptive regimen but became pregnant after a 5-day course of tetracycline [15]. In 1982, DeSano and Hurley described 16 pregnancies over a 2-year period in their private obstetric/gynecologic practices, all in patients who claimed to be compliant with their contraceptive regimen [16]. Antibiotics had been consumed in 13 of the cases; 5 patients had reported using ampicillin, 3 patients used penicillin, 3 patients had used sulfisoxazole or another sulfonamide antibiotic, 1 patient had used tetracycline, and 1 patient had used cephalexin. In 1986, a case report of an alleged antibiotic–oral contraceptive interaction appeared in the dental literature. Bainton reported a case of a 19-year-old who had taken an oral contraceptive for 18 months and received an intramuscular injection of a

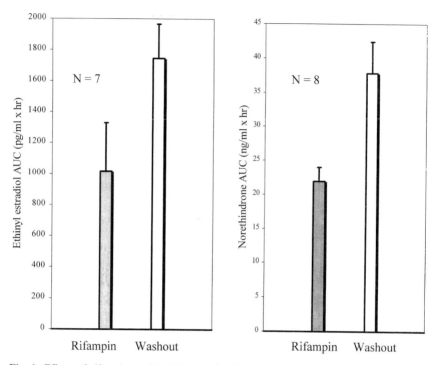

Fig. 1. Effects of rifampin on blood levels of ethinyl estradiol and norethindrone. Women received daily doses of 450–600 mg rifampin for up to 1 year from exposure to tuberculosis, followed by a 1-month washout period. A single dose of Minovlar® (50 ug ethinyl estradiol plus 1 mg norethindrone acetate) was administered after an overnight fast, toward the end of rifampin therapy and again 1 month after discontinuing rifampin. Blood samples for pharmacokinetic analyses were taken immediately before Minovlar® ingestion and then at 1, 2, 3, 4, 6, 8, 11, 14, and 24 hours after dosing. There was a significant decrease in area under the plasma concentration curves (mean ± SE) for both ethinyl estradiol (p < 0.01) and norethindrone (p < 0.01) during rifampin therapy compared with the control washout period as analyzed by Student t tests. (*Adapted from* Back DJ, Breckenridge AM, Crawford FE, et al. The effect of rifampicin on the pharmacokinetics of ethinyl estradiol in women. Contraception 1980;21(2):135–43; and Back DJ, Breckenridge AM, Crawford FE, et al. The effect of rifampicin on norhisterone pharmacokinetics. Eur J Clin Pharmacol 1979;15:193–7; with permission.)

long-acting penicillin combination during a surgical extraction procedure [17]. Three months later, she was found to be pregnant with twins.

Back et al published the most comprehensive report of potential antibiotic–oral contraceptive interactions [18]. They gathered data from the United Kingdom's Committee on Safety in Medicines between 1968 and 1984. During this time, 63 pregnancies were reported with simultaneous administration of oral contraceptives and antibiotics, excluding rifampin. Penicillins were implicated in 32 of these pregnancies, tetracyclines in 12, cotrimoxazole (sulfamethoxazole and trimethoprim) in 5, metronidazole in 3, erythromycin in 2, cephalosporins in 2, and either "unknown antibiotics" or antibiotics not commonly used in dentistry in the other 7 cases. In an effort to temper these findings, they also reported, that there were over 307 million prescriptions for these same antibiotics, and approximately 2.5 million regular users of oral contraceptives during this time period. Based on these figures, the actual number of reported pregnancies in England alleged to involve oral contraceptive interactions with antibiotics other than rifampin was extremely low.

In the United States, 29 reports of unintended pregnancies in oral contraceptive users who received penicillins or tetracyclines were listed in the United States Department of Health and Human Services' MEDWATCH Spontaneous Reporting System [19]. These numbers also should be tempered with the fact that over 11 million women per year use oral contraceptives in the United States [1].

The pharmacological basis of the interaction

A number of theories have been proposed to explain the occasional failures seen in oral contraceptive effectiveness when antibiotics are concomitantly ingested. The evidence-based support or "better, lack of support" for each theory is briefly reviewed below.

Hepatic microsomal enzyme induction

A number of drugs are capable of inducing liver microsomal enzymes, thereby increasing the rate of metabolism of both themselves and other drugs. This is certainly the case with rifampin, a potent inducer of the liver microsomal enzyme system. When ingested by women who are also oral contraceptive users, circulating estrogen and progestin concentrations may drop dramatically, below levels necessary to prevent ovulation. Decreased oral contraceptive effectiveness has been described with the concurrent use of other drugs known to induce microsomal enzymes, such as anticonvulsants and barbiturates [18,20]. None of the antibiotics currently used in outpatient dentistry, however, are liver microsomal enzyme inducers.

Interference with enterohepatic circulation of steroid metabolites

The ability of antibiotics to inhibit the enterohepatic recirculation of the estrogen component of oral contraceptives is probably the most widely promulgated theory of oral contraceptive failure. Ethinyl estradiol (EE) is well absorbed in humans, but the bioavailability of EE is approximately 40–50% because of a large first-pass metabolism in the gut and liver. Some of these inactive metabolites are sulfate and glucuronic acid conjugation products, which are subsequently excreted in the bile [21]. It is thought that these conjugates are then hydrolyzed by gut colonic bacteria, liberating the lipid-soluble and active parent compound, which is readily absorbed from the intestine into the bloodstream, providing the necessary additional serum concentrations to prevent ovulation (Fig. 2). This enterohepatic recirculation would be far more important for EE than for progestins because the latter undergoes significant phase 1 oxidative metabolism prior to conjugation. In theory, antibiotics that kill or inhibit the growth of the colonic bacteria involved in the deconjugation of EE can inhibit the enterohepatic recirculation of the active estrogen component. Animal studies do support the enterohepatic recirculation theory [22], but studies in humans fail to document the same interference. Some experts have speculated that there may be a subset of women that rely more heavily on enterohepatic recirculation of EE to maintain therapeutic serum levels. An atypical gut flora, which is highly sensitive to the administered antibiotic and/or a defective cytochrome p450 isoenzyme system where phase 2 metabolism (glucoronidation and sulfation) of the parent EE molecule is more heavily relied upon than initial phase 1 hydroxylation reactions, may contribute to this phenomena and the subsequent reduction in antiovulatory estrogen blood levels [22–24].

Interference with absorption from the gastrointestinal tract

There have been few studies concerning the absolute bioavailability of EE. Indirect evidence exists that EE is rapidly absorbed with the peak plasma concentration achieved at 120 minutes after dosing [24]. Interference with oral contraceptive absorption from the gastrointestinal tract has been demonstrated with ascorbic acid, but to date no interactions with antibiotics through this mechanism have been reported. Infective diarrhea because of increased gastrointestinal motility might reduce oral contraceptive

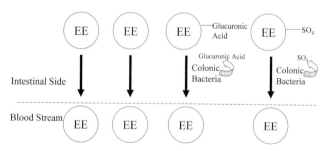

Fig. 2. Proposed action of colonic bacteria on the disposition of ethinyl estradiol (EE). EE undergoes a significant first-pass effect, and some of these inactive metabolites are conjugates of glucuronic acid and SO_4. These conjugated metabolites of EE would be inactive and lack sufficient lipid solubility to be absorbed into the blood stream, leading to a diminution of EE blood levels. It is hypothesized that bacteria, which are part of the normal intestinal flora, cleave the glucuronic acid and SO_4 groups from the metabolized EE molecules, liberating the active and lipid-soluble parent molecule that can be reabsorbed into the blood stream. By killing or inhibiting the growth of the normal intestinal microflora, antibiotics may interfere with this recycling process and result in the reduction of EE blood levels.

absorption. Although antibiotics can induce diarrhea, there are no published reports of such an event reducing the effectiveness of oral contraceptive agents.

Alterations in plasma protein binding

Ethinyl estradiol is 97% bound to plasma proteins, namely albumin, and plays a role in sex hormone-binding globulin capacity. As synthetic progestins are carried by sex hormone-binding globulin, various ratios of ingested hormones may produce alterations in binding, leading to significant changes in total plasma hormone concentrations. In general, protein-binding drug interactions are overemphasized for most drugs, and their effects are short lived. The only reported protein binding interactions with oral contraceptives involve anticonvulsants, not antibiotics [9,20].

Increased excretion of the contraceptive

Documented cases of increased urinary or fecal excretion of oral contraceptives by concomitant antibiotic use, including that caused by antibiotic-induced diarrhea, has not been substantiated in the literature.

Clinical studies evaluating the interaction

Although case reports should not be ignored and theoretically could indicate a rare interaction between antibiotics and oral contraceptives, a number of reviews have been published implying that the ability of commonly prescribed antibiotics to reduce the efficacy of oral contraceptives is an established, proven drug interaction [25–27]. An excerpt of such an article read, "The antibiotics that interfere with the ovulatory inhibiting effects of oral contraceptives are penicillin V potassium, amoxicillin, cephalexin, tetracycline and erythromycins" [27]. Unfortunately, these authors cited previously published case reports and not any controlled studies or pharmacokinetic data [28]. In 1991, the American Dental Association (ADA) Health Foundation Research Institute added "fuel to the fire" by publishing a statement that read "...Many antibiotics commonly used in dentistry interfere with the action of oral contraceptives, resulting in unexpected pregnancies" [29].

Many experts refer to the study published by Williams and Pulkinnen in 1971 as scientific proof of an interaction between antibiotics and oral contraceptives [30]. Although the authors reported reduced estrogen concentrations in pregnant patients taking ampicillin, this study did not evaluate the effect of ampicillin on blood levels of the estrogen or progestin component of oral contraceptives. Since then, a number of studies have looked directly at oral contraceptive blood levels in both the absence and presence of antibiotic treatment. All studies reached a similar conclusion. The concomitant

ingestion of ampicillin, tetracycline, doxycycline, metronidazole, erythromycin, clarithromycin, temafloxacin, or fluconazole did not reduce plasma levels of either the estrogen or progestin component of the oral contraceptive
[21,24,31–36]. The results of one such study with the antibiotic doxycycline
[36], a drug that is being widely employed in periodontal therapy, is illustrated in Fig. 3.

A second type of study addressing the interaction has analyzed unintended pregnancy rates as the outcome measure in oral contraceptive users
who consumed antibiotics. These studies have appeared in the dermatology
literature and are retrospective by nature. In a survey that evaluated pregnancy rates in 34 oral contraceptive users who were prescribed erythromycin, tetracycline, or minocycline, a pregnancy rate of 1.4% per year was
calculated [37]. This pregnancy rate did not differ from the accepted normal failure rate of oral contraceptives. In a larger retrospective study of
356 patients with a history of combined antibiotic-oral contraceptive use
and of 425 women taking oral contraceptives without antibiotic exposure,
Helms et al reported a yearly pregnancy rate of 1.6% in the antibiotic group
and 0.96% in the control group [4]. There was no significant difference

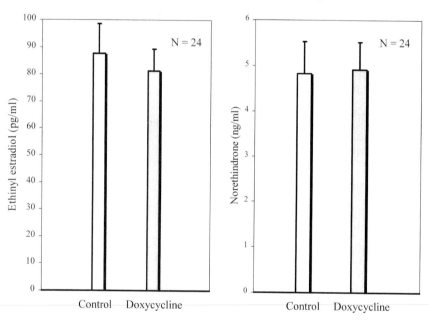

Fig. 3. Effects of doxycycline on blood levels of ethinyl estradiol and norethindrone. Women on
a steady dose of Ortho-Novum® (35 ug ethinyl estradiol plus 1 mg norethindrone; Ortho-
McNeil Pharmaceutical, Raritan, NJ) had serum concentrations of ethinyl estradiol and
norethindrone measure on days 18, 19, and 20 of the menstrual cycle, both in the absence and
presence of doxycycline therapy 100 mg twice daily. There were no significant reductions in
serum concentrations (mean ± SE) of either hormonal constituent during antibiotic therapy
($p = 0.49$ for ethinyl estradiol concentrations and $p = 0.36$ for norethindrone concentrations,
paired student t tests).

(P = 0.4) in pregnancy rates between the antibiotic and control groups, and both groups had pregnancy rates blow the 3% failure rate typically found in the United States.

Legal actions and opinions

Reports of at least two successful litigations (settled out of court) involving unintended pregnancies in oral contraceptive users prescribed antibiotics by dentists who failed to warn the patients of the possibility of reduced oral contraceptive efficacy continues to be emphasized by dental/legal experts [38]. Unfortunately, these legal proceedings cannot be researched or even substantiated. In the one published case where a plaintiff and her husband sued an army-based oral surgeon and gynecologist for malpractice and "wrongful life" for not warning her of a potential antibiotic/oral contraceptive interaction and the unintended pregnancy that allegedly occurred either during or shortly after she was prescribed penicillin V, the health professionals were exonerated [39]. In summarizing these legal proceedings, the patient and her husband lost the case for the following reasons:

(1) Her experts were unable to cite a single published scientific study that statistically demonstrated an association between penicillin use and oral contraceptive failure
(2) The scientific studies that her experts did cite all demonstrated a lack of interaction between commonly employed antibiotics and oral contraceptives
(3) All review articles cited by her experts supporting the interaction were not evidence-based
(4) Under California law, rare risks of drug therapy do not have to be discussed (ie, the risk of contraceptive failure during antibiotic therapy would have to be at least double the normal failure rate for the necessity of informed discussion)
(5) Her experts were unable to prove that she became pregnant either during or shortly after she was taking penicillin.

Summary

With the exception of rifampin-like drugs, there is a lack of scientific evidence supporting the ability of commonly prescribed antibiotics, including all those routinely employed in outpatient dentistry, to either reduce blood levels and/or the effectiveness of oral contraceptives. To date, all clinical trials studying the effects of concomitant antibiotic therapy (with the exception of rifampin and rifabutin) have failed to demonstrate an interaction. Like all drugs, oral contraceptives are not 100% effective with the failure rate in the typical United States population reported to be as high as 3%. It is thus possible that the case reports of unintended pregnancies during antibiotic therapy may simply represent the normal failure rate of these drugs. Considering that both drug classes are prescribed frequently to women of child-bearing potential, one would expect a much higher rate of oral contraceptive failure in this group of patients if a true drug:drug interaction existed. On the other hand, if the interaction does exist but is a relatively rare event, occurring in, say, 1 in 5000 women, clinical studies such as those described in this article would not detect the interaction. The pharmacokinetic studies of simultaneous antibiotic and oral contraceptive ingestion, and the retrospective studies of pregnancy rates among oral contraceptive users exposed to antibiotics, all suffer from one potential common weakness, ie, their relatively small sample size. Sample sizes in the pharmacokinetic trials ranged from 7 to 24 participants, whereas the largest retrospective study of pregnancy rates still evaluated less than 800 total contraceptive users. Still, the incidence of such a rare interaction would not differ from the accepted normal failure rate of oral contraceptive therapy.

The medico-legal ramifications of what looks like at best a rare interaction remains somewhat "murky." On one hand, we have medico-legal experts advising the profession to exercise caution and warn all oral contraceptive users of a potential reduction in efficacy during antibiotic therapy. These opinions are not evidence-based and rely heavily on one or two legal proceedings that cannot even be substantiated. On the other hand, there is one recently published legal proceeding in which the outcome was in favor of the oral surgeon. There is clearly a need for additional scientific research in oral contraceptive users that incorporates larger sample sizes, different time courses (prophylactic use versus standard 7–10 day use versus extended use), and different delivery systems (systemic administration versus local-controlled delivery) of antibiotic therapy. Though experts on this topic still recommend informing oral contraceptive users of the potential for a rare interaction, and for clinicians to advise them to employ additional barrier techniques of birth control during antibiotic therapy and for at least 1 week beyond the last dose [40], it is hoped that a set of guidelines regarding this controversy will eventually be published that is evidence-based, and not solely the results of anecdotal reports, expert opinions, and legal proceedings.

References

[1] Miller DM, Helms SE, Brodell RT. A practical approach to antibiotic treatment in women taking oral contraceptives. J Am Acad Dermatol 1994;30:1008–111.
[2] Goldfien A. The gonadal hormones and inhibitors. In: Katzung BG, editor. Basic and clinical pharmacology. 7th edition. Stamford: Appleton & Lange; 1998. p. 989–97.
[3] Weisberg E. Interactions between oral contraceptives and antifungal/antibacterials. Is contraceptive failure the result? Clin Pharmacokinet 1999;36(5):309–13.
[4] Helms SE, Bredle DL, Zajic J, et al. Oral contraceptive failure rates and oral antibiotics. J Am Acad Dermatol 1997;36:705–10.

[5] Sondheimer SJ. Update on oral contraceptive pills and postcoidal contraception. Curr Opin Obstet Gynecol 1992;4(4):502–5.

[6] Gillum LA, Mamidipudi SK, Johnston SC. Ischemic stroke risk with oral contraceptives: a meta-analysis. JAMA 2000;284(1):72–8.

[7] Reimers D, Jezek A. The simultaneous use of rifampicin and other antitubercular agents with oral contraceptives. Prax Pneumol 1971;25(5):255–62.

[8] Noche-Fink I, Breuer H, Reimers D. Effects of rifampicin on the menstrual cycle and on estrogen excretion in patients taking oral contraceptives. JAMA 1973;226(3):378.

[9] Szoka PR, Edgren RA. Drug interactions with oral contraceptives: compilation and analysis of an adverse experience report database. Fertil Steril 1988;29(5 suppl 2):31s–38s.

[10] Back DJ, Breckenridge AM, Crawford FE, et al. The effect of rifampicin on the pharmacokinetics of ethinyl estradiol in women. Contraception 1980;21(2):135–43.

[11] Back DJ, Breckenridge AM, Crawford FE, et al. The effect of rifampicin on norhisterone pharmacokinetics. Eur J Clin Pharmacol 1979;15:193–7.

[12] Barditch-Crovo P, Trapnell CB, Ette E, et al. The effects of rifampin and rifabutin on the pharmacokinetics and pharmacodynamics of a combination oral contraceptive. Clin Pharmacol Ther 1999;65(4):428–38.

[13] Michaelets EL. Update: clinically significant cytochrome p450 drug interactions. Pharmacotherapy 1998;18(1):84–112.

[14] Dosseter J. Drug interaction with oral contraceptives. Br Med J 1975;4(5994):467–8.

[15] Bacon JF, Shenfield GM. Pregnancy attributable to interaction between tetracyclines and oral contraceptives. Br Med J 1980;280(6210):293.

[16] DeSano EA, Hurley SC. Possible interactions of antihistamines and antibiotics with oral contraceptive effectiveness. Fertil Steril 1980;37(6):853–4.

[17] Bainton R. Interaction between antibiotic therapy and contraceptive medication. Oral Surg 1986;61:453–5.

[18] Back DJ, Grimmer SF, Orme ML, et al. Evaluation of Committee on Safety of Medicines yellow card reports on oral contraceptive-drug interactions with anticonvulsants and antibiotics. Br J Clin Pharmacol 1988;25(5):527–32.

[19] Donley TG, Smith RF, Roy B. Reduced oral contraceptive effectiveness with concurrent antibiotic use: a protocol for prescribing antibiotics to women of childbearing age. Compend Contin Educ Dent 1990;9(6):392–6.

[20] Shenfield GM. Drug interactions with oral contraceptives. Med J Aust 1986;144:205–11.

[21] Back DJ, Breckenridge AM, MacIver M, et al. The effects of ampicillin on oral contraceptive steroids in women. Br J Clin Pharmac 1982;14:43–8.

[22] Back DJ, Breckenridge AM, Cross KJ, et al. An antibiotic interaction with ethinyl estradiol in the rat and rabbit. J Steroid Biochem 1982;16(3):407–13.

[23] Back DJ, Orme ML. Pharmacokinetics drug interaction with oral contraceptives. Clin Pharmacokin 1990;18(6):472–84.

[24] Orme ML, Back DJ. Interactions between oral contraceptive steroids and broad-spectrum antibiotics. Clin Exp Dermatol 1986;11(4):327–31.

[25] Fazio A. Oral contraceptive drug interactions: important considerations. South Med J 1991;84(8):997–1002.

[26] Pyle MA, Faddoul FF, Terezhalmy GT. Clinical implication of drugs taken by our patients. Dent Clin North Am 1993;37(1):73–90.

[27] Wynn RL. The top 50 drugs dispensed by pharmacies in 1996. Gen Dent 1997;45(5):416–20.

[28] Hersh EV. Adverse drug interactions in dental practice: interactions involving antibiotics. J Am Dent Assoc 1999;130:236–51.

[29] ADA Health Foundation Research Institute, Department of Toxicology. Antibiotic interference with oral contraceptives. J Am Dent Assoc 1991;122(12):79.

[30] William K, Pulkkinen MO. Reduced maternal plasma and urinary estriol during ampicillin treatment. Am J Obstet Gynecol 1971;109(6):893–6.

[31] Back DJ, Tjia J, Martin C, et al. The interaction between clarithromycin and oral contraceptive steroids. J Pharm Med 1991;2(1):81–7.

[32] Back DJ, Tjia J, Martin C, et al. The lack of interaction between temafloxacin and combined oral contraceptive steroids. Contraception 1991;43(4):317–23.

[33] Joshi JV, Joshi UM, Sankholi GM, et al. A study of interaction of low-dose combination oral contraceptive with ampicillin and metronidazole. Contraception 1980;22(6):643–52.

[34] Lazar JD, Wilner KD. Drug interactions with fluconazole. Rev Infect Dis 1990;12(suppl 3):S327–33.

[35] Murphy AA, Zacur HA, Charche P, et al. The effect of tetracycline on levels of oral contraceptives. Am J Obstet Gynecol 1991;164(1):28–33.

[36] Neely JL, Abate M, Swinker M, et al. The effect of doxycycline on serum levels of ethinyl estradiol, norethindrone, and endogenous progesterone. Obstet Gynecol 1991;77(3): 416–20.

[37] London BM, Lookingbill DP. Frequency of pregnancy in acne patients taking oral antibiotics and oral contraceptives. Arch Dermatol 1994;130:392–3.

[38] Zinman EJ. Legal considerations. In: Newman MG, van Winkelhoff AJ, editors. Antibiotics and antimicrobial use in dental practice. 2nd edition. Chicago: Quintessence Publishing Co, Inc; 2001. p. 257–72.

[39] California court denies wrongful birth claim. J Law Med Ethics 1996;24(3):273–4.

[40] Burroughs KE, Chambliss ML. Antibiotics and oral contraceptive failure. Arch Fam Med 2000;9(1):81–2.

THE DENTAL
CLINICS OF
NORTH
AMERICA

Dent Clin N Am 46 (2002) 665–677

Periodontal therapy using local delivery of antimicrobial agents

Richard Niederman, DMD[a],*,
George Abdelshehid, BS[b],
J. Max Goodson, DDS, PhD[a]

[a]*Center for Evidence-Based Dentistry, The Forsyth Institute, 140 The Fenway, Boston, MA 02115, USA*
[b]*Harvard School of Dental Medicine, 188 Longwood Avenue, Boston, MA 02115, USA*

Periodontal diseases are bacterial infections that occur at or below the gingival margin. They occur in approximately 70% of the United States population and severely affect 20–30% of the United States population, who spend approximately $5 billion per year on therapy.

Optimum, cost-effective preventive therapy might logically lie in the elimination or control of the infection. Over the last century, numerous investigations attempted to define the etiologic agents of this disease. A small group of specific bacterial species are now considered to be the causative agents [1]. This group includes *Bacteroides forsythus, Porphyromonas gingivalis, Treponema denticola,* and *Actinobacillus actinomycetemcomitans.*

The recognition that specific microbes are the causative agents of periodontal disease stimulated the development of new tools to reduce the supra- and subgingival microbiota. Among the agents are chlorhexidine mouthwash, triclosan dentifrice, electronic toothbrushes, and systemic and local drug delivery. The purpose of these approaches is to attempt to disinfect pathogen reservoirs.

Local drug delivery is the focus of this article. Several treatments normally adjunctive to scaling and root planing have been tested. These include chlorhexidine disks, tetracycline fibers, and gels containing doxycycline, metronidazole, or minocycline microspheres. This article examines the efficacy of these local delivery systems.

This work was supported by DE 13850.
* Corresponding author.
E-mail address: rniederman@forsyth.org (R. Niederman).

A MEDLINE search strategy was developed and implemented to identify studies on the efficacy of local antimicrobial drug delivery systems for the treatment of periodontal disease (Table 1). The search included articles from 1966 to September 2001 week 1, and was executed on the Ovid interface for MEDLINE (http://gateway.ovid.com). The five antimicrobial agents included in this search were local delivery products containing metronidazole (MET) (Elyzol®, a gel that can be injected into the periodontal pocket), chlorhexidine (CHX) (PerioChip®, a flat disk that can be inserted into the pocket), tetracycline (TTC) (Actisite®, a fiber that can be placed into the periodontal pocket), doxycycline (DOX) (Atridox®, a gel that can be injected into the pocket), and minocycline (MNC) (Arestin®, a microsphere gel that can be injected into the pocket).

Inclusion criteria were randomized controlled trials, in vivo human trials, publications in English, and trials that compared one or more of these agents in local delivery systems with each other, to scaling and root planing (SRP) or to another control group. From the identified articles, the Food and Drug Administration (FDA) pivotal studies were selected for detailed analysis to determine the number needed to treat (NNT). When a new drug comes to market, the FDA standard has been to require two controlled clinical trials that demonstrate efficacy of the product. Generally, the applicant company conducts several trials. Although not commonly appreciated, the FDA selects the trials it considers "pivotal" and allows the applicant company to write the package insert using data from those trials. Hence, identification of pivotal trials was accomplished by determining the trials that were cited in the package insert of each product.

Table 1
MEDLINE search

Step	Search history	Results
1	Exp periodontics/	13494
2	Exp periodontal diseases/	40247
3	1 or 2	45576
4	Chlorhexidine.tw.	2856
5	Metronidazole.tw.	6572
6	Tetracycline.tw.	12948
7	Doxycycline.tw.	3408
8	Minocycline.tw.	2024
9	4 or 5 or 6 or 7 or 8	25701
10	Fiber.tw.	39794
11	Chip.tw.	1532
12	Gel.tw.	130288
13	10 or 11 or 12	170862
14	Local delivery.tw. or *drug delivery/	566
15	13 or 14	171394
16	3 and 9 and 15	187
17	Limit 16 to (human and english language)	165

NNT was determined using the percentage of patients, sites, or teeth with either a probing depth (PD) reduction or attachment level (AL) gain of ≥ 2 mm:

$$NNT = 1/(\%\text{experimental sites} \geq 2\,mm - \%\,\text{control sites} \geq 2\,mm)$$

We further analyzed the data to determine cost effectiveness for each drug:

$$\text{cost effectiveness} = (\text{estimated product cost} + \text{care cost}) \times NNT$$

Additional data for chlorhexidine and minocycline were obtained from their respective package inserts, and data for tetracycline were obtained from the author of the study.

The MEDLINE search (see Table 1) identified 165 articles, 52 of which fit the inclusion criteria. All 52 studies conducted randomized control trials examining the efficacy of five different local delivery systems for antimicrobial agents to treat periodontal disease.

Tables 2 through 6 provide details of the identified studies. Eighteen studies examined metronidazole (Table 2), with studies ranging in size from 10 to 206 subjects, and study lengths from 1.5 to 9 months. The chlorhexidine delivery system was examined in 12 studies (Table 3), with study sizes ranging from 10 to 418 subjects, and study length from 1 to 9 months.

Table 2
Metronidazole

Ref[a]	N	Experimental group—metronidazole	Control group (s)	Outcomes BP	PD	AL	PI	GI	M	Followup (m)
[2]	84	+SRP	SRP	+	+	+			+	6
[3]	12	±SRP	SRP; UC	+	+		+	+		2
[4]	10	Alone	Placebo	+	+	+			+	3
[5]	12	Alone	UC		+		+	+		6
[6]	46	Alone	SRP		+	+			+	4.5
[7]	18	+SRP	TC; SRP	+	+	+			+	6
[8]	84	+SRP	SRP	+	+	+				6
[9]	30	Alone	SRP	+	+				+	6
[10]	206	Alone	SRP	+	+					6
[11]	24	Alone	SRP	+	+				+	6
[12]	61	Alone	SRP	+	+					3
[13]	59	+SRP	SRP	+	+	+			+	9
[14]	84	+SRP	SRP	+	+	+				9
[15]	29	+SRP	SRP	+	+	+	+			3
[16]	54	+SRP	TC; MC; SRP	+	+	+	+	+		1.5
[17]	10	±SRP	SRP; UC		+	+	+	+	+	1.5
[18]	12	±SRP	SRP; UC		+	+	+	+	+	1.5
[19]	69	±SRP	TC; CX; SRP	+	+	+				3

[a] Ref, reference number; N, number of total subjects completing the study; BP, bleeding on probing; PD, probing depth; AL, attachment level; PI, plaque index; GI, gingival index; M, microbiota; m, months; SRP, scaling and root planing; TC, tetracycline; UC, untreated control; MC, minocycline.

Table 3
Chlorhexidine

Ref	N	Experimental group—chlorhexidine	Control group (s)	Outcomes						Followup (m)
				BP	PD	AL	PI	GI	M	
[19]	69	Alone	MT; TC; SRP	+	+	+				3
[20]	10	+SRP	SRP	+	+		+	+	+	2
[21]	10	Alone	Placebo	+	+		+	+	+	1
[22]	26	+SRP	TC; SRP	+	+	+	+	+		8
[23]	10	+SRP	SRP	+	+	+	+	+		8
[24]	418	+SRP	SRP ± Placebo	+	+	+	+	+		9
[25]	10	+SRP	SRP		+		+		+	8
[26]	22	+SRP	TC; SRP	+	+	+	+	+		3
[27]	10	+SRP	SRP + Placebo[a1]	+	+				+	9
[28]	42	+SRP	SRP ± Placebo		+	+				9
[29]	94	+SRP	SRP	+	+	+	+	+		6
[30]	58	+SRP	SRP[a2]		+		+	+	+	3

[a] Ancillary treatment: 1. Amine fluoride and stannous fluoride gels; 2. Chlorhexidine gluconate irrigation; H_2O irrigation.

Ref, reference number; N, number of total subjects completing the study; BP, bleeding on probing; PD, probing depth; AL, attachment level; PI, plaque index; GI, gingival index; M, microbiota; m, months; SRP, scaling and root planing; MT, metronidazole; TC, tetracycline.

Nineteen studies examined the efficacy of the tetracycline delivery system (Table 4), with study size ranging from 10 to 123 subjects, and study lengths ranging from 1-month to 5-year followup study. Five studies examined the efficacy of the doxycycline delivery system (Table 5) and engaged between 141 and 758 subjects, all with study lengths of 9 months. The minocycline delivery system was examined in five studies (Table 6), with study sizes ranging from 15 to 54 people and study lengths from 1.5 to 18 months.

Study outcomes and design varied considerably. For example, 85% of the studies examined bleeding on probing (BP), 96% examined pocket depth (PD), 77% examined attachment level (AL), 48% examined probing index (PI), 35% examined gingival index (GI), and 38% examined microbiota (M).

Because of variability in study design, we elected to examine in detail only the four agents with FDA pivotal trials. Table 7 summarizes the data derived from the FDA pivotal studies and articulates the NNT using this data. NNTs were calculated for change in probing depth (PD) and AL, with 2 mm selected as a statistically and clinically significant change. For pocket depth reduction, the efficacies of the products from most to least effective were, respectively, tetracycline fiber, chlorhexidine disk, and minocycline microspheres. For attachment level only the tetracycline delivery system study provided data that allowed us to determine NNT. For the doxycycline delivery system, the study design did not allow for a determination of NNT.

It should be noted that the pivotal studies all exhibited variability in clinical characteristics. For example, all of the studies lasted 9 months, except for the tetracycline delivery system studies, which lasted 6 months.

Table 4
Tetracycline

Ref	N	Experimental group—tetracycline	Control group (s)	BP	PD	AL	PI	GI	M	Followup (m)
[7]	18	+SRP	MT; SRP	+	+	+			+	6
[16]	54	+SRP	MT; MC; SRP	+	+	+	+	+		1.5
[19]	69	Alone	MT; CX; SRP	+	+	+				3
[22]	26	+SRP	CX; SRP	+	+	+	+	+		3
[26]	22	+SRP	CX; SRP	+	+	+	+	+		3
[31]	107	Alone	SRP; UC; Placebo	+		+				2
[32]	16	±SRP	SRP[a]	+	+	+	+		+	3
[33]	105	+SRP	SRP	+	+	+				6
[34]	116	±SRP	SRP	+	+	+	+			12
[35]	116	±SRP	SRP	+	+	+	+			12
[36]	26	+SRP	SRP	+	+	+				60
[37]	18	Alone	UC	+	+	+				1
[38]	10	±SRP	SRP; UC	+	+		+	+	+	2
[39]	107	Alone	SRP; UC; Placebo	+		+				2
[40]	10	±SRP	SRP; UC			+	+			12
[41]	123	+SRP	SRP	+	+	+				6
[42]	19	+SRP	UC	+	+	+		+		6
[43]	10	Alone	SRP; UC; Placebo	+	+	+	+			6.5
[44]	17	+SRP	SRP	+	+	+		+	+	2

[a] Ancillary treatment: citric acid.

Ref, reference number; N, number of total subjects completing the study; BP, bleeding on probing; PD, probing depth; AL, attachment level; PI, plaque index; GI, gingival index; M, microbiota; m, months; SRP, scaling and root planing; UC, untreated control; CX, chlorhexidine; MT, metronidazole; MC, minocycline.

The studies also varied in number of drug placements and use of scaling and root planing in the experimental groups. Thus, the interpretation of the NNT needs careful consideration.

Although clinical efficacy is a desired outcome, cost effectiveness is a concern of the provider and payer. We therefore estimated cost effectiveness for these agents. Determination of the care cost includes the following variables:

Table 5
Doxycycline

Ref	N	Experimental group—doxycycline	Control group (s)	BP	PD	AL	PI	GI	M	Followup (m)
[45]	758	Alone	SRP; Placebo; UC	+	+	+	+			9
[46]	141	Alone	SRP; UC	+	+	+				9
[47]	170	Alone	Placebo[a]	+	+	+	+			9
[48]	317	Alone	SRP	+	+	+				9
[49]	170	Alone	Placebo[a]	+	+	+	+			9

[a] Ancillary treatment: sanguinarium chloride.

Ref, reference number; N, number of total subjects completing the study; BP, bleeding on probing; PD, probing depth; AL, attachment level; PI, plaque index; GI, gingival index; M, microbiota; m, months; SRP, scaling and root planing; UC, untreated control.

Table 6
Minocycline

Ref	N	Experimental group—minocycline	Control group (s)	Outcomes						Followup (m)
				BP	PD	AL	PI	GI	M	
[16]	54	+SRP	TC; MT; SRP	+	+	+	+	+		1.5
[50]	26	+SRP	SRP + Placebo	+	+	+				3
[51]	20	+SRP	SRP + Placebo	+	+	+	+	+	+	18
[52]	15	Alone	SRP; SS	+	+	+			+	1.5
[53]	39	±SRP	SRP; UC	+	+	+	+	+	+	6

SS, supragingival scaling; TC, tetracycline; MT, metronidazole; UC, untreated control.

Ref, reference number; N, number of total subjects completing the study; BP, bleeding on probing; PD, probing depth; AL, attachment level; PI, plaque index; GI, gingival index; M, microbiota; m, months; SRP, scaling and root planing.

cost of the agent, cost of wastage, number of drug placements, cost of scaling and root planing, and cost associated with clinician time. Assuming the effectiveness is accounted for by the NNT values calculated for PD reduction of ≥2 mm, we estimated the treatment cost for each local delivery system for treatment of a single tooth and a complete quadrant (Table 8, Fig. 1). Table 9 uses these calculations to estimate cost effectiveness. When treating a single tooth, total cost per tooth was least for the tetracycline delivery system ($99). The tetracycline delivery system was also approximately 3–4 times more cost effective than either the chlorhexidine or minocycline delivery systems, respectively ($495 versus $1260–$2016).

When treating a quadrant as an additional procedure to another dental treatment, cost analysis indicated that total cost per tooth for the chlorhexidine and minocycline delivery systems was half that of the tetracycline delivery system. Cost effectiveness was similar for the tetracycline and chlorhexidine delivery systems ($195 and $200), however, both of which were approximately 1.5 times more cost effective than the minocycline delivery system ($320).

Because data submitted to the FDA for validation of the doxycycline delivery product considered only equivalence of the product compared with SRP, cost effectiveness could not be determined. Cost comparison, however,

Table 7
Number needed to treat

Drug	Delivery system	Brand	Study length (m)	# SRP (expt)[a]	# Drug placements (expt)	NNT PD[b]	NNT AL
Tetracycline	Fiber	Actisite	6	1	1	5	9
Chlorhexidine	Chip	PerioChip	9	1	3	10	NA
Minocycline	Microsphere	Arestin	9	1	3	16	NA
Doxycycline	Gel	Atridox	9	0	2	NA	NA

[a] Expt, SRP received by experimental group; NTT; number needed to treat.

[b] CHX, MNC mean values for PD ≥2 mm from the two FDA studies.

SRP, scaling and root planing; PD, probing depth; AL, attachment level; FDA, Food and Drug Administration; NA, not available.

Table 8
Treatment cost

Assumptions						
Product[a]	Cost/unit purchase[b]	Teeth treated/unit[b]	Treatment visits required	Non treatment visits	Placement time (min/tooth)	Total setup cost[c]
TTC	$24	2	1	1	15	$50
CHX	$12	1	3	0	3	$75
MNC	$12	1	3	0	3	$75
DOX	$24	6	2	0	2	$50

Treatment of one tooth					
Product	Used product cost	Waste product cost	Placement cost[c]	Cost/tooth	As an add-on[d]
TTC	$12	$12	$25	$99	$49
CHX	$36	$0	$15	$126	$51
MNC	$36	$0	$15	$126	$51
DOX	$8	$40	$7	$105	$55

Treatment of one quadrant[d]					
Product	Used product cost	Waste product cost	Placement cost	Cost/tooth	As an add-on[e]
TTC	$84	$12	$175	$46	$39
CHX	$36	$0	$105	$31	$20
MNC	$36	$0	$105	$31	$20
DOX	$36	$40	$49	$28	$20

[a] TTC, tetracycline; CHX, chlorhexidine; MNC, minocycline; DOX, doxycycline; SRP, scaling and root planing.

[b] Assumptions: Tetracycline @ $24 per fiber, 2 teeth per fiber, $12 per tooth, 15 min for placement per tooth, 1 treatment and 1 removal visit. Chlorhexidine @ $12 per chip, 1 tooth per chip, $12 per tooth, 1 min for placement per tooth, 3 treatment visits. Minocycline @ $12 per cartridge, 1 tooth per cartridge, $12 per tooth, 1 min per placement per tooth, 3 treatment visits. Doxycycline @ $24 per cartridge, 6 teeth per cartridge, $4 per tooth, 1 min per placement per tooth, 2 treatment visits

[c] Assumptions: Setup cost = $25 per visit (treatment or nontreatment). Chair time = $100 per h × (placement time per tooth/60 min).

[d] Assumptions: One quadrant = 7 teeth (treatment cost − $200/quadrant = $29/tooth).

[e] Assumptions: When used as an additional or addon procedure, setup costs have been covered by the first procedure.

revealed that total cost associated with the doxycycline delivery system alone was approximately $28 per tooth, whereas the cost associated with SRP alone was $29 per tooth (Table 8[C], Assumption 4).

This systematic review was conducted to identify the available literature and to determine cost effectiveness of locally delivered antimicrobial agents in the treatment of periodontal disease. All 52 articles found in our search examined the efficacy of at least one of five different local delivery systems to one another or to scaling and root planing. Because there was a significant variability among the studies, we chose to more closely examine the FDA pivotal studies, and because metronidazole is not approved for use in the United States, it was excluded from further evaluation. Because of the

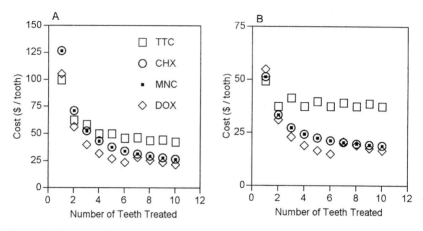

Fig. 1. (A) The cost of treatment of teeth ($/tooth) with periodontal disease by local delivery products as a visit scheduled solely for local delivery treatment. (B) The added cost of treatment of teeth ($/tooth) with periodontal disease by local delivery products.

variability in study design and reported results, a comprehensive product comparison was not possible. The available data only allowed for an NNT determination for pocket depth reduction, not for attachment level gain. The following comments speak to the overall results and their interpretation, based on study variability.

The FDA pivotal studies provided data for a determination of the NNT for three products: tetracycline fibers (Actisite), chlorhexidine disks (Perio-Chip), minocycline microspheres (Arestin). We were unable to make this determination for the doxycycline gel (Atridox) in that this product was not used as an adjunct to SRP. Inspection of the doxycycline gel data, however,

Table 9
Cost effectiveness[a]

	To treat one tooth		
Product[b]	Total cost ($)/tooth	NNT	Cost effectiveness ($)
TTC	99	5	$99 \times 5 = 495$
CHX	126	10	$126 \times 10 = 1260$
MNC	126	16	$126 \times 16 = 2016$
	Cost/tooth when treating one quadrant as an additional procedure		
Product[b]	Total cost ($)/tooth	NNT	Cost effectiveness ($)
TTC	39	5	$39 \times 5 = 195$
CHX	20	10	$20 \times 10 = 200$
MNC	20	16	$20 \times 16 = 320$

[a] Cost, over and above SRP, to have one additional pocket reduced by ≥2 mm.
[b] TTC, tetracycline; CHX, Chlorhexidine; MNC, minocycline.
SRP, scaling and root planing; NNT, number needed to treat.

demonstrated that the therapeutic effects of doxycycline gel alone were similar to those for SRP alone.

The NNTs suggest that at ≤9 months and compared with SRP alone, SRP plus the tetracycline fiber drug delivery system (Actisite) was most effective in reducing pocket depth (lowest NNT of five). This compares with an NNT of 10 and 16 for the chlorhexidine disk and the minocycline gel, respectively.

The NNT, although an awkward name and concept, has a useful clinical application. It allows one to provide a risk and benefit assessment to the patient. For example, for the tetracycline fiber, an NNT of five indicates the following risk and benefit. For every five teeth that are treated with SRP plus fibers (risk), one tooth will achieve ≥2 mm of pocket depth reduction when compared with SRP alone (benefit). Said differently, a patient may have five teeth treated with SRP plus fibers, but only one tooth will benefit by ≥2 mm more than SRP alone. Thus, the risk:reward ratio is 5:1.

As indicated, there were differing study designs. In addition, there were also differing drugs and drug delivery systems. Thus the differing results among the products may be attributable to study design, drug used, or drug delivery system. Although all three may be important, the available pharmacokinetic data suggest that the delivery system may have the greatest effect. The fibers sustain a constant high level of antibiotic in the gingival crevice for the week that they are in place. In contrast, the drug concentration for the other delivery systems decreases substantially over the first few days. Having a constant high level of drug in place over an extended period of time might account for the clinical effect.

The issue of study longevity could also have an impact on the results. The tetracycline fiber delivery system studies ranged from 2 to 6 months, whereas the other studies were 9 months in length (see Table 7). Thus one might suspect that the apparent efficacy of the tetracycline delivery system could degrade between 6 and 9 months. There is no evidence for or against this hypothesis.

The number of drug placements also varied within the studies being considered. The tetracycline delivery system was applied once, the doxycycline gel delivery system was applied twice, and the chlorhexidine disk and minocycline microsphere systems were applied three times (see Table 7). One would suspect that multiple placements would enhance the efficacy of the drug system, but this was not found to be the case.

Many complicating issues arise when attempting to determine the efficacy of these local delivery agents, most notably the cost effectiveness. The clinician and the patient must determine if the cost of the product is worth the possible benefit. The cost includes the price of the local delivery agent, the number of teeth treated, the number of drug placements required, the cost of product wastage, the cost associated with clinician time, and from the patient's perspective, the number of trips to the dentist.

Analysis revealed that when treating a single tooth, the tetracycline delivery system was the most cost effective, but when treating a quadrant the tetracycline and chlorhexidine delivery systems were equally cost effective. This is because of the relative balance of lower cost per tooth and higher NNT for chlorhexidine versus higher cost per tooth and lower NNT for tetracycline. From a patient's cost:benefit perspective, the cost per tooth to achieve a benefit from the tetracycline fibers is $195–$495 per tooth (Table 9). At the other end of the spectrum, following treatment by the minocycline delivery system, a patient would spend $320–$2,016 per tooth to obtain a clinically meaningful improvement in one tooth (see Table 9).

The results of the cost analysis clearly indicate that for all local delivery systems, the most expensive treatment occurred as a single tooth treated at a dedicated visit (Fig. 1, Table 8). Considerable economy could be realized by treating multiple teeth. Treatment of a quadrant was estimated to cost $30–$45 per tooth (see Fig. 1). Treatment of a quadrant as an added procedure costs as little as $20 per tooth. Clearly, the economic argument favors the adjunctive use of local delivery products as for periodontal maintenance. If multiple teeth are treated as an added procedure, even less effective treatments (ie, higher NNT) become cost effective (see Table 9).

As with all treatments, it is the clinician's responsibility to explain the treatment options available, their cost, and their expected efficacy to the patients so that the patient can decide the relative worth of their possible benefits. To some patients, maximizing effectiveness may be the primary objective irrespective of cost. For these patients, treatments with low NNT values would be preferred. To others, maximizing cost effectiveness may be the primary objective. For these patients, an appeal to multiple tooth treatments as an adjunctive procedure would be desirable. Still other patients may believe that any treatment beyond scaling and root planing is not worth the extra expenditure. Only by combining benefit and cost analysis can the needs of each individual patient be met.

References

[1] Socransky SS, Haffajee AD, Cugini MA, Smith C, Kent RL Jr. Microbial complexes in subgingival plaque. J Clin Periodontol 1998;25:134–44.
[2] Palmer RM, Matthews JP, Wilson RF. Adjunctive systemic and locally delivered metronidazole in the treatment of periodontitis: a controlled clinical study. Br Dent J 1998;184:548–52.
[3] Awartani FA, Zulqarnain BJ. Comparison of the clinical effects of subgingival application of metronidazole 25% gel and scaling in the treatment of adult periodontitis. Quintessence Int 1998;27:41–8.
[4] Needleman IG, Watts TLP. The effect of 1% metronidazole gel in routine maintenance of persistent furcation involvement in human beings. J Periodontol 1989;60:699–703.
[5] Sander L, Frandsen EVG, Arnbjerg D, Warrer K, Karring T. Effect of local metronidazole application on periodontal healing following guided tissue regeneration. Clinical findings. J Periodontol 1994;65:914–20.
[6] Rudhart A, Rurucker P, Kage A, Hopfenmuller W, Bernimoulin JP. Local metronidazole application in maintenance patients. Clinical and microbiological evaluation. J Periodontol 1998;69:1148–54.

[7] Lie T, Bruun G, Boe OE. Effects of topical metronidazole and tetracycline in treatment of adult periodontitis. J Periodontol 1998;69:819–27.

[8] Palmer RM, Matthews JP, Wilson RF. Non-surgical periodontal treatment with and without adjunctive metronidazole in smokers and non-smokers. J Clin Periodontol 1999;26: 158–63.

[9] Stelzel M, Flores-de-Jacoby L. Topical metronidazole application compared with subgingival scaling. A clinical and microbiological study on recall patients. J Clin Periodontol 1996;23:24–9.

[10] Ainamo J, Ellingsen BH, Hansen BF, Johansson LA, Darring T, Kisch J, et al. Clinical responses to subgingival application of a metronidazole 25% gel compared to the effect of subgingival scaling in adult periodontitis. J Clin Periodontol 1992;19:723–9.

[11] Pedrazzoli V, Kilian M, Karring T. Comparable clinical and microbiological effects of topical subgingival application of a 25% metronidazole gel and scaling in the treatment of adult periodontitis. J Clin Periodontol 1992;19:715–22.

[12] Klinge B, Attstrom R, Karring T, Kisch J, Lewin B, Stoltze K. Three regimens of topical metronidazole compared with subgingival scaling on periodontal pathology in adults. J Clin Periodontol 1992;19:708–14.

[13] Stelzel M, Flores-de-Jacoby L. Topical metronidazole application as an adjunct to scaling and root planing. J Clin Periodontol 2000;27:447–52.

[14] Griffiths GS, Smart GJ, Bulman JS, Weiss G, Schroweder J, Newman HN. Comparison of clinical outcomes following treatment of chronic adult periodontitis with subgingival scaling or subgingival scaling plus metronidazole gel. J Clin Periodontol 2000;27: 910–7.

[15] Riep B, Purucker P, Bernimoulin JP. Repeated local metronidazole-therapy as adjunct to scaling and root planing in maintenance patients. J Clin Periodontol 1999;26:710–5.

[16] Radvar M, Pourtaghi N, Kinane DF. Comparison of 3 periodontal local antibiotic therapies in persistent periodontal pockets. J Periodontol 1996;67:860–5.

[17] Noyan U, Yilmaz S, Kuru B, Kadir T, Acar O, Buget E. A clinical and microbiological evaluation of systemic and local metronidazole delivery in adult periodontitis patients. J Clin Periodontol 1997;24:158–65.

[18] Yilmaz S, Kuru B, Noyan U, Kadir T, Acar O, Buget E. A clinical and microbiological evaluation of systemic and local metronidazole delivery in early onset periodontitis patients. J Marmara Univ Dent Faculty 1996;2:500–9.

[19] Moran J, Addy M, Wade W, Newcombe R. The use of antimicrobial acrylic strips in the non-surgical management of chronic periodontitis. Clin Mater 1990;6:123–35.

[20] Quirynen M, Bollen CML, Vandekerckhove BNA, Dekeyser C, Papaioannou W, Eyssen H. Full- vs. partial-mouth disinfection in the treatment of periodontal infections: short-term clinical and microbiological observations. J Dent Res 1995;74:1459–67.

[21] Kalaitzakis CJ, Tynelius-Bratthall G, Attstrom R. Clinical and microbiological effects of subgingival application of a chlorhexidine gel in chronic periodontitis. A pilot study. Swed Dent J 1993;17:129–37.

[22] Unsal E, Walsh TF, Akkaya M. The effect of a single application of subgingival antimicrobial or mechanical therapy on the clinical parameters of juvenile periodontitis. J Periodontol 1995;66:47–51.

[23] Vandekerckhove BNA, Bollen CML, Dekeyser C, Darius P, Quirynen M. Full- versus partial-mouth disinfection in the treatment of periodontal infections. Long-term clinical observations of a pilot study. J Periodontol 1996;67:1251–9.

[24] Jeffcoat MK, Bray KS, Ciancio SG, et al. Adjunctive use of a subgingival controlled-release chlorhexidine chip reduces probing depth and improves attachment level compared with scaling and root planing alone. J Periodontol 1998;69:989–97.

[25] Bollen CML, Vandekerckhove BNA, Papaioannou W, Van Eldere J, Quirynen M. Full- versus partial-mouth disinfection in the treatment of periodontal infections. A pilot study: long-term microbiological observations. J Clin Periodontol 1996;23:960–70.

[26] Unsal E, Akkaya M, Walsh TF. Influence of a single application of subgingival chlorhexidine gel or tetracycline paste on the clinical parameters of adult periodontitis patients. J Clin Periodontol 1994;21:351–5.

[27] Oosterwaal PJM, Mikx FHM, van't Hof MA, Renggli HH. Comparison of the anti-microbial effect of the application of chlorhexidine gel, amine fluoride gel and stannous fluoride gel in debrided periodontal pockets. J Clin Periodontol 1991;18:245–51.

[28] Jeffcoat MK, Palcanis KG, Weatherford TW, Reese M, Geurs NC, Flashner M. Use of a biodegradable chlorhexidine chip in the treatment of adult periodontitis: clinical and radiographic findings. J Periodontol 2000;71:256–62.

[29] Soskolne WA, Heasman PA, Stabholz A, Smart GJ, Palmer M, Flashner M, et al. Sustained local delivery of chlorhexidine in the treatment of periodontitis: a multi-center study. J Periodontol 1997;68:32–8.

[30] Jolkovsky DL, Waki MY, Newman MG, Otomo-Corgel J, Madison M, Flemmig TF, et al. Clinical and microbiological effects of subgingival and gingival marginal irrigation with chlorhexidine gluconate. J Periodontol 1990;61:663–9.

[31] Goodson JM, Gugini MA, Kent RL, et al. Multicenter evaluation of tetracycline fiber therapy: II. Clinical response. J Periodontol Res 1991;26:371–9.

[32] Jeong S, Han S, Lee S, Magnusson I. Effects of tetracycline-containing gel and a mixture of tetracycline and citric acid-containing gel on non-surgical periodontal therapy. J Periodontol 1994;65:840–7.

[33] Newman MG, Kornman KS, Doherty FM. A 6-month multi-center evaluation of adjunctive tetracycline fiber therapy used in conjunction with scaling and root planing in maintenance patients: clinical results. J Periodontol 1994;65:685–91.

[34] Drisko CL, Cobb CM, Killoy WJ, et al. Evaluation of periodontal treatments using controlled-release tetracycline fibers: clinical response. J Periodontol 1995;66:692–9.

[35] Michalowicz BS, Pihlstrom BL, Drisko CL, et al. Evaluation of periodontal treatments using controlled-release tetracycline fibers: maintenance response. J Periodontol 1995;66:708–15.

[36] Wilson TG, McGuire MK, Greenstein G, Nunn M. Tetracycline fibers plus scaling and root planing versus scaling and root planing alone: similar results after 5 years. J Periodontol 1997;68:1029–32.

[37] Needleman IG, Gerlach RW, Baker RA, Damani NC, Smith SR, Smales FC. Retention, antimicrobial activity, and clinical outcomes following use of a bioerodible tetracycline gel in moderate-to-deep periodontal pockets. J Periodontol 1998;69:578–83.

[38] Heijl L, Dahlen G, Sundin Y, Wenander A, Goodson JM. A 4-quadrant comparative study of periodontal treatment using tetracycline-containing drug delivery fibers and scaling. J Clin Periodontol 1991;18:111–6.

[39] Goodson JM, Cugini MA, Kent RL, et al. Multicenter evaluation of tetracycline fiber therapy: I. Experimental design, methods, and baseline data. J Periodontol Res 1991; 26:361–70.

[40] Goodson JM, Hogan PE, Dunham SL. Clinical responses following periodontal treatment by local drug delivery. J Periodontol 1985;56:81–7.

[41] Tonetti MS, Cortellini P, Carnevale G, Cattabriga M, de Sanctis M, Pini Prato GP. A controlled multicenter study of adjunctive use of tetracycline periodontal fibers in mandibular class II furcations with persistent bleeding. J Clin Periodontol 1998;25: 728–36.

[42] Mombelli A, Lehmann B, Tonetti M, Lang NP. Clinical response to local delivery of tetracycline in relation to overall and local periodontal conditions. J Clin Periodontol 1997;24:470–7.

[43] Maze GI, Reinhardt RA, Agarwal RK, Dyer JK, Robinson DH, DuBois LM, et al. Response to intracrevicular controlled delivery of 25% tetracycline from poly (lactide/glycolide) film strips in SPT patients. J Clin Periodontol 1995;22:860–7.

[44] Yalcin F, Demirel K, Utku O. Evaluation of adjunctive tetracycline fiber therapy with scaling and root planing: short-term clinical results. Periodontal Clin Invest 1999;21:23–7.

[45] Garrett S, Johnson L, Drisko CH, et al. Two multicenter studies evaluating locally delivered doxycycline hyclate, placebo control, oral hygiene and scaling and root planing in the treatment of periodontitis. J Periodontol 1999;70:490–503.

[46] Garrett S, Adams DF, Bogle G, et al. The effect of locally delivered controlled-release doxycycline or scaling and root planing on periodontal maintenance patients over 9 months. J Periodontol 2000;71:22–30.

[47] Poson AM, Garrett S, Stoller NH, et al. Multi-center comparative evaluation of sub-gingivally delivered sanguinarine and doxycycline in the treatment of periodontitis. I. Study design, procedures, and management. J Periodontol 1997;68:110–8.

[48] Ryder MI, Pons B, Adams D, et al. Effects of smoking on local delivery of controlled-release doxycycline as compared to scaling and root planing. J Clin Periodontol 1999; 26:683–91.

[49] Polson AM, Garrett S, Stoller NH, et al. Multi-center comparative evaluation of subgingivally delivered sanguinarine and doxycycline in the treatment of periodontitis. II. Clinical results. J Periodontol 1997;68:119–26.

[50] Graca MA, Watts TLP, Wilson RF, Palmer RM. A randomized controlled trial of a 2% minocycline gel as an adjunct to non-surgical periodontal treatment, using a design with multiple matching criteria. J Clin Periodontol 1997;24:249–53.

[51] Timmerman MF, van der Weijden GA, van Steenbergen TJM, Mantel MS, de Graaff J, van der Velden U. Evaluation of the long-term efficacy and safety of locally-applied minocycline in adult periodontitis patients. J Clin Periodontol 1996;23:707–16.

[52] Yeom HR, Park YJ, Lee SJ, Rhyu IC, Chung CP, Nisengard RJ. Clinical and microbiological effects of minocycline-loaded microcapsules in adult periodontitis. J Periodontol 1997;68:1102–9.

[53] Jones AA, Kornman KS, Newbold DA, Manwell MA. Clinical and microbiological effects of controlled-release locally delivered minocycline in periodontitis. J Periodontol 1994; 65:1058–66.

The COX-2 inhibitors: new analgesic and anti-inflammatory drugs

Asma A. Khan, BDS, PhD[a,b],
Raymond A. Dionne, DDS, PhD[b,*]

[a]Department of Oral and Craniofacial Biological Sciences, Dental School,
University of Maryland, Baltimore, MD, USA
[b]Pain and Neurosensory Mechanisms Branch, National Institute of Dental and
Craniofacial Research, National Institutes of Health, 10 Center Drive, Room 1N-117,
Bethesda, MD 20892-1258, USA

One of the major challenges in dentistry is the management of pain. Pain not only signals tissue injury, but it also acts as an impediment to most dental procedures, delays the resumption of normal activities following dental surgical procedures, and lessens the likelihood of patients seeking dental procedures in the future. Although pain during therapy usually is controlled by local anesthesia, postoperative pain control is often inadequate either because of insufficient relief of pain or unacceptable side effects. Side effects such as drowsiness, nausea, and vomiting from opioids occur with greater frequency in ambulatory dental patients than in nonambulatory hospitalized patients. In addition, inadequate pain control during the immediate postoperative period may contribute to the development of hyperalgesia leading to greater pain later during recovery [1]. Pain associated with dentistry also is recognized as contributing to apprehension about future dental care such that patients frequently report themselves as nervous or terrified at the prospects of dental care [2]. These considerations indicate that optimal analgesic therapy for ambulatory dental patients should be efficacious, with a minimum incidence of side effects, and, ideally, should lessen the prospects for pain associated with future dental therapy.

Dentists largely rely on nonsteroidal anti-inflammatory drugs (NSAIDs) as alternatives to traditional combinations of aspirin or acetaminophen

This work was supported by Division of Intramural Research, NIDCR, and Training grant #T32DE07309.

* Corresponding author.
E-mail address: rdionne@dir.nidcr.nih.gov (R.A. Dionne).

with opioid analgesics such as codeine to treat pain in ambulatory patients. Although NSAIDs are remarkably effective in the management of pain and inflammation, their use is limited by several adverse effects including gastrointestinal bleeding and ulceration, impaired renal function, and inhibition of platelet aggregation. The mortality rate associated with NSAID administration is one of the highest attributable to any drug class [3]. Gastrointestinal toxicity associated with chronic NSAID use is estimated to result in more than 100,000 hospitalizations and 16,000 deaths per year in the United States alone [4]. It has been reported that geriatric patients are at an even greater risk for toxicity with chronic use of NSAIDs [5,6].

The new generation of selective cyclooxygenase-2 (COX-2) inhibitors holds promise for achieving the therapeutic effects of the traditional NSAIDs without the deleterious side effects associated with nonselective COX-1/COX-2 inhibitors. This article reviews the therapeutic use of selective COX-2 inhibitors with emphasis on the potential safety associated with their use.

Role of cyclooxygenase in pain

Numerous endogenous mediators are involved in nociception and in the inflammatory response. Among these are proinflammatory prostaglandins such as prostaglandin E_2 (PGE_2) and prostaglandin I_2 (PGI_2). Cyclooxygenase (COX) constitutes the rate-limiting step in the synthesis of these prostaglandins. It is commonly believed that NSAIDs exert their therapeutic effect by inhibiting the enzyme COX, which in turn inhibits the synthesis of prostaglandins. As prostaglandins are also involved in maintaining a broad spectrum of homeostatic functions such as cytoprotection of the gastric mucosa and control of renal function, inhibition of prostaglandin synthesis results in many adverse effects.

Elucidation of the two COX isoforms gave rise to the concept that the constitutive enzyme COX-1 is responsible for the production of the prostaglandins with homeostatic functions in tissues such as the stomach, kidney, and platelets, whereas COX-2, the inducible enzyme, is responsible for the production of the prostaglandins involved in inflammation [7]. Accordingly, it was postulated that the therapeutic effects of NSAIDs are attributable to inhibition of COX-2, whereas inhibition of COX-1 accounts for the adverse effects associated with NSAIDs. This led to the development of selective COX-2 inhibitors as a class of NSAIDs designed to selectively inhibit COX-2 and to have no effect on COX-1 at therapeutic doses. Celecoxib and rofecoxib are the first generation of selective COX-2 inhibitors approved by the Food and Drug Administration (FDA) for pain indications. Valdecoxib belongs to the second generation of selective COX-2 inhibitors and was recently approved by the FDA.

Selective COX-2 inhibitors

Analgesic efficacy and anti-inflammatory effect

Celecoxib was the first selective COX-2 inhibitor to be approved by the FDA and accounts for almost 25% of the anti-inflammatory drug market. Its indications include the management of rheumatoid arthritis, osteoarthritis, acute pain, and primary dysmenorrhea in adults (Table 1). Celecoxib has demonstrated a COX-1 sparing effect in both in vitro and ex vivo studies [8,9]. A study examining the in vivo selectivity of celecoxib demonstrated that administration of celecoxib 200 mg orally (PO) before the extraction of impacted third molars had no effect on thromboxane B_2 (a product of COX-1) and inhibited PGE_2 only at time points that are consistent with induction of COX-2 (Fig. 1) [10]. The time-action and peak analgesic effect of celecoxib is approximately half (much lower than) that of ibuprofen 600 mg PO. Another study using the oral surgery model demonstrated celecoxib to be superior to placebo, comparable to 650 mg of aspirin, but generally less effective than standard doses of naproxen [11].

Rofecoxib has been reported to be more selective for COX-2 than celecoxib using in vitro assays [12]. It is approved for the management of osteoarthritis, acute pain, and treatment of primary dysmenorrhea. Rofecoxib seems to have greater analgesic efficacy than celecoxib based on the results of studies in the oral surgery model. Rofecoxib 50 mg was compared with ibuprofen 400 mg and placebo in a single dose study in the oral surgery model of acute pain using traditional analgesic endpoints and the two-stopwatch method for estimating analgesic onset (Fig. 2). The total pain relief and sum of the pain intensity difference score over 8 hours following a single 50 mg

Table 1
Pharmacokinetics and drug interactions of celecoxib and rofecoxib

	Celecoxib	Rofecoxib
Onset of analgesia	60 min	30 min
Drug interaction		
ACE enzyme converting inhibitors	Y	Y
Antacids	Y	?
Codeine and oxycodone	Y	N
Frusemide and thiazides	Y	Y
Inhibitors of CYP2D9	Y	N
Lithium	Y	Y
Methotrexate	N	Y
Substrates of CYP2D6	Y	N
Warfarin	Y	Y
Approved doses (mg/day)		
For acute pain	200–400	Up to 50
For osteoarthritis	100–200	Not approved
For rheumatoid arthritis	200–400	12.5–25

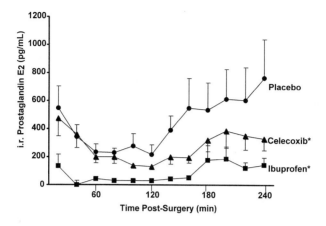

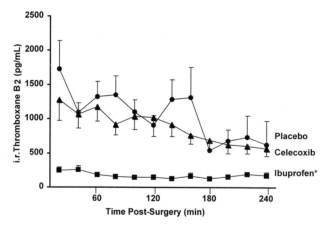

Fig. 1. Comparison of immunoreactive levels of (A) prostaglandin E_2 (i.r.PGE_2) and (B) thromboxane B_2 (i.r.TxB_2) at the surgical site after extraction of impacted third molars. Ibuprofen suppressed levels of PGE_2 and TxB_2, whereas celecoxib suppressed only PGE_2 ($P < 0.001$), thus demonstrating a COX-1 sparing effect. (*Adapted from* Khan AA, Dionne RA, Capra NF. In vivo selectivity of a selective cyclooxygenase-2 inhibitor in the oral surgery model. Clin Pharmacol Therap 2002;72:44–9; with permission.)

dose of rofecoxib was superior to placebo but not distinguishable from ibuprofen 400 mg [13]. The median time to onset of pain relief was indistinguishable for rofecoxib (0.7 hour) and ibuprofen (0.8 hour), but significantly fewer subjects in the rofecoxib group required additional analgesic within 24 hours of study drug than in the placebo or ibuprofen groups. In a second study comparing rofecoxib in doses of 12.5, 25, and 50 mg to naproxen 550 mg and placebo, a clear dose analgesic response was demonstrated [14]. The 25- and 50-mg doses of rofecoxib were statistically indistinguishable from naproxen for pain relief and pain intensity difference. In both studies, the incidence of clinical and laboratory adverse experience were similar. A single-dose study

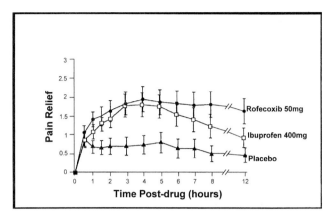

Fig. 2. Comparison of the analgesic effects of a single dose of rofecoxib 50 mg to ibuprofen 400 mg and placebo.

using the oral surgery model demonstrated that the analgesic effect of rofecoxib 50 mg lasts up to 24 hours, ibuprofen 400 mg lasts approximately 9 hours, and celecoxib 200 mg has an estimated duration of 5 hours [15].

Valdecoxib has been approved for the treatment of osteoarthritis, rheumatoid arthritis, and for the management of primary dysmenorrhea. Using the oral surgery model, the efficacy of valdecoxib 400 mg was compared with that of rofecoxib 50 mg [16]. The results of this clinical trial demonstrated that valdecoxib 40 mg has a quicker onset of action than that of rofecoxib 50 mg. The administration of valdecoxib resulted in better pain relief and lower pain intensity as compared with rofecoxib. Valdecoxib was not approved for the management of acute pain at this initial FDA review.

Management of acute orofacial pain with selective COX-2 inhibitors

Several studies have examined the analgesic efficacy of rofecoxib and celecoxib using the oral surgery model of acute inflammation [10,15,17]. There are, however, no published reports examining the efficacy of rofecoxib in acute orofacial pain of other etiologies such as endodontic pain, pain resulting from orthodontic treatment, and pain following periodontal surgery.

Limitations of orally administered selective COX-2 inhibitors and the nonselective NSAIDs for dental pain include delayed onset when compared with an injectable opioid and the inability to consistently relieve severe pain. The analgesic dose of rofecoxib 50 mg as a single dose over 24 hours is greater than the recommended dose for rheumatoid and osteoarthritis 12.5–25 mg, owing to concern for a greater incidence of side effects with repeated doses, such as extremity edema. This could present a problem if pain occurs before the recommended remedication time, (ie, a second dose of rofecoxib should not be administered until 24 hours after the initial dose). In such a situation it would be safer to administer acetaminophen with or without an opioid.

The best strategy for minimizing pain onset is administration of an NSAID before the postoperative induction of COX-2. The use of COX-2 inhibitors in preemptive analgesia has been evaluated in patients undergoing spinal fusion surgery [18]. The preoperative oral administration of rofecoxib 50 mg or celecoxib 200 mg resulted in lower pain scores and decreased use of morphine during the postoperative period as compared with placebo. Preoperative administration of rofecoxib provided a more sustained analgesic effect compared with preoperative treatment with celecoxib. The administration of rofecoxib 50 mg 1 hour before arthroscopic knee surgery resulted in lower incidental pain score and less opioid use in the 24-hour post surgical period [19]. It is reasonable to assume that administration of a COX-2 inhibitor before induction of COX-2 will not only suppress pain in the immediate postoperative period but will also prevent peripheral and central sensitization, thus preventing hyperalgesia.

Management of chronic orofacial pain with selective COX-2 inhibitors

A review of the primary literature reveals little scientific support that the daily use of NSAIDs offers benefit for chronic orofacial pain [20]. The results of two placebo-controlled studies suggest that NSAIDs are ineffective for chronic orofacial pain. The analgesic effects of ibuprofen, 2400 mg per day for 4 weeks, could not be separated from placebo in a group of patients with chronic myogenous orofacial pain [21]. A similar comparison of piroxicam, 20 mg daily for 12 days, to placebo for pain associated with temporomandibular disorders (TMD) also failed to demonstrate any therapeutic advantage for the NSAID [22]. Although little evidence from randomized clinical trials exists regarding the efficacy of NSAIDS in chronic orofacial pain, standard texts and summaries of expert opinion often provide recommendations for specific drugs and doses but either do not provide support for these recommendations or extrapolate from chronic inflammatory conditions such as arthritis [23,24]. A short trial of an NSAID may be considered for patients with an inflammatory component to their TMD. The development of selective COX-2 inhibitors offers an alternative for use of NSAIDs without the adverse effects associated with dual COX-1/COX-2 inhibitors.

Clinical and animal studies suggest that tolerance to NSAIDs can develop with repeated administration. In a group of subjects with chronic lower back pain, the mean reduction in chronic lower back pain intensity following an initial dose of 1200 mg per day ibuprofen was 23% [25]. After 2 weeks of 2400 mg per day of ibuprofen or placebo, the mean reduction in pain intensity for the last dose was fourfold lower in the drug group. The initial low level of response suggests that lower back pain is not particularly sensitive to ibuprofen and may explain, in part, the poor response seen for chronic musculoskeletal pain in the orofacial area. The development of tolerance over 2 weeks would suggest a similar process for TMD pain that could make the analgesic response negligible over the course of a chronic condition. Tolerance to diflunisal with repeated administration has been demonstrated in animals without a reduction in the amount of drug in the blood over time following administration of the first dose in comparison with a dose given following 3 days of diflunisal [26]. This suggests a functional change in the pharmacologic response rather than enhanced pharmacokinetic disposition such that the same amount of drug elicits less analgesia. Long-term administration of selective COX-2 inhibitors for chronic orofacial pain should be evaluated for initial analgesic efficacy, the development of tolerance, and safety with repeated dosing.

Adverse effects

Numerous recent studies have suggested that the original paradigm regarding the roles of COX-1 and COX-2 was overly simplistic. Findings from animal studies have demonstrated constitutive expression of COX-2 in specialized cell types or tissues including the kidney, brain, ovary, and uterus [27–29]. There is also evidence that COX-1 can be induced by stressful stimuli such as radiation injury to the intestine, and may play a protective role in this circumstance [30].

It has been suggested that although COX-2 is proinflammatory in the early stages of inflammation, it may aid in the resolution of inflammation in the later stages [31]. This effect of COX-2 may be by way of the generation of anti-inflammatory prostaglandins of the cyclopentone family. Studies on the gastric mucosa in mice have demonstrated that inhibition of COX-2 delays the healing of ulcers [32]. It has also been demonstrated that COX-2 inhibition exacerbates the inflammation associated with colonic injury [33]. Newberry et al [34] reported that COX-2 dependent metabolites are essential in the development and maintenance of intestinal immune homeostasis. This emerging information clearly demonstrates that COX-1 and COX-2 have more complex physiologic and pathophysiologic roles than originally thought.

Gastrointestinal effects

Two large, randomized clinical trials have examined the risk for gastrointestinal complications following the use of these drugs, the Celecoxib Long-Term Arthritis Safety Study (CLASS) and the Vioxx Gastrointestinal Outcomes Research (VIGOR). The CLASS trial consisted of two studies: Celecoxib 400 mg twice daily (BID) was compared with diclofenac 75 mg BID in one study and with ibuprofen 800 mg three times daily (TID) [35]. The primary end points were ulcer, perforation, gastric-outlet obstruction, and upper gastrointestinal bleeding. The duration of the study was 13 months. The published data from only the first 6 months demonstrated that the incidence of GI effects in the celecoxib group (0.8%) was numerically lower than the

NSAID group (1.5%). No comparison was made to placebo because of the duration of the study. A subsequent report [36] indicates that after reviewing the entire study data, the FDA's Arthritis Advisory Committee concluded that celebrex offered no proven safety advantage over the other two drugs (diclofenac and ibuprofen) in reducing the risk for ulcer complications.

In the VIGOR trial, rofecoxib 50 mg once daily (QD) was compared with naproxen 500 mg BID in patients with rheumatoid arthritis (N = 8076) [37]. The median of the total treatment time was 9 months. The incidence of gastrointestinal (GI) perforation, GI hemorrhage, or symptomatic peptic ulcer was 4.5 per 100 patient-years in the naproxen group and 2.1 per 100 patient-years in the rofecoxib group, a difference of 54% (P < 0.001) between the two groups. A similar study conducted over a 12 month period comparing rofecoxib 12.5, 25, or 50 mg/day to ibuprofen 800 mg/3 times daily, diclofenac 50 mg/3 times daily, and nabutmatone 1500 mg/day in osteoarthritic patients (N = 5435) demonstrated that the incidence of GI effects following the use of rofecoxib (1.3%) was slightly lower than with the conventional NSAIDs (1.8%) [38]. These data indicate that selective rofecoxib seems to be associated with fewer gastrointestinal events than the nonselective NSAIDs. Subjects who have preexisting risk factors such as history of peptic ulcers and gastrointestinal bleeding, however, are likely to be at a higher risk for developing GI events following the use of selective COX-2 inhibitors.

Cardiovascular effects

Thromboxane A_2 (TxA$_2$) and prostacyclin I_2 (PGI$_2$) are products of the cyclooxygenase pathway that are involved in platelet-vascular homeostasis. PGI$_2$ is a vasodilator and inhibits platelet aggregation and leukocyte adherence, whereas TxA$_2$ is a vasoconstrictor and promotes platelet aggregation. Selective COX-2 inhibitors suppress the synthesis of PGI$_2$ and have no effect on TxA$_2$, shifting the hemostatic balance toward a prothrombotic state [39] with greater potential to initiate adverse occlusive vascular events.

The results of the CLASS trial demonstrated that there was no significant difference in the rates of major cardiovascular events between the treatment groups. The results of the VIGOR trial showed that the risk for developing a thrombotic cardiovascular event following treatment with rofecoxib as compared with naproxen was 2.38 (P = 0.002). It is not clear at this point whether these results reflect a beneficial effect of naproxen to decrease platelet aggregation or a prothrombotic effect of rofecoxib.

A comparison of the cardiovascular effects of celecoxib and rofecoxib using the data from the two trials is difficult because they had distinctly different patient populations and the NSAIDs used as controls were different. It is likely that the CLASS trial failed to reveal the increased risk for cardiovascular events following celecoxib administration, as 21% of the subjects in this trial were permitted to take aspirin <325 mg/day, whereas its use was not permitted in the VIGOR study. All the subjects in the VIGOR trial had rheumatoid arthritis, whereas only 11% of the subjects in the CLASS trial had rheumatoid arthritis, a risk factor for myocardial infarction [40].

Renal effects

Although both COX isoforms are constitutively expressed in the kidneys, the effect of COX-2 inhibition on renal function remains unknown. As COX-2 is involved in the regulation of the renin-angiotensin system, inhibition of COX-2 has the potential to cause hypertension and renal failure [28]. The results of a study by Rossat et al [41] using healthy salt-depleted male volunteers demonstrated that selective COX-2 inhibition causes water and salt retention with a transient decrease in glomerular filtration rate. Analyses of the post marketing data for celecoxib and rofecoxib reveal that the incidence of hypertension and edema is similar to that of the nonselective NSAIDs [42].

Drugs in the pipeline

Parecoxib, an injectable prodrug of valdecoxib, holds the promise of an effective means of managing severe acute pain, including postoperative pain. Desjardins et al [43] demonstrated that the preoperative administration of parecoxib 40 and 80 mg is effective and safe for treating postoperative pain. It has been demonstrated that parecoxib 40 mg IV and IM provides effective analgesia in a postoral surgery model with the analgesic relief provided by parecoxib being comparable to 60 mg of ketorolac [44]. Etoricoxib is yet another selective COX-2 inhibitor that is currently being reviewed by the FDA. It has been demonstrated to be highly selective for COX-2 (Table 2). It has also been reported to be a potent COX-2 inhibitor in various animal models including carrageenan-induced paw-edema and hyperalgesia, and adjuvant-induced arthritis. JTE-522, a selective COX-2 inhibitor also being developed for the management of pain, has been demonstrated to selectively inhibit the synthesis of PGE_2 in the inflammatory tissue at doses having no effect on PGE_2 production in the gastric mucosa [45].

Table 2
Ratios of COX-1 IC_{50}/COX-2 IC_{50} values of NSAIDs in human whole blood assays

Drug	IC_{50} ratios
Etoricoxib	106
Rofecoxib	35
Valdecoxib	30
Celecoxib	7.6
Diclofenac	3.0
Ibuprofen	0.2

A high ratio of Cox-1 IC_{50}/Cox-2 IC_{50} implies that the agent is relatively selective for COX-2. Data from Riendeau D, Percival MD, Bridean C, et al. Etoricoxib (MK-0663): preclinical profile and comparison with other agents that selectively inhibit cyclooxygenase-2. J Pharmacol Exp Ther 2001;296(2):558–66.

Summary

Selective COX-2 inhibitors offer a therapeutic alternative to the conventional nonselective NSAIDs. Rofecoxib has been demonstrated to be a valuable therapeutic agent in the management of acute orofacial pain. Selective COX-2 inhibitors are also indicated in patients who are likely to undergo surgery or invasive procedures in the near future because these drugs do not prolong the bleeding time. The efficacy of these drugs in the management of chronic orofacial pain is yet to be evaluated. The pharmacoeconomic impact of COX-2 inhibitors must also be considered, as the cost of selective COX-2 inhibitors is considerably higher than the other commonly used NSAIDs.

Although it is clear that COX-2 inhibitors offer some advantages over the nonselective NSAIDs in terms of a lower risk of GI toxicity with long-term use, the effects following short-term use are still unclear. Until more data are available, COX-2 inhibitors should be avoided or used with the same caution as for conventional NSAIDs in patients with compromised renal and cardiac function.

References

[1] Gordon SM, Dionne RA, Brahim J, et al. Blockade of peripheral neuronal barrage reduces postoperative pain. Pain 1997;70:209–15.

[2] Dionne RA, Gordon SM, McCullagh LM, et al. Assessment of clinical needs for anesthesia and sedation in the general population. J Am Dent Assoc 1998;129:167–73.

[3] Kremer J. From prostaglandin replacement to specific COX-2 inhibition: a critical appraisal. J Rheumatol 2000;27(Suppl 60):9–12.

[4] Singh G, Triadafilopoulos G. Epidemeology of NSAID induced gastrointestinal complications. J Rheumatol 1999;26:18–24.

[5] Carson JL, Strom BL, Morse ML. The relative gastrointestinal toxicity of the nonsteroidal anti-inflammatory drugs. Arch Int Med 1987;147:1054–9.

[6] Hersh EV, Moore PA, Ross G. Over-the-counter analgesics and antipyretics: a critical assessment. Clin Ther 2000;22:500–48.

[7] Vane JR, Bakhle YS, Botting RM. Cyclooxygenases 1 and 2. Annu Rev Pharmacol Toxicol 1998;38:97–120.

[8] Penning TD, Talley JJ, Berteshaw SR, et al. Synthesis and biological evaluation of the 1, 5′diarypyraziol class of cyclooxygenase inhibitors: identification of 4-{5-(4-Methylphenyl)-3-(trifloromethyl)-1H-pyrazol-1-yl] benzenesulfonamide (SC-68735, celecoxib). J Med Chem 1997;40:1347–65.

[9] Schwartz B, Hurley SM, Hubbard RC, et al. A pilot study of the platelet effects of SC-58635, a novel COX-2 inhibitor. ILAR Congress of Rheumatology; 1997. p. 159.

[10] Khan AA, Dionne RA, Capra NF. In vivo selectivity of a selective cyclooxygenase-2 inhibitors in the oral surgery model. Clin Pharmacol Ther 2002;72:44–9.

[11] Hubbard RC, Jasper DR, Nugent MJ, et al. SC-58635, a highly selective inhibitor of COX-2, is an effective analgesic in an acute post-surgical pain model. J Invest Med 1996;44:293A.

[12] Matheson AJ, Figgit DP. Rofecoxib: a review of its use in the management of osteoarthritis, acute pain and rheumatoid arthritis. Drugs 2001;61:833–65.

[13] Brown J, Morrisson BW, Christensen S, et al. MK-0966 50 mg versus ibuprofen 400 mg in post-surgical dental pain [abstract]. Clin Pharmacol Ther 1999;645:118.

[14] Fricke JF, Morrison BW, Fite S, et al. MK-966 versus naproxen sodium 550 mg in post-surgical dental pain [abstract]. Clin Pharmacol Ther 1999;645:119.

[15] Malmstrom K, Daniels S, Kotey P. Comparison of rofecoxib and celecoxib, two cyclooxygenase-2 inhibitors, in post-operative dental pain: a randomized placebo- and active-comparator controlled clinical trial. Clin Ther 1999;21:1653–63.

[16] Fricke J, Varkalis J, Zwillich S, Adler R, Forester E, Recker DP, et al. Valdecoxib is more efficacious than rofecoxib in relieving pain associated with oral surgery. Am J Ther 2002;9(2):89–97.

[17] Morrison BW, Christensen S, Yuan W, Brown J, Amlani S, Seidenberg B. Analgesic efficacy of the cyclooxygenase-2-specific inhibitor rofecoxib in post-dental surgery pain: a randomized, controlled trial. Clin Ther 1999;21(6):943–53.

[18] Reuben SS, Connelly NR. Postoperative analgesic effects of celecoxib or rofecoxib after spinal fusion surgery. Anesth Analg 2000;91:1221–5.

[19] Reuben SS, Fingeroth R, Krushell R, Maciolek H. Evaluation of the safety and efficacy of the perioperative administration of rofecoxib for total knee arthroplasty. J Arthroplasty 2002;17(1):26–31.

[20] Truelove EL. The chemotherapeutic management of chronic and persistent orofacial pain. Dent Clin N Am 1994;38:669–88.

[21] Singer EJ, Sharav Y, Dubner R, et al. The efficacy of diazepam and ibuprofen in the treatment of chronic myofascial orofacial pain. Pain 1987;(Suppl 4):S83.

[22] Gordon SM, Montgomery MT, Jones D. Comparative efficacy of piroxicam versus placebo for temperomandibular pain [abstract]. J Dent Res 1990;69:218.

[23] Dworkin SF, Truelove EL, Bonica JJ, et al. Facial and head pain caused by myofascial and temperomandibular disorders. In: Bonica JJ, editor. The management of pain. Philadelphia: Lea and Febiger; 1990. p. 727–45.

[24] McNeill C. Temperomandibular disorders. Chicago: Quintessence 87;1993.

[25] Pownall R, Pickvance NJ. Does treatment timing matter? A double blind crossover study of ibuprofen 2400 mg per day in different dosage schedules in treatment of lower back pain. Br J Clin Pract 1985;39:267–75.

[26] Walker JS, Levy G. Effect of multiple dosing on the analgesic action of diflunisal in rats. Life Sci 1990;46:737–42.

[27] Yamagata K, Andreasson KI, Kaufmann WE, Barnes CA, Worley PF. Expression of mitogen-inducible cyclooxygenase in brain neurons: regulation by synaptic activity and glucocorticoids. Neuron 1993;11:371–86.

[28] Harris RC, McKanna JA, Akai Y, et al. Renal effects of cyclooygenase-2 selective inhibitors. J Clin Invest 1994;93:2504–10.

[29] Lim H, Gupta RA, Ma W, et al. Cyclo-oxygenase-2 derived prostacyclin mediates embryo implantation in the mouse via PPARδ. Genes Dev 1999;13:1561–74.

[30] Houchen CW, Stenson WF, Cohn SM. Disruption of cyclooxygenase-1 gene results in an impaired response to radiation injury. Am J Physiol Gastrointest Liver Physiol 2000; 279:G858–65.

[31] Gilroy DW, Colville-Nash PR, Willis D, et al. Inducible cyclooxygenase may have anti-inflammatory properties. Nat Med 1999;5:698–701.

[32] Mizuno S, Sakamoto C, Matsuda K. Induction of cyclooxygeanse-2 in gastric mucosal ulcers and its inhibition by the specific agonist delays healing in mice. Gastroenterology 1997;112:387–97.

[33] Reuter BK, Asfaha S, Buret A, et al. Exacerbation of inflammation-associated colonic injury in rat through inhibition of cyclooxygenase-2. J Clin Invest 1996;98:2076–85.

[34] Newberry RD, Stenson WF, Lorenz RG. Cyclooxygenase-2-dependent arachidonic acid metabolites are essential modulators of the intestinal immune response to dietary antigen. Nat Med 1999;5:900–6.

[35] Silverstein FE, Faich G, Goldstein JL, et al. Gastrointestinal toxicity with celecoxib vs nonsteroidal antiinflammatory drugs for osteoarthritis and rheumatoid arthritis: the CLASS study: a randomized controlled trial. JAMA 2000;284:1247–5.

[36] Okie S. Missing data on celebrex. The Washington Post: A11, August 5, 2001.

[37] Bombardier C, Laine L, Reicin A, et al. Comparison of upper gastrointestinal toxicity of rofecoxib and naproxen in patients with rheumatoid arthritis. N Engl J Med 2000; 343:1520–8.

[38] Langman MJ, Jensen DM, Watson DJ, et al. Adverse upper gastrointestinal effects of rofecoxib compared with NSAIDs. JAMA 1999;282:1929–33.

[39] Hennan JK, Huang J, Barret TD, et al. Effects of selective COX-2 inhibition on vascular responses and thrombosis in the canine coronary arteries. Circulation 2001;104:820–5.

[40] Wallberg-Jonsson S, Johansson H, Ohman ML, et al. Extent of inflammation predicts cardiovascular disease and overall mortality in seropositive rheumatoid arthritis: a retrospective cohort study from disease onset. J Rheumatol 1999;26:2562–71.

[41] Rossat J, Maillard M, Nussberger J, et al. Renal effects of selective cyclooxygenase-2 inhibition in normotensive salt-depleted subjects. Clin Pharmacol Ther 1999;66:76–84.

[42] Whelton A. Renal aspects of treatment with conventional non-steroidal anti-inflammatory drugs versus cyclooxygenase-2 specific inhibitors. Am J Med 2001;110(Suppl 1):S33–42.

[43] Desjardins PJ, Grossman EH, Kuss ME, Talwalker S, Dhadda S, Baum D, et al. The injectable cyclooxygenase-2-specific inhibitor parecoxib sodium has analgesic efficacy when administered preoperatively. Anesth Analg 2001;93(3):721–7.

[44] Daniels SE, Grossman EH, Kuss ME, et al. A double-blind, randomized comparison of intramuscularly and intravenously administered parecoxib sodium versus ketorolac in a post-surgery pain model. Clin Ther 2001;23:1018–31.

[45] Wakitani K, Tazaki H, Matsushita, et al. JTE-522 selectively inhibits cyclooxygenase-2-derived prostaglandin production in inflammatory tissue. Inflam Res 2000;49:117–22.

THE DENTAL
CLINICS OF
NORTH
AMERICA

Dent Clin N Am 46 (2002) 691–705

Rational use of analgesic combinations

James C. Phero, DMD[a],*, Daniel Becker, DDS[b,c]

[a]University of Cincinnati Physicians Pain Center, Anesthesia Department,
University of Cincinnati College of Medicine, 231 Albert Sabin Way,
Post Office Box 670531, Cincinnati, OH 45267-0531, USA
[b]Allied Health Technology, Sinclair College, 444 West Third Street, Dayton,
OH 45202, USA
[c]Miami Valley Hospital, One Wyoming Street, Dayton, OH 45409, USA

Current techniques for analgesic management of pain have benefited from recent pharmacologic advances and a better understanding of the mechanisms of action of the older analgesic agents. Practitioners commonly use commercially available analgesics that take advantage of incorporating opioid agents with nonopioids such as acetaminophen (APAP) or non-steroidal anti-inflammatory agents (NSAID). Opioid and APAP combinations account for 5 of the top 200 prescription medications sold in the United States based on total number of prescriptions written. Hydrocodone combined with APAP was the single most commonly written United States prescription in 2000 [1]. This field is growing with the newest commercially available compounded analgesic not containing an opioid, but incorporating two nonopioid analgesics with distinctly different analgesic actions, tramadol and APAP. Though the practitioner and patient typically find commercially available analgesic combinations convenient, certain pain management situations are optimized by compounding analgesics from separate prescriptions for each analgesic agent. This article will focus primarily on the use of oral analgesics for acute pain management.

Analgesic drugs interrupt nociceptive pathways that transmit impulses destined to be interpreted as pain in the central nervous system (CNS). Analgesics are classified as opioids and nonopioids, but the older terms "narcotic" and "non-narcotic" are used interchangeably. Conventional thought has credited opioids as acting within the brain and spinal cord, whereas the action of nonopioids is confined to the periphery, ie, the site of injury. Both have been shown, however, to act centrally and peripherally

* Corresponding author.
E-mail address: james.phero@uc.edu (J.C. Phero).

to varying degrees [2]. Therefore, the principal feature that distinguishes these two classes of analgesics is their mechanism of action.

Opioids act on specific receptors. The three major opioid receptors include the μ, κ, and δ receptors. Current knowledge indicates that opioid analgesia is mediated primarily by binding to the μ receptor. This results in postsynaptic membrane hyperpolarization following activation of inwardly rectifying potassium channels and presynaptic depolarization secondary to the inhibition of voltage-dependent calcium channels. But some opioids, ie, methadone and levorphanol, have N-methyl-d-aspartate (NMDA) receptor antagonist properties and inhibit the reuptake of serotonin and noradrenaline, which may make them useful in the treatment of complex regional pain syndromes (CRPS). Opioids have no dose limit or ceiling dose, ie, the patient can increase the dose until analgesia is obtained or limiting side effects occur. The agonist-antagonist, pentazocine, and weak mμ receptor binding agent, propoxyphene, are also listed in the opioid category. Pentazocine and propoxyphene are labeled as Drug Enforcement Administration (DEA) schedule IV agents. Tramadol, though binding weakly to mμ opioid receptors, is not scheduled by the DEA and is covered in the nonopioid section of this article.

The largest class of nonopioids is the NSAIDs, which interrupt prostaglandin synthesis and have a maximal dose or ceiling; greater NSAID doses provide no additional analgesia. Other commonly used nonopioid analgesics are acetaminophen and tramadol, which do not have anti-inflammatory properties.

It is rational for the practitioner to combine these classes when managing pain. To select combination regimens wisely, it is important first to understand the significant pharmacologic features of each category alone.

Nonopioids

The nonopioids include NSAIDs, APAP, and tramadol. NSAIDs demonstrate good analgesic efficacy for mild to moderate orofacial pain. NSAIDs are recommended for the initial management of orofacial pain with an inflammatory component and musculoskeletal pain. Acetaminophen and tramadol are options to be considered in place of, or in addition to NSAID therapy.

NSAIDs

Actions, side effects, and contraindications

NSAIDs include a large group of synthetic compounds having analgesic, anti-inflammatory, and antipyretic efficacy. These therapeutic effects, as well as their most notable side effects, are presumably the result of inhibiting cyclooxygenases that catalyze the synthesis of prostaglandins and thromboxanes.

The most frequent side effects attributed to NSAIDs are gastrointestinal in nature and include dyspepsia, erosions, and ulcerations. Interestingly, patient complaint of dyspepsia (upset stomach) is usually unrelated to mucosal injury. The incidence of dyspepsia with the newly released COX-2 inhibitors is similar to that of other NSAIDs (see article in this issue on COX-2 agents). The anti-platelet effect of conventional NSAIDs is a consideration, but aspirin is the only NSAID that prolongs bleeding time to a significant extent. This is because aspirin's anti-platelet action is irreversible, lasting the lifespan of the platelet (10–14 days). Other NSAIDs bind weakly and reversibly to platelet cyclooxygenases with their influence completely lost after drug elimination.

All NSAIDs shunt the arachidonic pathway toward leukotriene synthesis. These substances mediate a variety of tissue responses, including those associated with bronchospasm and anaphylaxis [3]. It has been suggested that certain individuals may be extremely sensitive to even subtle elevations in leukotriene synthesis, which may induce signs and symptoms of an allergic response. It has been suggested that the term "aspirin intolerance" should be used to distinguish this reaction from true hypersensitivity responses. Acetaminophen and/or tramadol can be recommended for patients reporting allergic reactions to any NSAID, unless the patient can identify a particular NSAID they have tolerated in the past.

Several medical conditions present relative and/or absolute contraindications for routine use of NSAIDs. These include: a current history of nephropathy, erosive or ulcerative conditions of the gastrointestinal (GI) mucosa, anticoagulant therapy, hemorrhagic disorders, pregnancy, and a prior history of intolerance or allergy to any NSAID. Several drug interactions involving NSAIDs are noteworthy and require a thorough drug history [4] (Table 1). Acetaminophen and/or tramadol are the primary alternatives when NSAIDs are contraindicated.

Efficacy, selection, and dosages

All NSAIDs have greater potency as analgesics and antipyretics than as anti-inflammatory agents. For example, a single 325–1000 mg dose of aspirin may reduce pain and fever, but daily doses of 4–6 gm are required to suppress inflammation effectively. This is not to say that NSAIDs have poor anti-inflammatory efficacy; it merely illustrates the fact that the clinician must consider the desired outcome when determining an appropriate dose.

The analgesic dose-response curves for NSAIDs, as well as acetaminophen, demonstrate a ceiling effect. A point is reached where increasing the dose further provides no improvement in pain relief. For aspirin, this ceiling response occurs at approximately 1000 mg, and for ibuprofen, 400 mg. A

Table 1
Drug interactions of clinical concern related to patient pain management

Prescribed drug	Interaction agent	Interaction explanation
NSAID	Antihypertensives	Effectiveness of most classes of antihypertensive drugs is reduced following prolonged use of most NSAIDs. If NSAIDs are required for longer than 4 days, patient's blood pressure control should be assessed. Calcium channel blockers have not been implicated.
NSAID	Hypoglycemics (eg, glyburide/ Micronase, glipizide/ Glucotrol)	Avoid aspirin and phenylbutazone as combined therapy with insulin and oral hypoglycemics may result in hypoglycemia. Other NSAIDs have not been implicated.
NSAID	Lithium (Lithobid®)	Lithium excretion is reduced and toxic blood levels of lithium may develop over 5–10 days of NSAID therapy. Limit NSAID use to 2 or 3 days.
NSAID	Methotrexate (Rheumatrex®)	Increasing methotrexate serum levels leading to systemic toxicity an increased incidence of stomatitis.
NSAID	Warfarin (Coumadin®)	Antiplatelet effects of NSAIDs may add to anticoagulant effect of warfarin. Gl erosive effects may be more prone to hemorrhage.
Other NSAIDs	Combining NSAIDs, especially ASA	Diminishes serum levels of each.
Acetaminophen	Ethanol/Hydantoins (eg, phenytoin/ Dilantin®)	Chronic use of alcohol or phenytoin increases risk of hepatotoxicity. Reduce daily dose limit from 4 grams to 2 grams.
Acetaminophen	Warfarin (Coumadin®)	Acetaminophen may inhibit metabolism of warfarin leading to elevated INR. Use caution if prescribing APAP for more than 3 days.
Acetaminophen	Carbamazepine (Tegretol®)	Increases metabolite of acetaminophen, decreasing its analgesic effect but increasing accumulation of hepatotoxic metabolite
Propoxyphene	Carbamazepine (Tegretol®)	Increased serum levels of carbamazepine leading to toxicity.
Tramadol	Opioid dependency	May reinitiate physical dependence. Agents that lower seizure threshold (eg, SSRI, TCA, Neuroleptics) increase risk of seizures.
Pentazocine	Opioid dependency	May precipitate withdrawal.
Opioids (all)	Sedatives	Profound sedation and respiratory depression may occur with any drug class having a sedative effect.
Opioids (all)	H2 Blockers (eg, ranitidine/ Zantac and climetidine/ Tagamet®)	May delay opioid metabolism. Use caution in determining opioid dose and duration of use.

Table 1 (*continued*)

Prescribed drug	Interaction agent	Interaction explanation
Codeine derivatives	SSRI antidepressants (eg, fluoxetine/ Prozac® and paroxetine/ Paxil®)	Some SSRI antidepressants inhibit demethylation of prodrug to active metabolite, rendering analgesic ineffective. Drugs that inhibit hepatic CYP2D6 enzymes are implicated. See H2 blockers above.
Meperidine	MAO inhibitors (eg, phenelzine/Nardil®)	Mechanism of interaction unclear, but seizures and coma have been reported.

GI, gastrointestinal; INR, international normalization ratio; MAO, monoamine oxidase; SSRI, selective serotonin reuptake inhibitor; TCA, tricyclic anti-depressant; NSAID, nonsteroidal anti-inflammatory drugs.

ceiling for their anti-inflammatory response cannot be ascertained because at higher dosages, side effects become prohibitive. As typically higher NSAID doses are required to suppress inflammation than to provide analgesia, many NSAIDs are marketed in several dosages (ie, ibuprofen is available in dosages ranging from 200–800 mg). When prescribing a NSAID, select low dose ranges for noninflammatory pain and reserve higher dosages for those situations in which inflammation and swelling are a consideration.

Compared with other NSAIDs, aspirin not only produces a greater incidence of side effects but also has been shown to have slightly less analgesic efficacy. Thus, aspirin is a questionable choice for managing postoperative pain. All NSAIDs have the potential to produce side effects similar to aspirin, but most exhibit a lower frequency. In particular, ibuprofen is one of the safest. It produces GI symptoms in less than 3% of patients treated, and its antiplatelet activity is considerably less than aspirin and most other NSAIDs.

Clinical trials comparing NSAIDs, including the COX-2 inhibitors (ie, rofecoxib [Vioxx®] and celecoxib [Celebrex®]) have not identified substantive differences in their anti-inflammatory or analgesic efficacy. Conclusions from clinical trials, however, are based on summaries of data from large groups of patients. The clinician must appreciate that there can be considerable variation among individual patients in terms of clinical response and GI tolerance. In a given patient, an unsatisfactory response with one NSAID does not preclude therapeutic success with another. Considering its low cost and side-effect profile, ibuprofen is a logical first-line agent. The COX-2 agent rofecoxib does offer the advantage of once-a-day dosing, no increase in bleeding times, and minimal GI issues (see COX-2 article in this issue). But the practitioner must weigh the patient benefits against the increase in COX-2 drug cost over generic NSAIDs when prescribing. Regardless of the drug selected initially, one should optimize agent dosage before assuming the response is inadequate and switching to another agent.

The preoperative use of NSAIDs has been demonstrated repeatedly to decrease the intensity of postoperative pain and swelling [5]. This is not surprising because NSAIDs inhibit the "formation" of prostaglandins; they do not destroy or inhibit those already formed. More recent understanding of pain mechanisms has found that benefits of this practice are evident as long as prostaglandin synthesis is inhibited before local anesthesia wanes. Otherwise, prostaglandins trigger nociceptive impulses that travel to the brain and "wind up" the brain's interpretation of pain intensity. When an extensive surgical procedure is planned, optimal serum levels of an NSAID should be established either preoperatively or prior to patient discharge and while tissues remain anesthetized. This use of "pre-emptive analgesia" may also be useful for endodontic and extensive restorative procedures as well.

Acetaminophen

The action of acetaminophen is poorly defined but is believed to interrupt the influence of prostaglandins within CNS pathways. Acetaminophen is approximately as active as aspirin in inhibiting prostaglandin synthetase (cyclooxygenase) within the CNS but has little influence on peripheral prostaglandin synthesis. This is one of several explanations for it lacking anti-inflammatory efficacy and sharing none of the peripheral side effects common to NSAIDs. As an analgesic and antipyretic, however, acetaminophen is equal in potency and efficacy to aspirin, achieving its analgesic ceiling at 1000 mg. This would suggest that it is somewhat inferior to ibuprofen and other NSAIDs.

The major adverse effect of acetaminophen is hepatotoxicity. This is attributed to a metabolite that is not adequately conjugated following acute doses of 10–15 g (150–250 mg/kg). A lower dose may be toxic for patients having depleted storage of glycogen such as that associated with dieting, anorexia, and those suffering primary liver dysfunction or receiving hepatotoxic medications. For example, patients suspected of chronic alcoholism should limit their daily acetaminophen intake to 2 gm rather than the normal daily maximum of 4 gm [6].

Tramadol

Tramadol, though not classified as a controlled substance by the DEA, is a central analgesic with binary action (CABA). Tramadol binds weakly to mµ opioid receptors and inhibits the reuptake of norepinephrine and serotonin. Tramadol's principal metabolite (M1) demonstrates, however, a more significant agonist action on mµ receptors than the parent agent. Tramadol-induced analgesia is only partially antagonized by the opiate antagonist naloxone. Because of the dual mechanism of action, the adverse-event profile of tramadol differs from that of NSAIDs (eg, gastrointestinal or renal/cardiovascular considerations) or traditional opioids. Tramadol is marketed as an effective and safe analgesic for moderate to moderately severe pain. It was available in Europe and Asia for over a decade before being approved for use in the United States. Nausea, vomiting, and dizziness may occur with the use of tramadol. Tramadol should be used with caution in patients with a history of seizure disorder. Tramadol is considered to have a low incidence for abuse (0.5–1.0 case per 100,000 patients) and is not a scheduled drug. But tramadol is not recommended for patients with a tendency for opioid abuse or dependence [7,8]. A single dose of tramadol as the sole analgesic has been shown to provide pain relief within 1 hour that continues for at least 6 hours [9]. Tramadol offers the clinician the potential to reduce the incidence of somnolence and constipation commonly seen with opioid use, but tramadol monotherapy may not be safer or more effective than mild opioid/acetaminophen combinations [10]. Consequently, the practitioner may find tramadol useful when added for breakthrough pain to NSAID, COX-2, and/or acetaminophen used for baseline acute pain management.

In situations where the practitioner wishes to avoid opioid therapy, the rationale for prescribing an NSAID for baseline inflammation and pain management with consideration of tramadol, acetaminophen, or the tramadol/acetaminophen combination for breakthrough pain in acute, postoperative orofacial pain management has been suggested [11]. The use of the tramadol/APAP combination tablet in patients with dental pain has been shown to have more rapid onset and greater efficacy than tramadol alone, without an apparent increase in adverse events [12]. In a comparison of tramadol/acetaminophen tablets with codeine/acetaminophen capsules for chronic pain, the pain rating scores for onset, duration, and relief were similar. The incidence of somnolence, however, was 17% with tramadol/acetaminophen, and 24% with codeine/acetaminophen. The incidence of constipation was 11% with tramadol/acetaminophen and 21% with codeine/acetaminophen. Headache was more common in the tramadol/acetaminophen group (11%) than the codeine/acetaminophen group (7%). Both groups had an 8% incidence of discontinuance from allergic reactions, primarily rash or pruritus [13].

Summary of nonopioids

In most cases, postoperative dental pain includes an inflammatory component. For this reason, NSAIDs are rational first-line agents, often superior to conventional dosages of opioids. Should a patient present a contraindication to NSAIDs, acetaminophen and/or tramadol are the only alternatives in this category of agents. Nonopioids exhibit a ceiling to their analgesic response, and optimal doses should be established before assuming the NSAID has failed.

In pain management situations involving acute pain and inflammation, where the practitioner wishes to avoid or limit opioid therapy, there is the consideration of using a NSAID for baseline inflammation and pain management with the option of adding APAP, tramadol, or the combination of tramadol/APAP for baseline and/or breakthrough pain control.

Data relevant for prescribing the more commonly used nonopioids is summarized below (Table 2).

Table 2
Selected nonopioid analgesics useful for reducing postoperative pain and inflammation

Nonsteroidal anti-inflammatory drugs (NSAIDs)	Dosage (70 kg adult)	Clinical characteristics (hours)		
		Onset	Peak	Duration
Ibuprofen (Motrin®)	400–800mg tid/qid	0.5	1–2	4–6
Naproxen (Anaprox®)	275–550mg bid/tid	1	2–4	5–7
Celecoxib (Celebrex®) COX-2	200 mg bid	0.5	1–2	11–15
Rofecoxib (Vioxx®)	25–50mg qd	1	1–2	17–24
Valdecoxib (Bextra®)	20–40mg qd	0.5	1–2	24
Non-NSAID analgesics				
Acetaminophen (Tylenol®)	500–1000mg qid[a]	0.5	0.5–2	4–6
Tramadol (Ultram®)[b]	25–100mg qid	1	1–2	4.66

[a] Daily total dose not to exceed 4 gm on healthy 70 kg adult.

[b] Considered nonopioid because mechanism of action is by serotonin/norepinephrine reuptake inhibition in addition to weak opioid μ binding.

(*Adapted from* American Pain Society: Principles of analgesic use in the treatment of acute pain and cancer pain, 4th edition. Glenview (IL): American Pain society; 1999. p 5–10; with permission.)

Opioid analgesics

Actions and effects

Opioids produce the majority of their therapeutic and adverse effects by acting as agonists at μ and/or κ opioid receptors. Unlike the nonopioids, which exhibit a ceiling effect, the analgesic response to opioids acting at mμ receptors continues to improve as their dose is increased. Although their analgesic efficacy is unlimited, side effects often preclude the use of doses adequate to completely relieve severe pain. These include sedation, respiratory depression, dependence, nausea, miosis, and constipation. Following prolonged use, patients develop tolerance to most opioid effects. Constipation and miosis are notable exceptions, however. For this reason, patients suffering chronic and/or terminal illnesses may require astonishing doses to achieve analgesia, but constipation and visual impairment are troublesome. Similar doses, if administered to patients who have not developed tolerance, so-called "opioid-naive" patients, would be lethal because of respiratory depression. Use caution when considering newer high-dose, sustained-release opioids designed for tolerant patients.

Therapeutic use of opioids

Patients and practitioners are often concerned with the potential for addiction, which may limit prescribing and use, leading to inadequate management of pain [13]. This can be attributed to confusion regarding drug dependence and drug addiction. Patients consuming opioids regularly for more than 1 week may develop a degree of drug dependence. This may require gradual tapering of the dosage to avoid withdrawal symptoms.

Drugs do not produce addiction, however. This is a compulsive pattern of behavior in which an individual continues to seek the drug for effects they perceive as pleasurable. Addictive behavior is a psychiatric condition that can be reinforced by a particular drug, but it is not a pharmacodynamic property. Obviously, opioids must be prescribed cautiously for patients who demonstrate addictive personality.

The practitioner should carefully consider the use of opioid therapy for the short-term management of breakthrough pain in acute, orofacial pain that is moderate to severe. Despite popular belief, all of the traditional opioids have unlimited efficacy. This is to say that, at equipotent doses, opioids provide the same degree of pain relief. It is a misconception that pain unresponsive to codeine will respond to oxycodone, meperidine, or morphine. It may be desirable to change to one of these medications, but the decision should not be based on delusions regarding efficacy. A more likely explanation would be that an equianalgesic dose of one agent could not be achieved without significant side effects. Issues in opioid dosage are predicated on the pharmacokinetic profiles of the various agents, not their efficacy at opioid receptors.

Equianalgesic doses have been confirmed for opioids administered by parenteral routes. Those following oral administration are problematic because of altered bioavailability attributed to first-pass metabolism into inactive metabolites. Opioids used for treating moderate to moderately severe pain are compared below by equipotent dose, DEA schedule, and clinical duration (Table 3).

Genetic predisposition for patient conversion of opioids can lead to poor analgesia in certain patients. Codeine has very little affinity for the mμ receptor and may be considered a prodrug because 10% of the drug is metabolically converted to morphine by cytochrome P450 CYP2D6. Morphine is analgesic and codeine is antitussive. Approximately 7% of the Caucasian population metabolizes codeine and hydrocodone poorly because they have inherited two nonfunctional alleles for cytochrome P450 CYP2D6. In these individuals, analgesia resulting from codeine, oxycodone, or hydrocodone will be less than expected with the general population.

Specific opioid considerations

Codeine

Morphine 10 mg and codeine 120 mg are equipotent following intramuscular (IM) administration. The lower potency and greater incidence of nausea attributed to codeine can be explained by the following information. The only difference in their molecular structure is a methyl group that prevents their binding to mμ receptors. Codeine and its derivatives are prodrugs, meaning that they are inactive in the form administered. Approximately 10% of a parenterally administered dose of codeine is demethylated to morphine, and this is responsible for its analgesic influence. This accounts for low analgesic

Table 3
Commonly prescribed opioids in the United States shown with oral doses that are equipotent to morphine 10 mg IM

Drug	DEA Schedule	PO dose equivalent to 10 mg morphine IM (mg)	Clinical duration (hours)	Comments
Morphine	II	60[a]	4–6	M-6-G and M-3-G can accumulate in renal failure
Meperidine	II	300	2–3	Poor choice for oral use because of 25% bioavailability. Normeperidine, a neurotoxin, can accumulate.
Oxycodone	II	20	4–6	Available commercially combined or separately
Hydrocodone	III	30	3–4	Only available commercially combined
Codeine	II as separate agent; III when commercially combined	200	3–4	Concerns with itching and nausea
Propoxyphene	IV	200	6	Available commercially combined or separately. Norpropoxyphene, a neurotoxin, can accumulate.
Pentazocine	IV	50	4	Agonist-antagonist—not to be used in presence of other opioids or narcotic dependent patient. PO only available combined commercially with APAP.

APAP, acetaminophen; DEA, Drug Enforcement Agency; PO, oral.

These doses should be viewed as maximum for outpatient use and seldom required for acute orofacial pain management, especially when combined with a non-opioid for baseline pain control. Initial dose should be a fourth to half these maximums.

[a] 60 mg PO is appropriate only for the initial dose. Subsequently, equipotent doses are 30–40 mg.

(From Baumann TJ. Pain management. In: DiPiro JT, Talbert RL, Yee GC, et al, editors. Pharmacotherapy: a pathophysiologic approach. Stamford (CT): Appleton and Lange; 1997. p. 1259–78; and Kastrup EK. Opioids. In: Olin BR, Hebel SK, editors. Drug facts and comparisons 2000, 54th edition. St. Louis: Facts and Comparisons; 2000. p. 784-806.)

potency because 90% remains as the methylated parent drug having little or no analgesic efficacy but retaining useful antitussive properties. Unfortunately, this parent molecule also produces nausea and constipation, and for this reason, codeine is used only in lower doses (eg, 30–90 mg) for managing milder pain intensity.

It is not uncommon for patients to report prior episodes of nausea as an "allergic reaction." IgE antibodies, however, have been detected that react with several opioids, including codeine, and nearly all opioids are capable of triggering degranulation of mast cells leading to the direct release of histamine. Until issues regarding cross reactivity among opioids are resolved, a prudent approach would be to select alternatives that are molecularly dissimilar. For example, when a patient reports clinical signs that are allergic in nature, eg, rash or pruritis, one should select an agent that is not derived from codeine, eg, propoxyphene or meperidine. Drug interactions involving opioids are summarized below (see Table 1). The influence of certain antidepressants on the effectiveness of codeine and its derivatives has significant efficacy implications.

Hydrocodone and oxycodone

Hydrocodone and oxycodone are attractive analgesics because they have oral bioavailability comparable to codeine (ie, 60%, and their greater potency reduces the portion of an administered dose contributing to nausea and constipation). Unfortunately, equianalgesic doses were initially poorly understood and spawned the release of combination products that contain irrational formulations.

Like codeine, oxycodone, and hydrocodone are methylated molecules having little or no analgesic efficacy. Presumably, 10% of a dose administered parenterally is demethylated to its respective morphine counterpart, hydromorphone and oxymorphone. Evaluation of the information (see Table 3) reveals that the oral dose for codeine is approximately $20\times$ the IM dose of morphine. (200 mg versus 10 mg). This table indicates that 200 mg codeine, 30 mg hydrocodone, and 20 mg oxycodone are equipotent oral doses and are equianalgesic to morphine 10 mg IM. Clinical studies that have attempted to address equianalgesic doses of codeine derivatives are sparse, but they support this opinion. Beaver et al found that oxycodone 10 mg was comparable to codeine 100 mg, and this would extrapolate to oxycodone 20 mg and codeine 200 mg. Studies by Hopkinson and by Beaver have shown that hydrocodone 10 mg was approximately equipotent to codeine 60 mg, and this would extrapolate to 33 mg hydrocodone and 200 mg codeine [15].

Meperidine

Meperidine 75 mg is equianalgesic to morphine 10 mg following IM administration. A significant portion of an IM dose of meperidine is converted to normeperidine, a metabolite that has no analgesic properties but is a noted CNS stimulant. Furthermore, this metabolite has a 15–20-hour elimination half-life, compared with 3 hours for the parent drug. For hospitalized patients, meperidine is used only for a day or two; otherwise, normeperidine will accumulate. This issue becomes even more problematic following oral administration. The oral bioavailability for meperidine is approximately 25%, which requires a 300 mg dose to be equianalgesic to its IM dose of 75 mg. This introduces an even greater risk for accumulation of normeperidine. Poor oral absorption and accumulation of normeperidine make meperidine a very poor choice as an oral analgesic.

Propoxyphene

Propoxyphene is available only for oral administration. Its equianalgesic dose compared with morphine has not been established, but its potency is low. By convention, 100 mg is considered equipotent to oral codeine 60 mg. It is similar to meperidine in that it is converted to norpropoxyphene, a CNS stimulant having an elimination half-life of 30 hours. Propoxyphene is a DEA class IV agent. Its use should be limited to short-term management of mild to moderate pain.

Pentazocine (opioid agonist-antagonist)

Pentazocine is the only oral agonist-antagonist analgesic available in the United States. Pentazocine in the United States is available for oral use compounded with naloxone, a narcotic antagonist, presumably to prevent parenteral injection abuse issues. When taken by mouth as intended, naloxone does not inactivate the pentazocine, as naloxone has no bioavailability when taken orally. Additionally, pentazocine is available compounded with APAP. Though this agent can provide agonist analgesia when administered as the sole analgesic, pentazocine should not be used in the presence of other opioids. When other opioids are present, pentazocine will serve as an opioid antagonist, thus reducing the patient's analgesia. Additionally, it should not be prescribed for patients who are at risk for opioid withdrawal for the same reason. Pentazocine is a DEA schedule IV agent. It can be considered for the limited short-term management of mild to moderate pain.

Adjunctive therapy

A final consideration is the use of adjuvant agents that complement the opioid and nonopioid agents. Local anesthetics and GABAergic drugs are two examples of agents in this group that can be used to control pain. Longer-acting local anesthetics such as bupivacaine (Marcaine®) can be useful as part of a compound approach to patient pain control. Additionally, where muscle spasm, sleep disturbance, and/or anxiety are a consideration, the use of benzodiazepines such as lorazepam (Ativan®) can be added to the pain management combination.

Analgesic regimens

Mild and moderate pain can frequently be managed effectively using optimal doses of nonopioids (eg, 400–800 mg ibuprofen, 1000 mg acetaminophen, and 25–50 mg rofecoxib). Though it is unwise to combine NSAIDs, adding acetaminophen to an NSAID would be sensible considering their different sites of action [16]. Regardless of pain severity, one should optimize dosages of these agents and then, if necessary, add an opioid to the regimen. This practice will generally reduce the amount of opioid required, sometimes to only a fraction of the maximum doses listed in Table 3. Ideally, one should maintain the regular nonopioid dosing schedule and add an opioid product as needed for breakthrough pain.

Table 4
Management of mild, moderate and severe acute, orofacial pain in a healthy 70 kg adult

Indication	Regimen (70 KG adult examples)
Mild pain eg, root planning, routine endodontics	Ibuprofen: initial dose 400–800 mg, then 400–600 mg qid for 1–2 days, then PRN or Rofecoxib: Initial dose 50 mg, then 25–50 mg for 1–2 days then PRN and/or Acetaminophea: Initial dose 1000 mg, then 500–1000 mg q6h hours for 1–2 days, then PRN and/or Tramadol/acetaminophen[a]
Moderate pain eg, routine implant surgery, Soft tissue impactions	Baseline pain management with nonopioid: Establish regimen as per Mild Pain above plus Control breakthrough pain with Codeine 30–60 mg q4h PRN or Hydrocodone 5–10 mg q4h PRN or Oxycodone 5–10 mg q4h PRN or Pentazocine 25 mg q4h PRN and/or Tramadol 37.5–100 mg q4–6 hours PRN
Severe pain eg, bony impactions, complex implant surgery	Baseline pain management nonopioid: Establish regimen as per Mild Pain above, using maximum doses and continuing for 3–5 days before allowing PRN dosing plus Control breakthrough pain with: Hydrocodone 10–20 mg q4hours PRN or Oxycodone 5–15 mg q4h PRN or Pentazocine 50 mg q4h PRN and/or Tramadol 37.5–100 mg q4-6h prn

NSAID, nonsteroidal anti-inflammatory agent.

[a] NSAID use permits the use of tramadol/APAP combination with either q 4–6 h dosing or PRN.

When moderate to severe pain is anticipated with an inflammatory component, as NSAID should be used preoperatively. The practitioner should consider using a loading-dose for the initial NSAID, which is usually double the maintenance dose. Where concerns are present with exceeding the recommended daily ceiling dose of APAP- or NSAID-containing compounds, the practitioner can consider prescribing tramadol or an opioid that is not compounded, ie, oxycodone or codeine as a separate prescription. The practitioner must remember that titration to clinical response is necessary. Recommended doses do not apply to patients with renal or hepatic insufficiency or other medical conditions affecting drug metabolism. Elderly patients generally require lower doses, titrated slowly to the desired effect or side effects that are intolerable. Opioids for breakthrough pain may be prescribed commercially compounded. The nonopioid (generally APAP) compounded with the opioid must be considered when the baseline pain management analgesic is chosen to avoid nonopioid overdose and/or system toxicity. If tramadol is chosen as the initial breakthrough agent, another opioid may be added in addition if analgesia is inadequate at the maximum recommended dose of tramadol. Pentazocine should not be used if other opioids have been administered.

Based on this logic, it is not surprising that such a large number of commercially compounded analgesics have prepared containing both a non-opioid and an opioid ingredient. The opioid contained in most of these products is either codeine or one of its derivatives, eg, hydrocodone. It's unfortunate that some of these compounds were formulated with little consideration given to equianalgesic dosage strategies. Also, several products contain quantities of acetaminophen that preclude the use of multiple tablets to achieve an adequate amount of opioid for patients who experience severe pain. When prescribing combination products, the clinician must pay particular attention to the amount of acetaminophen in each compounded tablet so that the maximum daily dose is not exceeded. In some cases the clinician may choose to write separate prescriptions for the opioid and non-opioid analgesic needs of the patient to avoid acetaminophen overdose. Suggested regimens are presented in Table 4.

Summary

Careful selection of an effective analgesic regimen based on the amount and type of pain the patient is expected to have can prevent the stress and anxiety associated with breakthrough pain. When analgesics fail, it is not unusual for patients to go to desperate lengths to seek relief. The clinician can and should develop a variety of effective, safe analgesic regimens based on estimates of anticipated pain intensity that apply sound pharmacologic principles.

References

[1] RxList. The Internet drug index. The top 200 prescriptions for 2000 by number of prescriptions dispensed. Available at: http://www.rxlist.com/00top.htm. Accessed September 10, 2002.

[2] Stein C. The control of pain in peripheral tissue by opioids. N Engl J Med 1995;332(25): 1685–90.

[3] Babu KS, Salvi SS. Aspirin and asthma. Chest 2000;118(5):1470–6.

[4] Beaver WT, Wallenstein SL, Rogers A, Houde RW. Analgesic studies of codeine and oxycodone in patients with cancer: comparisons of oral with intramuscular codeine and of oral and intramuscular oxycodone. J Pharmacol Exp Ther 1978;207:92–100.

[5] Jackson DL, Moore PA, Hargreaves KM. Preoperative nonsteroidal anti-inflammatory medication for the prevention of postoperative dental pain. JADA 1989;119:641–7.

[6] Whitcomb DC, Block GD. Association of acetaminophen toxicity with fasting and ethanol. JAMA 1994;272(23):1845–50.

[7] Cicero TJ, Adams EH, Geller A, et al. A postmarketing surveillance program to monitor Ultram (tramadol) abuse in the United States. Drug Alcohol Depend 1999;57:7–22.

[8] Ultram. (tramadol). In: Physician's desk reference. 55th edition. Montvale (NJ): . Medical Economics Co; 2001. p. 2398–401.

[9] Katz WA. Pharmacology and clinical experience with tramadol in osteoarthritis. Drugs 1996;52(Suppl 3):39–47.

[10] Moore PA, Crout RJ, Jackson DL, et al. Tramadol hydrochloride: analgesic efficacy compared with codeine, aspirin with codeine, and placebo after dental extraction. J Clin Pharmacol 1998;38(6):554–60.

[11] Moroz BT, Ignatov YD, Kalinin VI. Use of tramadol hydrochloride in therapeutic operative dentistry: clinical investigation. Curr Ther Res 1991;49:371–5.

[12] Medve RA, Wang J, Karim R. Tramadol and acetaminophen tablets for dental pain. Anesth Prog 2001;48(3):79–81.

[13] Mullican WS, Lacy JR. Tramadol/acetaminophen combination tablets and codeine/ acetaminophen combination capsules for the management of chronic pain: a comparative trial. Clin Ther 2001;23(9):1429–45.

[14] Savage SR. Opioid use in the management of chronic pain. Med Clin North Am 1999; 761–86.

[15] Hopkinson JH. Hydrocodone-aunique challenge for an established drug: comparison of repeated or doses of hydrocodone (10 mg) and codeine (60 mg) in the treatment of postpartum pain. Curr Ter Res 1978;24:503–16.

[16] Breivik EK, Barkvoll P, Skowlund E. Combining diclofenac with acetaminophen or acetaminophen-codeine after oral surgery: a randomized, double-blind, single-dose study. Clin Pharmacol Ther 1999;66(6):625–35.

Further reading

Cooper SA, Engel J, Ladov M, et al. Analgesic efficacy of an ibuprofen-codeine combination. Pharmacotherapy 1982;2:162–7.

Cooper SA, Precheur H, Rauch D, et al. Evaluation of oxycodone and acetaminophen in treatment of postoperative dental pain. Oral Surgery. Oral Medicine and Oral Pathology 1980;50:496–501.

Dionne RA. Additive analgesic effects of oxycodone and ibuprofen in the oral surgery model. American Journal of Oral and Maxillofacial Surgeons 1999;57:673–8.

Dionne RA, Campbell RA, Cooper SA, et al. Suppression of postoperative pain by preoperative administration of ibuprofen in comparison to placebo, acetaminophen and acetaminophen plus codeine. J Clin Pharmacol 1983;23:37–43.

Doroschak AM, Bowles WR, Hargreaves KM. Evaluation of the combination of flurbiprofen and tramadol for management of endodontic pain. J Endod 1999;25:660–3.

Forbes JA, Bates JA, Edquist IA, et al. Evaluation of two opioid-acetaminophen combinations and placebo in postoperative oral surgery pain. Pharmacotherapy 1994;14:139–46.

Palangio M, Damask MJ, Morris E, et al. Combination hydrocodone and ibuprofen versus combination codeine and acetaminophen for the treatment of chronic pain. Clin Ther 2000; 22:879–92.

Piletta P, Porchet HC, Dayer P. Central analgesic effect of acetaminophen but not aspirin. Clin Pharmacol Ther 1991;49(4):350–4.

University of Michigan Health Sciences Center - Pain Management. Equianalgesic table. Available at: http://www.med.umich.edu/pain/apainmgt.htm#table. Accessed May 10, 2002.

Wideman GL, Keffer M, Morris E, et al. Analgesic efficacy of a combination of hydrocodone with ibuprofen in postoperative pain. Clin Pharmacol Ther 1999;65:66–76.

THE DENTAL
CLINICS OF
NORTH
AMERICA

Dent Clin N Am 46 (2002) 707–717

Dental postoperative pain management in children

Anupama Rao Tate, DMD[a],*,
George Acs, DMD, MPH[b]

[a]Department of Dentistry, Children's National Medical Center,
111 Michigan Avenue Northwest, Washington, DC 20010, USA
[b]Department of Pediatrics, George Washington University School of Medicine,
2300 Eye Street Northwest, Washington, DC 20037, USA

In the past 20 years nearly all healthcare professional groups have evolved their understanding of childhood pain. Surgeons, anesthesiologists, and nursing professionals have reassessed commonly held beliefs that children somehow differed from adults in their response to noxious stimulus and their need to relieve them of such stimuli, as may have accompanied invasive procedures [1]. During this time, significant controversies existed over the use of only paralytic drugs for general anesthesia techniques, the use of narcotic agents in postoperative management of children, and even preoperative and postoperative management of children undergoing circumcision [2].

Interest in pain control in children has blossomed over the past decade, but there remains an incongruity between pain management theory and clinical practice. Possible reasons for this difference include incorrect assumptions about pain and children, individual and social attitudes toward pain, and the complexity of assessing pain in children.

The pain experience in children is not necessarily a response to tissue damage. Children may experience pain in the absence of tissue injury and are also capable of experiencing multiple types of pain from the same injury because of the plasticity of a child's nociceptive system [3]. The child's pain system also allows the practitioner to modify the pain experience of the child. Many clinicians do not give serious consideration to postoperative pain relief for children because of the unfounded beliefs that children do not experience pain to the same degree as adults and that children are perceived to bounce back from painful procedures. Furthermore, in the weeks that

---

* Corresponding author.
E-mail address: atate@cnmc.org (A.R. Tate).

elapse between invasive dental procedures and subsequent appointments, there is infrequent effort to query the child or parent about the post-treatment experience. The passage of time certainly serves to heal and forget.

There are many pain reducing strategies available to clinicians who are willing to accept that children do experience pain following dental procedures and can benefit from its relief. Strategies may include preoperative and postoperative approaches. Ultimately, pain assessment and its treatment in children should be an integral part of clinical practice for every dental professional.

Changing philosophy of pain management

The first studies of pain management in children found that children often did not receive any medication after surgery. In 1974, Eland conducted a study of 25 children after surgery, of which 16% had no prescription for pain medication after surgery, and 52% received pain medication [4]. In 1983, Mather and Mackie conducted a study with 170 children and also found that 16% did not have analgesic prescriptions for postoperative pain [5]. Over time the views about children and the need for postoperative pain management improved. By 1994, Asprey replicated Eland's 1974 study. With all 25 children matched by type of surgery and age, all children had a prescription for and received pain medication after surgery [6].

Historically, when comparing pain management in children with adults, children have been less likely to have narcotic medication prescribed. In 1968, in a 4-month study, Swafford and Allan reported that only 26 of 180 pediatric patients in the intensive care unit received narcotics and that no pain medications were given to children in the recovery room [7]. At the same time, however, 54 injections of pain medication were given to 107 adult patients in the recovery room in 1 week. In 1977, Eland and Anderson reported that 18 adults with identical diagnoses as 25 children who had surgery received 671 doses of pain medication, whereas the children received only 24 doses [4]. In 1983, Beyer studied postoperative pain management in 50 children and 50 adults after cardiac surgery. Six children received no pain prescriptions [8]. Overall, children were prescribed significantly fewer potent narcotics. During the observation period, children received 30% of all analgesic administrations, whereas adults received 70%. In 1992, Elander et al reported the mean number of pain medication doses administered to infants, children, and adults during the 5 days after heart surgery [9]. They reported that on average, infants had fewer doses (10 doses) when compared with children (15 doses) and adults (26 doses).

When researchers compared doses of analgesic prescribed it was noted that children often received subtherapeutic doses compared with adults. A study by Burokas in 1985 found that 38% of 40 children who had major surgery had subtherapeutic doses of analgesics prescribed and only two children received all the pain medication that had been prescribed [10].

Definition of pain

Pain is a highly personalized state accompanying tissue damage as a result of an adequate stimulus. It is a construct including an individual's past experiences, learned responses, and expectations in addition to species-specific physiologic responses. Pain may fluctuate in intensity and quality as a consequence of the passage of time. Pain is a signal of enormous biologic importance. A measure of the biologic and social importance of pain is evident in the more than 300 commercially available over-the-counter analgesics [11]. Physiologically, pain involves signals that are transmitted over specialized neural pathways. When these signals terminate, they induce a host of secondary responses that may become organized in the central nervous system. At the physiologic level, some of these responses involve further transmission of neural signals and the releases of neurotransmitters and humorally active chemicals (gamma-aminobutyric acid, GABA) and endogenous opioids [11].

The spinothalamic tract is the anatomic system designed for the central transmission of pain information. It is often thought of as a conduit for sensory messages from pain-specific receptors in the periphery. Two classes of afferent nerve fibers convey pain information. Small, lightly myelinated nerve fibers (A-delta class) carry afferent sensory information at 5–30 m/second. Unmyelinated C fibers, less than 2 μm in diameter, conduct at only 0.5–2.0 m/second. The cell body for all primary sensory afferents lies in the dorsal root ganglion, and the proximal axon segment enters the spinal cord to synapse. Substance P is believed to be the neurotransmitter for the C fibers. Physiologists often speak of two kinds of pain: fast pain and slow pain. Appreciation of a pinprick is rapid, quick to decay, and fairly localizable; this is followed by a persistent, noxious sensation that is usually more diffuse. Often, this is the pain that keeps people awake at night. The slow pain resides in the C fibers and the spinoreticular pathway [11].

In 1965 Melzak and Wall introduced the gate theory that was an important step forward in the understanding of pain control [12]. The gate theory proposed that a gate control system modulated sensory input from the skin before it evoked pain perception and response. The gate theory suggests that pain phenomena are determined by interactions among different neurologic systems. Control over transmission is postulated to be affected by the afferent impulses acting on a gating mechanism and by impulses descending from the brain. Impulses in large diameter fibers were assumed to decrease the effectiveness of afferent volleys, whereas small afferents increase it. The substantia gelatinosa was suggested as the actual control mechanism and the presynaptic terminals of afferent fibers as the site of action. It was also proposed that the signal that triggered the action system responsible for pain perception and response occurred when the output of transmission cells reached or exceeded a preset threshold level. Since the introduction of this theory, revisions have been made in recognition of new or better understanding of physiology. Perhaps the most significant addition to the gate control theory is a level of control that is proposed to be through higher central nervous system processes, such as the evolution of input in past experiences, that may exert control over activity in discriminative and motivational systems. Melzack clearly stated that physiologic processes alone are inadequate to explain the perception of pain. Their work lead to investigations into the "emotional" components involved in the perception of pain [13].

A major advance in the understanding of pain came in 1975 when the mechanism of narcotic analgesia became better understood. Derivatives of the opium poppy such as morphine have been available for the relief of pain since the mid-nineteenth century. The discovery of the opiate receptor lead to the discovery of endogenous opiates such as the enkephalins and endorphins. The receptor-mediated effect helped in the understanding of the relationship of morphine and reversal agents such as naloxone [11].

Children and pain

Numerous lines of evidence suggest that even in the human fetus, pain pathways and cortical centers necessary for pain perception are well developed late in gestation. Anand showed in 1987 that marked nociceptive activity clearly constitutes a physiologic and perhaps even a psychologic form of stress in neonates [14]. Studies suggest that developmental changes in response to painful stimuli occur early in infancy. In fact, anticipatory fears of sharp objects can be seen in children approximately 1 year of age [15]. As a child matures, develops a broader vocabulary, and witnesses a variety of environments, the ability to communicate feelings becomes increasingly adept and sophisticated. In general, pain sensitivity increases and self-management of pain becomes more effective with increasing age [16].

It was not until recently that the dental literature started to discuss the presence of pain and its management in children. In 1986, Acs reported that 37.6% of children ages 6 to 13 years reported postoperative pain after having dental extractions [17]. In 1992, in a more broad study evaluating dental postoperative pain in children, 31.5% of the children treated reported pain following routine restorative dentistry procedures. There were no age-related differences in the report of pain, and female patients were significantly more likely to report pain following invasive restorative treatment [18].

The extent of injury caused by the surgical procedure is also a key factor in evaluating the need for postoperative pain management [19]. In 1988, a postextraction pain study in children indicated that as the "degree of difficulty," as measured by the amount of remaining unresorbed root structure of the extracted tooth increased, the report of pain increased. Therefore the dentist may consider the number of teeth extracted together with the degree of difficulty in determining the potential for postextraction pain and the need for analgesia [20].

Local anesthetics

Local anesthesia has been important to "painless" dentistry ever since cocaine local anesthesia in 1886 and procaine in 1904 were introduced. In the 1940s a new group, the amides, were introduced [21]. The first amide, lidocaine, changed the course of pain management in dentistry worldwide. The primary role of local anesthetic is to block the propagation of nerve impulses. Each anesthetic varies in its potency, onset time, and duration of action. Procaine has the lowest intrinsic potency; lidocaine, prilocaine, and mepivacaine have intermediate potency. Duration of anesthesia is one of the most important clinical properties to consider when choosing an appropriate agent. Lidocaine and prilocaine (with epinephrine) have an intermediate duration of 60–90 minutes of pulpal anesthesia and 3–5 hours of soft tissue anesthesia. Mepivacaine plain is often reported to have a shorter duration of soft tissue anesthesia, although a recent investigation suggests that anesthetic duration of mepivacaine plain and lidocaine with epinephrine are nearly identical [22].

A study done by Kohli surveyed pediatric dentists about their use of local anesthetics; 83% of the responding dentists stated that lidocaine was used most often, whereas mepivacaine was used most frequently by 11% of the dentists [23]. Articaine was first prepared in 1969, and recent reports by Wright show articaine's excellent pediatric safety and efficacy profile [24]. A study done by Malamed in 2000 comparing lidocaine with articaine indicated that articaine was a safe and effective local anesthetic in children. Articaine 4% with epinephrine 1:100,000 was demonstrated to have a time to onset and duration appropriate for clinical use in children, although no significant difference in pain relief was observed between articaine and lidocaine [21]. Previous reports of longer pulpal anesthesia and duration of articaine with vasoconstrictor when compared with lidocaine with vasoconstrictor have not been demonstrated [25]. Articaine has recently been approved for use in the United States and may be considered part of the armamentarium for use with pediatric dental patients in appropriate cases.

Analgesics

Since its introduction in 1899, aspirin, a salicylate, has been used widely for its analgesic, antipyretic, and anti-inflammatory properties. The most significant side effects of aspirin include alteration of coagulation by inhibition of platelet aggregation. The anticoagulation properties of aspirin are rarely a problem for children; however, because a single dose can increase bleeding time, aspirin should not be used before any surgical procedure. The possible association of aspirin with certain viral illnesses and the development of Reye syndrome has resulted in many practitioners opting for aspirin substitutes [16].

Acetaminophen is the most common analgesic used in pediatrics in the United States. Unlike aspirin it does not inhibit platelet function and causes less gastric upset. The primary disadvantage is that it has no clinically significant anti-inflammatory properties. Toxicity as a result of overdose may result in acute liver failure. Allergic reaction is rare [16].

The newer nonsteroidal anti-inflammatory drugs (NSAIDs) are principally derivatives of phenylalkanoic acid and exert their analgesic effects peripherally by inhibiting prostaglandin synthetase. These agents possess analgesic and anti-inflammatory properties that are superior to those of aspirin and are effective for the treatment of acute pain following minor surgery or trauma [16]. Ketorolac tromethamine and ibuprofen are common examples of NSAIDs. In 1987, McGraw studied the efficacy of ibuprofen suspension and acetaminophen elixir in children after dental extractions. The ibuprofen elixir was superior in the management of postextraction pain in children [26]. Most pain associated with dental procedures is inflammatory in nature; therefore usually agents with anti-inflammatory properties are most desirable for the treatment of dental pain.

Tramadol hydrochloride is a synthetic, centrally acting analgesic agent with spinal and supraspinal sites of action. Tramadol has been found to be effective and well-tolerated when administered postoperatively to children older than 1 year of age. Its negligible effect on respiration, despite equi-analgesic potency to morphine shown in adults would suggest that tramadol offers advantages over traditional opioids such as morphine for the relief of postoperative pain in children [27]. Pendeville reported on the post-tonsillectomy use of tramadol drops (2.5 mg/kg) versus acetaminophen suppositories (15 mg/kg) in children and showed postoperative pain scores to be significantly lower in patients managed with tramadol [28]. Roelose studied preoperative tramadol efficacy in children following multiple dental extractions. In children 4–6 years of age, 19.4% of the tramadol group required postoperative agents, compared with 82.8% of the placebo control group [29]. As further studies validate the pediatric use of tramadol, its use might increase.

Recent literature suggest that the preoperative administration of an analgesic, rather than the traditional postoperative use on an as-needed basis, was more effective in reducing postextraction pain, because the drug preceded rather than followed the inflammatory response and subsequent pain [30–32]. In 1995, however, Primosch compared preoperative ibuprofen, acetaminophen, and placebo administration on the parental report of postextraction pain in children [33]. Although there was a trend toward reduced postextraction pain reported by the parents, the preoperative administration of neither analgesic was found to be statistically superior to the placebo in children.

Narcotic analgesia such as opioids has been shown to act on opioid receptors in the central nervous system. These actions result in analgesia, sedation, and cough suppression. They carry the serious drawback of respiratory depression. Codeine is the standard oral narcotic used most commonly in children for moderate to severe pain. It is indicated for severe pain that is not responsive to acetaminophen or NSAIDs. Codeine is best used when combined with optimum analgesic doses of acetaminophen or ibuprofen. When choosing an analgesic agent in the management of postoperative dental pain in children, it is rare that the recommended dose of acetaminophen or NSAIDs does not control the dental pain. In fact, in a study evaluating the use of postextraction analgesics in children, few reported severe pain. In that study, when pain was reported, it was equally well relieved by ibuprofen or acetaminophen with codeine [34]. The combination of codeine and acetaminophen usually provides the needed relief in the rare cases when acetaminophen and NSAIDs are not sufficient to manage the pain. Rarely is the pain refractory to these agents; in these limited cases meperidine may be indicated [16].

Recommendations

The pain experience often determines whether an individual seeks or avoids healthcare. The thoughtful management of pre- and postoperative pain can increase the use of dentistry for routine care.

The first goal of the caregiver should be management of preoperative fears and anxieties. Acs reported on the effect of age and postoperative pain reporting. When comparing children of different ages, 6–9 years versus 10–13 years, it has been seen that the older group reports pain more frequently, yet the use of analgesic agents is the same for both groups. The report of postoperative pain is therefore tied to the mental awareness that comes from maturity. The postoperative pain of these older children is also affected by their past experiences and fears and even the expectations of their parents. The use of preoperative antianxiolytics, such as nitrous oxide and midazolam, can be helpful for children. Nitrous oxide can play a role in modifying perception of fear that may be related to anticipation of pain. This heightened preoperative perception of pain can affect postoperative pain relief needs; therefore the use of preoperative antianxiolytics can be critical to a pain management protocol. The use of these drugs should reduce the anxiety by decreasing awareness of the patient during the procedure. In addition, the appropriate use of topical and local anesthesia is critical for the management of pain during the procedure and after.

The selection and dosage of analgesics varies because of the changes in body weight and composition that occur throughout childhood. The first choice in most cases is the least potent analgesic with the fewest side effects. When postoperative pain is expected in young children, the analgesic agent should not be given on an "as needed" basis because of the difficulty in childhood reporting of pain. Table 1 shows common pediatric pain management agents and the appropriate dosage schedule. All medications should be prescribed in sufficient dosage and for an adequate duration to alleviate postoperative pain for the child. By being familiar with the duration of the

Table 1
Medications and dosage for oral pediatric postoperative pain management

Medication	Availability	Dosage	40 lb child	80 lb child
Acetaminophen	Elixir 160 mg/5 cc 325-mg tabs, 160 mg chewable	10–15 mg/kg/dose given at 4–6 h intervals	160 mg = 1 tsp 160 mg = 1 chewable	325 mg = 1 tab 320 mg = 2 chewables
Ibuprofen	Suspension 100 mg/5 cc 200-,300-,400-, 600-,800-mg tabs	4–10 mg/kg/dose given at 6–8 h intervals	100 mg = 1 tsp	200 mg = 2 tsp 200 mg = 1 tab
Tramadol	50 mg, 100 mg tabs	1–2 mg/kg/dose given at 4–6 h intervals— maximum: 100 mg	25 mg = ½ tab	50 mg = 1 tab
Codeine and acetaminophen	Suspension 12 mg/ 5 cc	0.5–1.0 mg codeine/kg/dose given at 4–6 h intervals	12 mg = 1 tsp	24 mg = 2 tsp
Meperidine	Syrup 50 mg/5 cc 50-mg, 100-mg tabs	0.5–0.8 mg/lb given at 4–6 h intervals	25 mg = ½ tsp	50 mg = 1 tsp

local anesthetic, the dentist can advise the parent to administer any analgesics before loss of local anesthesia-induced analgesia.

The practitioner should choose their pre- and postoperative pain management plan based on the type of procedure done. Table 2 categorizes common pediatric dental procedures based on their invasiveness. In general, pediatric dental procedures range from simple operative not requiring local anesthesia to the extraction of abscessed permanent teeth. Each case should be considered individually. For simple restorative dental procedures, one might choose a shorter-acting local anesthetic to reduce the chance of postoperative soft tissue damage by cheek or lip biting, although clinical research has not proven this relationship to be true. The use of a quick onset local anesthetic with shorter duration is appropriate when there is little anticipation for postoperative discomfort. Additionally, quick onset provides potential practice efficiencies. When considering lengthy procedures such as stainless steel crown and pulpotomies, the use of nitrous oxide and an intermediate duration anesthetic followed by ibuprofen might be indicated.

Table 2
Dental postoperative pain management protocol

	Local anesthesia	Preoperative medication	Postoperative medication[a]
Restorative procedures			
Simple operative	None		Acetaminophen
Operative	Mepivacaine/ articaine/lidocaine		Acetaminophen
Complex—SSC/pulp	Articaine/lidocaine		Acetaminophen
Extractions			
Primary, nonabscessed	Articaine/lidocaine		Ibuprofen
Primary, abscessed	Articaine/lidocaine		Ibuprofen
Multiple primary	Articaine/lidocaine	Ibuprofen	Acetaminophen or ibuprofen
Permanent teeth, Ankylosed teeth	Articaine/lidocaine	Ibuprofen	Acetaminophen with/without codeine

[a] Additional risk factors, such as patient age, previous report of pain, or use of analgesics should be considered before the decision to prescribe any analgesics is made.

More invasive procedures, such as extractions, should be categorized and considered based on the degree of difficulty of the procedure. Simple extraction of nonabscessed primary teeth with only half of the root structure remaining likely does not require the same management compared with the extraction of multiple abscessed primary teeth. In emergent cases there is often no opportunity to give preoperative analgesics; however, if one is going to extract multiple nonabscessed teeth then the use of preoperative ibuprofen might help alleviate or minimize the postoperative pain. Although the adult oral surgery literature supports treatment protocol that uses presurgical nonsteroidal anti-inflammatory agents, there is no evidence that such protocols are necessary in the pain management of children undergoing dental extractions [32,33].

It has been reported that 17% of children undergoing invasive restorative treatment and 22% of children needing tooth extraction require postoperative analgesia [18]. Studies have shown that children feel pain much the same way as adults and experience the need for postoperative pain management. It is also known that pain medications alleviate pain successfully in children. Therefore, one must have a plan for pain management in all pediatric patients. It is recognized that in a dental setting most pediatric procedures are less invasive or extensive compared with adult procedures. One must start with the unquestioned effectiveness of any administered local anesthesia, with sufficiently long lasting duration. In addition, instructions must be clearly given to the caregiver regarding postoperative medication. One should also note that certain factors may affect the need for postoperative medication: extent of invasiveness of procedure, age of the patient, and child's past pain history, along with parental expectations for pain.

Summary

Misconceptions about the need for pain management in pediatric patients have been shown to be wrong. We now understand that children feel pain and respond to pain medication in much the same way as adults. With this new understanding, practitioners must recognize all the factors that affect the feeling of pain. Pain can be variable and each patient brings a unique set of characteristics to be evaluated. The first objective should be to assess the patient's previous treatment history, medical condition, extent of treatment needed, and age. An effective pain management protocol begins with preoperative pain and anxiety control, with the use of agents such as nitrous oxide and local anesthetics. Postoperative pain medication should be given at the correct dosage and time intervals for the appropriate duration. With our commitment to pain management in children, these protocols should easily translate into improved clinical practice.

References

[1] Helgadottir HL. Pain management practiced in children after surgery. J Pediatr Nurs 2000;15(5):334–40.
[2] Walco GA, Cassidy RC, Schechter NL. Pain, hurt, and harm—the ethics of pain control in infants and children. N Engl J Med 1994;331(8):541–4.
[3] Barrett EJ. Pain management for children. Ont Dent 1997;74(8):34–6.
[4] Eland JM, Anderson JE. The experience of pain in children. In: Jacox A, editor. Pain: a source book for nurses and other health professionals. Brown & Compan: Boston: Little; 1977. p. 453–76.
[5] Mather L, Mackie J. The incidence of postoperative pain in children. Pain 1983;15:271–81.
[6] Asprey JR. Postoperative analgesic prescription and administration in a pediatric population. J Pediatr Nurs 1994;9(3):150–7.
[7] Swafford LI, Allan D. Pain relief in the pediatric patient. Med Clin N Am 1968;52(1): 131–6.
[8] Beyer JE, Degood DE, Ashley LC, Ressell GA. Pattern of postoperative analgesic use with adults and children following cardiac surgery. Pain 1983;17(1):71–81.
[9] Elander G, Hellstrom G. Analgesic administration in children and adults following open heart surgery. Scand J Caring Sci 1992;6:17–21.
[10] Burokas L. Factors affecting nurses' decision to medicate pediatric patients after surgery. Heart Lung 1985;14(4):373–9.
[11] Sudarsky L. Pathophysiology of the nervous system. Boston: Little, Brown & Company; 1990. p. 79–91.
[12] Melzack R, Wall PD. Pain mechanisms: a new theory. Science 1965;150:971.
[13] Melzack R, Casey KL. Sensory, motivational and central control determinants of pain: a new conceptual model. In: Kenhalo D, editor. The skin sense. Spingfield (IL): Thomas; 1968.
[14] Anand KJS, Phil D, Hickey PR. Pain and its effect in the human neonate and fetus. N Engl J Med 1987;317(21):1321–9.
[15] Barr RG. Pain in children. In: Wall PD, Melzack R, editors. Textbook of pain. New York: Churchill Livingstone; 1989.
[16] Pinkham JR. Pediatric dentistry. In: Pinkham JR, Fields Jr HW, editors. Infancy through adolescence. 2nd edition. Philadelphia: WB Saunders Company; 1994. p. 98–105.
[17] Acs G, Moore PA, Needleman HL, Shusterman S. The incidence of post-extraction pain and analgesic usage in children. Anesth Prog 1986;33:147–51.

The lipid solubility characteristics of a local anesthetic best predicts potency. Procaine is one of the least lipid-soluble and least potent local anesthetics, whereas bupivacaine is very lipid-soluble and therefore the most potent. Protein binding characteristics are a primary determinant of the duration of anesthesia. Agents that attach to protein components of nerve membranes are less likely to diffuse from the site of action and into the systemic circulation. Lidocaine's short duration and bupivacaine's long duration are caused, in part, by their distinctly different protein binding characteristics [4].

It is clear that lipid solubility, ionization, and protein-binding properties contribute to the clinical characteristics of local anesthetics. But factors such as the site injection, drug and vasoconstrictor concentration, volume of injection, and inherent vasoconstrictive properties of the anesthetic will also influence the clinical performance of a local anesthetic.

Ester anesthetics: procaine/propoxycaine

A combination of ester anesthetics, procaine and propoxycaine, was available in dental cartridges until 1989. The formulation in dental cartridges was the combination of 0.4% propoxycaine (Ravocaine®) and 2% procaine (Novocain®) with 1:20,000 levonordefrin as a vasoconstrictor. As stated earlier, ester anesthetics are generally less effective than amides because they have poor diffusion properties. Additionally, procaine has significant allergenicity and has been known to affect both the patient and practitioners. Procaine is a potent vasodilator and is not effective if used without a vasoconstrictor.

The termination of effect is through hydrolysis by plasma and tissues cholinesterases to para-aminobenzoic acid (PABA) and diethylamino alcohol. The PABA appears to be the allergen associated with procaine's allergenicity.

In the 1980s, there was some concern about the use of amide anesthetics with patients diagnosed with "malignant hyperthermia." This rare genetic syndrome causes a rapid and potentially fatal rise in body temperature during general anesthesia. Ester anesthetics at one time were considered to be the local anesthetic agents of choice for these patients. Recent evidence has determined, however, that this concern is unfounded and the use of an amide anesthetic for patients at risk for malignant hyperthermia is no longer contraindicated [5].

Lidocaine hydrochoride

Lidocaine hydrochloride (Xylocaine®, Octocaine®) was introduced into practice in the 1950s and, because of its excellent efficacy and safety, has become the prototypic dental local anesthetic in North America. Besides having excellent anesthetic efficacy, lidocaine has limited allergenicity with fewer than 20 reports of allergic reactions in the literature in the past 50 years. Given the frequent use of local anesthesia in dentistry (500,000–1,000,000 injections a day in the United States and Canada), the rare incidence of hypersensitivity reactions is an extremely important clinical advantage.

Lidocaine is formulated in cartridges as 2% lidocaine with 1:50,000 epinephrine, 2% lidocaine with 1:100,000 epinephrine, and 2% lidocaine with 1:200,000 epinephrine. The 2% lidocaine with 1:100,000 epinephrine is considered the standard for comparison with newer anesthetics. Lidocaine with epinephrine rapidly induces oral anesthesia and provides surgical anesthesia that last 90–180 minutes.

Mepivacaine hydrochloride

Mepivacaine hydrochloride (Carbocaine®, Polocaine®) has an important place in dental anesthesia because it has minimal vasodilating properties and can therefore provide profound local anesthesia without being formulated with a vasoconstrictor such as epinephrine or levonordefrin. The availability of a 3% formulation not containing a vasoconstrictor is a valuable addition to a dentist's armamentarium. It is available in dental cartridges as 3% mepivacaine plain or 2% mepivacaine 1:20,000 levonordefrin. Mepivacaine plain is often reported to have a short duration of soft tissue anesthesia, although a recent investigation suggests that although pulpal durations of mepivacaine plain are shorter than 2% lidocaine with epinephrine, soft tissue anesthesia for mepivacaine and lidocaine with epinephrine are nearly identical [6].

Prilocaine hydrochloride

Prilocaine hydrochloride (Citanest®) can provide excellent anesthesia with or without a vasoconstrictor. One of its metabolic products, toluidine, has been associated with the development of methemoglobinemia (see following article "Adverse reactions to local anesthetics"). It is available in preparations of 4% prilocaine plain and 4% prilocaine with 1:200,000 epinephrine. The formulation containing epinephrine has anesthetic characteristics similar to 2% lidocaine 1:100,000 epinephine. The 4% prilocaine plain formulation provides a slightly shorter duration of surgical anesthesia. Although the pH of the solution in dental cartridges is somewhat less acidic, there is little indication that prilocaine causes less discomfort upon injection [7].

Articaine hydrochloride

The local anesthetic articaine hydrochloride (Ultracaine®, Septocaine®) has been available in Europe (1976) and Canada (1982) for several decades. Recently, the United States Food and Drug Administration (FDA) approved use of articaine in the United States. Because of its unique chemistry and pharmacologic profile, 4% articaine with epinephrine may provide practitioners with an alternative to the currently available dental local anesthetics. In Canada, articaine is marketed under the brand name of Ultracaine® and Septanest®, and in the United States as Septocaine®. The United States formulation contains 4% articaine hydrochloride 1:100,000 epinephrine bitartrate in a sterile 1.7 mL. glass cartridge.

Similar to most dental anesthetics available to the dental practitioner, articaine is classified as an amide anesthetic. The molecular structure of articaine additionally contains a thiophene (sulfur-containing) ring and an ester side chain (Fig. 1). As articaine is absorbed from the injection site into the systemic circulation, it is rapidly inactivated by hydrolysis of the ester side chain to articainic acid and therefore has an extremely short plasma half-life (27 minutes) [8].

The onset time, duration, and anesthetic profundity of articaine is comparable to 2% lidocaine with 1:100,000 epinephrine [9]. Articaine and prilocaine have been associated with a slightly higher incidence of mandibular and lingual paresthesia [10]. Articaine does not appear to have a greater allergenicity than other available dental anesthetic agents, probably because the ester metabolite is not the allergen PABA. Reports of toxicity reactions following the use of articaine for dental anesthesia are extremely rare. The rapid inactivation of articaine by plasma esterases may explain the apparent lack of overdose reactions reported following its administration, even though it is marketed as a 4% solution.

Clinical studies indicate that 4% articaine 1:100,000 epinephrine is an effective and useful local anesthetic for dental procedures. When reinjection

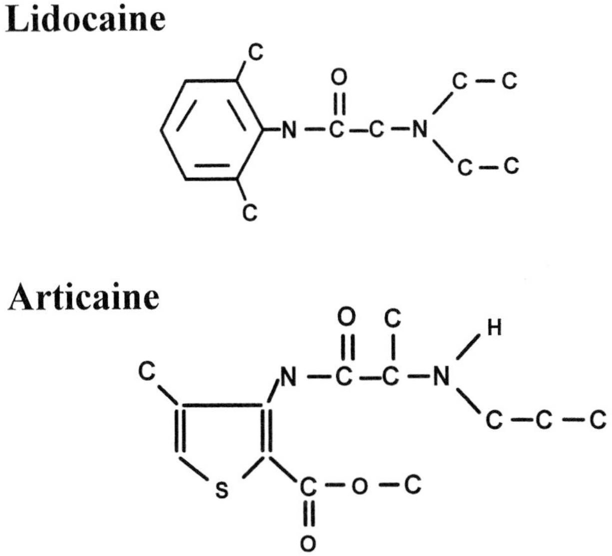

Fig. 1. Molecular structures of lidocaine and articaine.

of anesthesia is anticipated because of long appointments required for cosmetic dentistry, full mouth restoration, full mouth periodontal surgery, or multiple implant placements, articaine may be considered as a desirable anesthetic.

The 4% articaine solution with epinephrine has been reported to have an onset of 1.5–3.0 minutes for maxillary infiltrations, and only slightly longer for inferior alveolar blocks. The duration of soft tissue anesthesia ranges from 2–3 hours for maxillary infiltration anesthesia and 3–4 hours for mandibular block anesthesia [11].

There is little data to support the claim that articaine has superior diffusion properties or that lingual/palatal anesthesia can be induced following buccal infiltration. The establishment of maxillary and mandibular pulpal anesthesia following buccal infiltration with articaine has been compared with prilocaine using electrical stimulation of tooth pulp and lingual soft tissue. Results showed no statistically significant differences between articaine and prilocaine in their ability to induce anesthesia for any tissue at any of the sites tested [12,13].

Long-acting amide anesthetics: bupivacaine and etidocaine

In the past few decades, two long-acting amide local anesthetics, bupivacaine and etidocaine, have found a place in the dentists' armamentarium. These agents play a valuable role in the overall management of surgical and postoperative pain associated with dental care. As illustrated (Fig. 2), etidocaine and bupivacaine are chemical analogues of lidocaine and mepivacaine. Bupivacaine (1-butyl-2', 6'pipecoloxylidide) (Marcaine®) is identical to mepivacaine except for a butyl (4 carbon) substitution of the methyl (1 carbon)

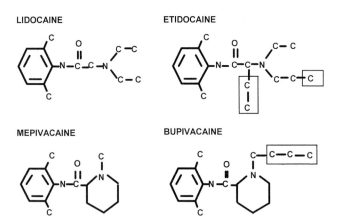

Fig. 2. Comparison of the molecular structures of standard anesthetics to long-acting anesthetics.

group at the aromatic amine. Etidocaine (2-N-ethylpropylamino-2′ butyroxylidide) (Duranest®) is identical to lidocaine except for a propyl (3 carbon) substitution and an ethyl (2 carbon) addition. These additions to the chemical structures of lidocaine and mepivacaine provide enhanced lipid solubility and, especially, protein-binding properties as compared with their shorter-acting analogues [14,15].

Although both bupivacaine and etidocaine may provide adequate surgical anesthesia, they are most useful for postoperative pain management. Clinical trials have shown that bupivacaine has a slightly longer onset time than conventional anesthetics [4]. The profundity of anesthesia, however, appears to be comparable. Onset times and profundity are optimized when preparations of bupivacaine include epinephrine [16]. Etidocaine, although less well studied in dentistry, appears to have a slight advantage over bupivacaine with regard to onset times. Onset times for etidocaine have been found to be slightly more rapid than bupivacaine (less than 1 minute difference) when the agents were compared in endodontics and oral surgery [17,18]. The profundity of mandibular anesthesia provided by etidocaine with epinephrine appears to be equivalent to conventional agents. The profundity of etidocaine anesthesia following maxillary infiltrations may be somewhat less [19].

When duration of soft-tissue anesthesia is evaluated, inferior alveolar blocks using bupivacaine have durations 2–3 times those of lidocaine and mepivacaine [20,21]. As might be expected, durations are somewhat shorter when maxillary infiltrations are evaluated. Bupivacaine provided soft tissue anesthesia for 4–5 hours after infiltration, and 5–8 hours following nerve blocks. Etidocaine provides similar increases in soft-tissue anesthesia duration following block injections. Because the epinephrine concentrations are lower in formulations of bupivacaine and etidocaine, increased bleeding during surgery has been demonstrated.

The use of long-acting local anesthetics to alleviate pain following third molar extractions has been consistently and repeatedly demonstrated [4, 22–24]. Patients undergoing third molar extractions involving bone removal were administered 0.5% bupivacaine without epinephrine, 0.5% bupivacaine 1/200,000 epinephrine, or 3% mepivacaine. The patients receiving bupivacaine with epinephrine had a mean duration of anesthesia of 7.0 hours (versus 2.9 hours for mepivacaine) and required the fewest doses of postoperative narcotic analgesics [24]. A combination strategy for managing postoperative pain using a nonsteroidal anti-inflammatory drug (NSAID) prior to surgery and a long-acting anesthetic may provide maximal comfort [23].

Additionally, it has been noted that some patients may be concerned about prolonged anesthesia. If a clear explanation of expectations is not provided, some patients may worry about possible dysesthesias caused by surgical trauma. Delays in recovery following local anesthetic using long-acting agents beyond 10 hours are not uncommon. Patient preparation and a thorough explanation of this pain control strategy are essential [19].

Bupivacaine and etidocaine have been used in the overall management of chronic pain either as symptomatic, diagnostic, or definitive therapy. Prolonged anesthesia and pain relief may facilitate physical therapy of certain skeletal muscle disorders. Some myofascial pain dysfunction syndromes may benefit from injection of a long-acting local anesthetic into "trigger points." Injections of long-acting agents, sometimes repeatedly over a course of weeks, may be useful in stimulating complete recovery from postherpetic neuralgias and reflex sympathetic dystrophies [25].

Advances in local anesthetic techniques

Dental patients have become increasingly less tolerant of a dentist who hurts them. The control of intra- and postoperative pain presents an age-old challenge: Will there ever be a perfect local anesthetic technique or delivery system? Through the past 3 decades, it appears that attempts to increase success rates, especially in the mandible with its dense, infiltration-resistant cortical bone, have accelerated.

The conventional inferior alveolar nerve block (IANB) sometimes misnamed as a mandibular block, has served the dental profession admirably since being formally documented by Halstead in 1905. In view of the fact that there were no anatomically proven alternatives until 1973 (Gow-Gates Condylar Neck Mandibular Block) and 1977 (Akinosi Closed Mouth Mandibular Block), the conventional approach offered advantages such as standardized landmarks, reasonable success (69–85%), relative simplicity, and almost universal practitioner acceptance from institutional teaching standards.

Disadvantages include, however, inadequate anesthesia for some patients, obscure and visually obstructuive landmarks (ie, buccal fat pad and tongue), risk of dysesthesia or paresthesia, and high vascularity enhancing local anesthesia and vasoconstrictor systemic absorption. The reasons for failure may include local anesthesia solution or vasoconstrictor, pK_a–pH incompatibility, needle-jaw size discrepancy, tissue vector forces, inadequate volume of solution, anatomical variations (hard tissue anatomy, neuroanatomy), and the uncooperative patient.

Some of the most recent advances in anesthetic techniques that provide alternatives to conventional methods include lingual infiltration, periodontal ligament injections, intraosseous anesthesia, computer-controlled injections, needleless injections, and electronic dental anesthesia.

Lingual infiltration

A relatively new concept, lingual infiltration of the mandible, theoretically and practically has merit but may also pose some disadvantages (Table 2). As with any technique, patient (anatomical) selection is important. It should be reinforced that, although mandibular infiltration is

Table 2
Advantages and disadvantages of local anesthetic techniques

Technique	Advantages	Disadvantages
Lingual infiltration injection	Thin cortical plate Lingual foramina Patient acceptance	Ballooning of tissue Avoiding submandibular salivary gland

Periodontal ligament injection	Immediate onset of anesthesia
	No collateral anesthesia
	Operate bilaterally in
	  the mandible
	Less volume
	Abscessed tooth
		Post-operative pain
		Decrease in pulpal blood flow
		Decrease in pulpal blood flow
		Presence of periodontal
		  disease
		Pressure required to inject
		Multiple injections for
		  multi-rooted teeth
		Access to posterior areas

Intraosseous injections	Immediate onset of anesthesia
	No collateral anesthesia
	Operate bilaterally in
	  the mandible
		Short duration of anesthesia
		"Intravascular" injection/
		  toxicity
		Palpitations
		Access to posterior areas
		Periodontal disease
		3 steps (Stabident®)
		Anatomical limitations

Computer controlled injection devices	Controlled pressure/volume
	  ratio
	Operator confidence
	Practice builder
	PDL injections
		Set-up time
		Cost (disposable items)
		Loss of volume (Wand®)
		Needle remains in tissue for
		  longer time
		Aspiration

PDL, periodontal ligament injection.

generally regarded as not reliably successful, certain conditions may establish profound anesthesia via the combination of facial (buccal) and lingual injection. A demonstration of this technique may be researched on the web at www.septocaine.com.

Periodontal ligament injections

The introduction of the intraligamentary injection techniques, an actual intraosseous delivery of local anesthesia, provides a supplement to routine submucosal anesthesia. For the route of administration commonly known as the periodontal ligament injection (PDL), it must be understood that the PDL space is simply the anatomical medium to deliver an intraosseous injection. Popularized by the Ligmaject® in the 1970s, the advantages and disadvantages are summarized below (see Table 2).

With a special syringe, the solution is introduced into the periodontal tissue. Success rates with the intraligamentary technique are variable, depending on practitioner experience, volume of solution injected, and the tooth being anesthetized [26]. Malamed has reported a success rate of 63% following first injection and an overall success rate of 92% with this technique [27].

Although intraligamentary injections appear to have a slightly lower success rate, their use for diagnostics in referred pain states, with uncontrolled hemophiliacs and as an adjunct following failed mandibular blocks, appears quite valuable.

Initially, injection into the PDL tissue occurs by advancement of a 30- or 27-gauge short needle to the point of obtaining significant back pressure on injection, a criterion required for the local anesthesia successfully to penetrate the cribiform plate and circumferentially anesthetize even in an abscessed or "hot" tooth. The volume of solution required is approximately 0.4–0.9 mL per administration, and recommendations for mandibular molars include a 2-site approach (mesial lingual and distal lingual). The duration will vary from 5 to 25 minutes, depending on volume, clearance, protein binding, and vasoconstrictor concentration. Reports of temporary cessation of pulpal blood flow suggest a potential introgenic result from this approach for vital or pediatric scenarios. But for endodontic treatment this is obviously not an issue.

Intraosseous anesthesia

Intraosseous anesthesia is often characterized as anesthetizing "a single tooth" by injecting local anesthesia directly into cancellous bone. This technique also offers both advantages and disadvantages (see Table 2). There are two standardized systems that perform the essentials of perforating (in this order) the epithelium (keratinized gingiva), connective tissue, periosteum, and cortical (compact) plate of bone.

Stabident® (Fairfax Dental, Miami, FL)

The principles of intraosseous anesthesia have been in the literature since the turn of the century. The procedure involved using a #1/2–#1 round bur to penetrate cortical bone, followed by the introduction of a slightly smaller circumference needle. Dr. Frank Dillon introduced the technologic concept of a perforator needle compatible with the injection of local anesthesia directly into the cancellous bone, thereby anesthetizing individual (and often multiple) teeth and adjacent hard tissue and soft tissue.

Understandably, with groundbreaking technology, this system has had some scrutiny. "Finding-the hole" seems to be the chief complaint among practitioners of this technique, although certain adjustments to visual acuity may reduce the hole-finding variable. Onset is almost instantaneous and duration may be from 15–30 minutes, depending on the site and choice of local anesthesic formulation.

X t.i.p.® (x t.i.p. Technologies, Lakewood, NJ)

Interest in intraosseous anesthesia escalated in 1999 with the introduction of the "cannula-insert" system marketed as the X t.i.p. (Dr. Arthur "Kit" Weathers, Griffin, GA). Initial anesthesia of the attached gingiva, via the mucobuccal fold or infiltration of the gingiva directly, must preclude the contra-angle guide sleeve. Leaving the guide sleeve in place, the ultra-short 27-gauge needle (0.5 inches) is introduced into the lumen and local anesthesia in the volume of 0.7–1.7 mL is slowly injected. Whether there is a need to use an anesthetic formulation containing epinephrine is controversial. Except for a potential rapid systemic uptake, the vasoconstrictor seems to be only minimally responsible for duration and efficacy. Post-op sequelae seem to be infrequent and are rarely reported (see Table 2).

Computer controlled injections

There are currently a number of computer-controlled injection devices available. Computer systems offer a variety of advantages and disadvantage (see Table 2). Compared to a standard syringe, computer-controlled injection devices are larger, require more operatory space, and are more expensive. Because the needle and handle generally appear less threatening and are more aesthetic, patient acceptance is generally high. The ability of the computer to control and limit the rate of the injection and subsequently limit patient discomfort has created considerable popularity for these devices.

The Wand® (Milestone Scientific, Inc, Livingston, NJ)

When first introduced, the Wand® was the first computer-controlled dental anesthetic delivery system. Product promotion and training has inundated the profession with suggestions that slow, controlled injections could be an "efficient practice builder and time saver." The lightweight and easily manipulative hand piece is a significant asset. A bidirectional rotation technique has been shown to eliminate needle deflection and is suggested to reduce discomfort of mucogingival penetration. True to the resolve of Milestone Scientific, Inc, the Wand Plus® introduced improvements requested by dental practitioners. These included verbal prompts, aspiration time reduction from 14 to 5 seconds, and streamlining and simplifying the technology.

The technique-enhancing suggestions include the Anterior Middle Superior Alveolar Block (AMSA), Palatal Anterior Superior Alveolar Nerve Block (PASA), and the modified PDL-Local Anesthesia Delivery, all of which the author (JMH) has received and has found personally impressive with respect to comfort of the injection delivery.

Comfort Control Syringe® (Midwest Dentsply, Des Plaines, IL)

This preprogrammed local anesthesia delivery system offers a selectable choice of rate of administration by technique. A unique concept developed by Dr. Mark Smith of Ontario, Canada, uses a hand-activated drive unit (as opposed to a foot-activated rheostat) for preprogrammed delivery of slow injection, increased speed of injection, and aspiration modes. Once the injection format and flow rate is selected, 10 seconds allows the initial slow-solution deposition. Then subsequently, the flow rate will increase to the preselected speed.

Needleless local anesthesia: Madajet®/Syrijet®
(Mada Equipment Company, Inc, Carlstadt, NJ)

Over 30 years ago, Mada Equipment Company, Inc, developed a revolutionary "no needle" technology that successfully captured a portion of the dental local anesthesia market. Based on a piston/pressure expulsion principle, the system offered demonstrable patient acceptance of "no invasiveness" and very effective soft tissue and possibly hard tissue anesthesia. But because of factors such as the armamentarium not accepting a standard dental local anesthesia cartridge, the "one setting" force of injection, and the necessity of priming the system to eliminate air, it appears that the professional market for this device is hesitant yet still active. The Madajet® and Syrijet® nonetheless have made a successful presence in the dental anesthesia field.

Electronic dental anesthesia (EDA)

One of the latest developments in local pain-control techniques in dentistry is electronic dental anesthesia (EDA). Manufacturers have been involved with many electrical wave forms and voltage/amperage parameters. According to the literature, there is some merit to the strategy, though the success rates, particularly for the more painful procedures seen in dental practice, seem not to be satisfactory for routine use in dentistry.

The documentation of EDA is well known, although the therapeutic results are reportedly varied. Based on the transcutaneous electronic nerve stimulation (TENS) principle, its use in medicine is widely documented (back pain, sports injuries). The successful transfer to the acute pain seen in dental practice has been questioned. Allowing patient control of the level of EDA needed for minor periodontal scaling, noninvasive restorative dentistry and other procedures depends on the so-called "Gate-Control Theory." In essence, a path of nerve impulses to the brain delivered by an electrical stimulation can gridlock a highway potentially capable of trafficking pain impulses from dental sources. It is also surmised that pain threshold may be elevated by naturally occurring biochemicals such as endorphins, enkephalins, serotonin, or even a placebo effect.

Research is ongoing in the quest for efficient delivery and effective results in many local anesthesia categories. The safety and patient acceptance have enhanced the development of this science, and the future will surely demonstrate the answers to questions such as "Will a perfect local anesthsia/vasoconstrictor/system ever be found?" and "Will traditional block anesthesia ever become obsolete?"

References

[1] Yagiela J, Malamed SF. Injectable and topical local anesthetics. In: Ciancio SG, editor. ADA guide to dental therapeutics. Chicago: ADA Publishing Co; 1998.

[2] Covino BG, Vassallo HG. Local anesthetics: mechanisms of action and clinical use. New York: Grune & Stratton; 1976.

[3] Moore PA. Manual of local anesthesia in dentristry. 4th edition. Rochester (NY): Eastman-Kodak Co; 1996.

[4] Moore PA. Bupivaciane: a long-lasting local anesthetic for dentistry. Oral Surg 1984; 58:369–74.

[5] Malignant Hyperthermia Association of the United States (MHAUS). Malignant hyperthermia—a concern in dentistry and oral & maxillofacial surgeryAvailable at: http://www.mhaus.org/dentoral.htmL. Accessed December 28, 2001.

[6] Hersh EV, Hermann DG, Lamp CL, Johnson PD, MacAfee K. Temporal assessment of soft tissue anesthesia following mandibular block injection. JADA 1995;126:1531–5.

[7] Wahl MJ, Overton D, Howell J, Siegel E, Schmitt MM, Muldoon M. Pain on injection of prilocaine plain vs. lidocaine With epinephrine: a prospective double-blind study. J Am Dent Assoc 2001;132:1396–1401.

[8] Oertel R, Rahn R, Kirch W. Clinical pharmacokinetics of articaine. Clin Pharmacokinet 1997;33(6):417–25.

[9] Malamed SF, Gagnon S, Leblanc D. Efficacy of articaine: a new amide local anesthetic. J Am Dent Assoc 2000;131(5):635–42.

[10] Haas DA, Lennon D. A 21 year retrospective study of reports of paresthesia following local anesthetic administration. J Can Dent Assoc 1995;61(4):319–30.

[11] Donaldson D, James-Perdok L, Craig BJ, Derkson GD, Richardson AS. A comparison of Ultracaine DS (articaine HCl) and Citanest forte (prilocaine HCl) in maxillary infiltration and mandibular nerve block. J Can Dent Assoc 1987;53(1):38–42.

[12] Haas DA, Harper DG, Saso MA, Young ER. Comparison of articaine and prilocaine anesthesia by infiltration in maxillary and mandibular arches. Anesth Prog 1990;37(5):230–7.

[13] Haas DA, Harper DG, Saso MA, Young ER. Lack of differential effect by Ultracaine (articaine) and Citanest (prilocaine) in infiltration anaesthesia. J Can Dent Assoc 1991: 57(3):217–23.

[14] Aberg G, Dhuner KG, Sydnes G. Studies on the duration of local anesthesia: structure/activity relationships in a series of homologous local anesthetics. Acta Pharacol Toxicol 1977;41:432–43.

[15] Tucker T, Mather LE. Clinical pharmacokinetics of local anesthetics. Clin Pharmacokinet 1979;4:241–78.

[16] Laskin JL, Wallace WR, DeLeo B. Use of bupivacaine hydrochloride in oral surgery—a clinical study. J Oral Surg 1977;35:25–9.

[17] Dunsky JL, Moore PA. Long-acting local anesthetics: a comparison of bupivacaine and etidocaine in endodontics. J Endodont 1984;10:457–60.

[18] Giovannitti JA, Bennett CR. The effectiveness of 1.5% etidocaine HCL with epinephrine 1:2000,000 and 2% lidocaine HCL with epinephrine 1:100,000 in oral surgery: a clinical comparison. J Am Dent Assoc 1983;107:616–8.

[19] Moore PA, Dunsky JL. Bupivacaine anesthesia: a clinical trial for endodontic therapy. Oral Surg 1983;55:176–9.

[20] Feldman G, Nordenram A. Marcaine in oral surgery. Acta Anaethesiol Scand 1966;23: 409–13.

[21] Nespaca JA. Clinical trials with bupivacaine in oral surgery. Oral Surg 1976;42:301–7.

[22] Davis WM, Oakley J, Smith E. Comparison of the effectiveness of etidocaine and lidocaine as local anesthetic agents during oral surgery. Anesth Prog 1984;31:159–64.

[23] Dionne RA, Wirdzek PR, Fox PC, Dulber R. Suppression of postoperative pain by the combination of a nonsteroidal anti-inflammatory drug, flurbiprofen and a long-acting local anesthetic, etidocaine. J Am Dent Assoc 1984;108:598–601.

[24] Trieger N, Gillen GH. Bupivacaine anesthesia and postoperative analgesia in oral surgery. Anesth Prog 1979;20:23–7.

[25] Burney RG, Moore PA, Duncan GH. Management of head and neck pain. Int Anes Clin 1983;21(40):79–96.

[26] Kaufmen E, Dworkin SF, LeResche L, Truelove EL, Sommers E. Intraligamentary anesthesia: a double-blind comparative study. J Am Dent Assoc 1984;108:175–8.

[27] Malamed SF. The periodontal ligament (PDL) injection: an alternative to inferior alveolar nerve block. Oral Surg 1982;53(2):117–21.

THE DENTAL
CLINICS OF
NORTH
AMERICA

Dent Clin N Am 46 (2002) 733–746

Vasoconstrictors: indications and precautions

Lenny W. Naftalin, DDS, John A. Yagiela, DDS, PhD*

*Section of Anesthesiology, Division of Diagnostic and Surgical Sciences,
University of California Los Angeles School of Dentistry,
10833 Le Conte Avenue, Box 951668, Los Angeles, CA 90095, USA*

Since 1901, when Braun first combined cocaine and epinephrine, vaso-constrictors have been added to local anesthetic solutions to increase the quality and duration of anesthesia, to aid in hemostasis, and, presumptively, to reduce toxicity of the local anesthetic. With the exception of cocaine, all local anesthetics are potential vasodilators, and vasoconstrictors are combined with them to counteract this effect. Epinephrine (Adrenaline®) and levonordefrin (Neo-Cobefrin®) are the most widely used vasoconstrictors in the United States. Felypressin, a noncatecholamine vasoconstrictor, is also available in Canada and many other countries [1–3].

Mechanism of action

Epinephrine and levonordefrin stimulate adrenergic receptors (also referred to as adrenoceptors) that are responsible for their vasoconstrictive and other properties. There are two basic categories of adrenergic receptors: α, which usually have excitatory actions, and β, which stimulate the heart but otherwise are mostly inhibitory. The α and β adrenoceptors have been further divided into α_1 (α_{1A}, α_{1B}, α_{1D}) and α_2 (α_{2A}, α_{2B}, α_{2C}), and β_1, β_2, and β_3 subtypes, respectively. Some important actions subserved by these adrenoceptors are listed below (Table 1) [2].

Vasoconstrictors differ in their affinity for adrenergic receptors (Table 2) [2]. One might assume that a vasoconstrictor added to a local anesthetic would ideally have only α-agonistic activity, because it is this activity that

* Corresponding author.
E-mail address: johny@dent.ucla.edu (J.A. Yagiela).

Table 1
Adrenergic receptor activities

Effector organ or function	Receptor[a]	Response
Cardiovascular system		
Heart rate	β_1, β_2	Increased[b]
Contractile force	β_1, β_2	Increased
Coronary arterioles	α_1, α_2/β_2	Constriction/dilation[c]
Automaticity	β_1, β_2	Increased
Conduction velocity	β_1, β_2	Increased[b]
Peripheral resistance	α_1, α_2/β_2	Increased/decreased
Capacitance veins	α_1/β_2	Constriction/dilation
Respiratory system		
Bronchial smooth muscle	β_2	Relaxation
Bronchial glands	α_1/β_2	Decreased secretion/increased secretion
Pulmonary arterioles	α_1/β_2	Constriction/dilation[c]
Gastrointestinal tract		
Motility and tone	α_1, α_2, β_1, β_2	Decreased
Sphincters	α_1	Contraction
Visceral arterioles	α_1/β_2	Constriction/dilation
Liver		
Glucose metabolism	α, β_2	Glycogenolysis, gluconeogenesis
Arterioles	α_1/β_2	Constriction/dilation
Fat		
Lipolysis	α, β_1, β_3	Lipolysis
Arterioles	α_1/β_2	Constriction/dilation
Pancreas		
Insulin secretion	α_2/β_2	Decreased/increased
Genitourinary system		
Urinary bladder sphincter	α_1	Contraction
Detrusor muscle	β_2	Relaxation
Trigone muscle	α_1	Contraction
Uterine tone	α_1/β_2	Contraction/relaxation[d]
Renal arterioles	α_1, α_2, β_1, β_2	Constriction/dilation
Skeletal muscle		
Neuromuscular transmission	α, β_2	Increased
Arterioles	α/β_2	Constriction/dilation
Salivary glands		
Secretion	β	Mucous secretion
Arterioles	α_1, α_2	Constriction
Skin and mucosa		
Arterioles	α_1, α_2	Constriction

[a] Primary receptors mediating pharmacologic response. Receptors separated by commas yield complementary actions; receptors separated by a slash have differing or opposing actions.

[b] Direct effects on the heart may be blocked or reversed by compensatory vagal reflex activity.

[c] Local regulatory processes largely govern blood flow.

[d] Effect depends on stage of menstrual cycle, sexual hormone concentrations, and other factors.

Table 2
Relative receptor potencies of adrenergic vasoconstrictors

	α_1	α_2	β_1	β_2
Epinephrine	+++	+++	+++	+++
Levonordefrin	+	++	++	+

Symbols indicate the relative potency: +++ = high, ++ = intermediate, + = low.

causes vasoconstriction. But epinephrine, the most commonly used vaso-constrictor, is also the least selective, exerting both strong α and β actions. Epinephrine is a highly effective vasoconstrictor for intraoral use in con-centrations of 1:200,000–1:50,000 (5–20 µg/mL) because of the predom-inance of α adrenoceptors in the oral mucosa, submucosa, and peridontium.

Levonordefrin is relatively specific for the α_2 receptor. It has about one sixth the vasoconstrictor potency of epinephrine and is therefore marketed in a 1:20,000 concentration (50 µg/mL) [1]. Felypressin, a nonsympathomi-metic vasoconstrictor, is a synthetic analogue of vasopressin, otherwise known as antidiuretic hormone. Felypressin stimulates V_{1a} receptors on vascular smooth muscle. Because it does not significantly influence the heart directly and invokes other effects that limit increases in peripheral resistance (eg, by inhibiting sympathetic neurotransmitter release), felypressin in standard doses has little effect on blood pressure, heart rate, or cardiac rhythm. It may, however, cause clinically significant coronary vasoconstric-tion in patients with heart disease. Felypressin is relatively ineffective as a hemostatic agent [2,3].

Indications

Several benefits accrue from adding vasoconstrictors to local anesthetic solutions. Most important for dentistry is the enhancement of local anesthe-sia in quality and duration. Vasoconstrictors have also been used to assist in hemostasis. Finally, it has been suggested that inclusion of a vasoconstrictor increases local anesthetic safety.

Enhancement of local anesthesia

Most local anesthetics cause vasodilation clinically, and the addition of a vasoconstrictor opposes this effect [4]. The vasodilating properties of local anesthetics increase local blood flow and their own absorption into the sys-temic circulation. These effects are especially true in dentistry, where local anesthetics are injected into highly vascular tissues. Lidocaine produces unre-liable pulpal anesthesia without a vasoconstrictor. With the addition of epi-nephrine, however, at a concentration of 1:100,000, 2% lidocaine blocks pulpal nerve fibers for 60–90 minutes, depending on the site of injection [2,3,5]. Procaine is similarly ineffective for pulpal anesthesia without a vaso-constrictor.

Several local anesthetics, most notably mepivacaine and prilocaine, are available without a vasoconstrictor. These two local anesthetics cause less vasodilation than lidocaine or procaine and can be used without a vasoconstrictor for short procedures. A maxillary tooth can be reliably blocked for about 20 minutes after supraperiosteal injection. But with the addition of a vasoconstrictor, the duration of pulpal anesthesia rises to 40 minutes with prilocaine and 50 minutes with mepivacaine. The effect durations of clinically available local anesthetics with and without vasoconstrictors after inferior alveolar nerve block are listed below (Table 3).

Bupivacaine, a long-acting local anesthetic, is also a powerful vasodilator. Because it is highly lipid-soluble (or hydrophobic) and tends to be sequestered in nerve membranes for a prolonged period, it is capable of providing protracted pulpal anesthesia without a vasoconstrictor. Even so, the addition of a vasoconstrictor increases its duration of anesthesia [6].

Hemostasis

Intraoperative hemostasis is important for optimal results when performing surgical procedures in the oral cavity. Infiltration of a local anesthetic containing epinephrine can help reduce blood loss during surgery and improve visualization of the operative field [7,8]. For local hemostasis, an epinephrine concentration of 1:50,000 with 2% lidocaine is more effective than a 1:100,000 strength [9]. Unfortunately, lidocaine partially counteracts the vasoconstrictive effect of epinephrine and enhances its systemic absorption [10]. A more rational, if less convenient, approach to control bleeding may be to inject less concentrated solutions of epinephrine without local anesthetic. Practitioners should also be aware that rebound hyperemia can occur (primarily from tissue ischemia and the accumulation of vasodilatory metabolites) once the vasoconstriction has dissipated, which can accentuate postoperative blood loss [3].

Epinephrine-impregnated gingival retraction cord is still used by some practitioners as a hemostatic agent. Such retraction cord may contain racemic epinephrine in amounts up to 1 mg/inch. When the retraction cord is placed in the gingival sulcus, especially in abraded, inflamed tissue, the potential exists for systemic uptake of large quantities of epinephrine [11,12].

Table 3
Effect of catecholamine vasoconstrictors on the duration of pulpal anesthesia after inferior alveolar nerve blockade

Local anesthetic	Duration (min)
2% Lidocaine	40 (unreliable)
2% Lidocaine with 1:100,000 epinephrine	85
3% Mepivicaine	40
2% Mepivicaine with 1:20,000 levonordefrin	75
4% Prilocaine	55
4% Prilocaine with 1:200,000 epinephrine	60

Increased safety

It has been suggested that the addition of a vasoconstrictor can protect against systemic local anesthetic toxicity [13]. By decreasing blood flow in the injected tissues, a vasoconstrictor slows the rate at which the local anesthetic enters the circulation. It is presumed that metabolic inactivation of the local anesthetic is more able to keep pace with absorption, and that the resulting smaller peak plasma concentrations of drug elicit fewer adverse effects. These presumptions are reflected in the fact that the maximum manufacturer's recommended dose of lidocaine is 4.5 mg/kg up to a maximum of 300 mg without a vasoconstrictor but 7 mg/kg up to a maximum of 500 mg with epinephrine [2].

Peak plasma concentrations of lidocaine are reduced by about 30–40% when it is coadministered intraorally with epinephrine [14–16]. Levonordefrin, however, has little significant effect on mepivacaine concentrations [15,16]. In neither case is there evidence of a reduction in local anesthetic toxicity with vasoconstrictor use [17–19]. Animal studies suggest that vasoconstrictors increase the relative distribution of large doses of local anesthetics into the brain even as they retard drug absorption from the injection site [20]. Thus, there is little direct proof that the addition of a vasoconstrictor makes a local anesthetic safer by retarding systemic absorption.

Even though the addition of a vasoconstrictor may not moderate maximum plasma concentrations of a local anesthetic, it may be useful in reducing the amount of local anesthetic needed for adequate pain relief. In the case of mepivacaine, a 2% solution is highly effective when combined with levonordefrin, but a 3% solution—representing 50% more drug—is needed in the absence of a vasoconstrictor. Furthermore, because a local anesthetic solution with vasoconstrictor often provides a longer duration of effect, there is a diminished need for reinjection and less likelihood for drug accumulation.

Precautions

As with any medication being considered for use, the potential risks of vasoconstrictors must be weighed against their expected benefits. For adrenergic vasoconstrictors, the greatest potential for adverse effects resides in patients with cardiovascular disease and who are taking certain interacting drugs. Concerns are also sometimes expressed about vasoconstrictor usage during pregnancy and in patients with sulfite intolerance.

Cardiovascular disease

There has been enduring debate about the potential risks of epinephrine and related vasoconstrictors to patients with cardiovascular disease. Arguments have been expressed that the amounts of catecholamines released endogenously in response to inadequate pain relief and/or the stress of dental treatment are much greater than those commonly injected for dental procedures [13,21]. It has also been suggested that a local anesthetic with vasoconstrictor is desirable in patients with cardiovascular disease because of the greater pain relief afforded by the combination [22].

Historical progression of this issue is reflected in several official pronouncements. In 1955, a special committee of the New York Heart Association (AHA) recommended 0.2 mg as the maximum dose of epinephrine that should be used in local anesthesia for patients with heart disease [23]. In 1964, the American Dental Association and the AHA jointly stated that vasoconstrictors were not contraindicated for patients with cardiovascular disease when administered carefully, slowly, and with preliminary aspiration to avoid intravascular injection [24]. The maximum strength of epinephrine that should be used was 1:50,000. Lastly, in 1986, the AHA emphasized safety by concluding, "Vasoconstrictor agents should be used in local anesthesia solutions during dental practice only when it is clear that the procedure will be shortened or the analgesia rendered more profound. When a vasoconstrictor is indicated, extreme care should be taken to avoid intravascular injection. The minimum possible amount of vasoconstrictor should be used" [25].

Epinephrine is normally released from the adrenal medulla at a basal rate of 2.5–7.5 ng/kg per minute [21] This endogenous amount may rise twenty- to fortyfold in times of stress [21]. The plasma concentrations of epinephrine associated with several injected doses and various physical activities are depicted here (Fig. 1) [2]. The data represented suggest that a single cartridge of 2% lidocaine with 1:100,000 epinephrine significantly increases plasma epinephrine over resting values, and that two cartridges yield a concentration equivalent to that of mild physical exertion. It is logical to conclude that ambulatory patients, including those with cardiovascular disease, should be able to tolerate these doses of vasoconstrictor because they are already doing so during the course of daily life.

Unfortunately, certain individuals have special risk for cardiovascular problems during dental treatment. These patients include those with unstable angina pectoris (chest pain without exertion), a recent heart attack or stroke (within 6 months), severe untreated or uncontrolled hypertension, and uncontrolled or untreated congestive heart failure. The American Society of Anesthesiologists' (ASA) physical status score classifies patients from ASA I (healthy patients with no systemic disease) to V (moribund patients with little chance of survival over the next 24 hours). The patients listed above would mostly be ranked as ASA IV, having severe systemic disease that is constantly life-threatening. Patients in this category should not receive invasive dental treatment until they have been stabilized medically [12]. Even then, vasoconstrictors should be avoided if at all possible because of the threat posed by accidental intravascular injection or rapid systemic absorption of the drug.

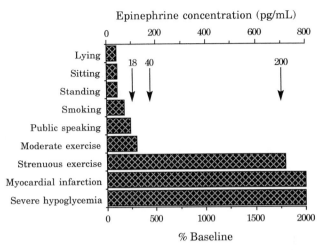

Fig. 1. Influence of various activities and conditions on venous plasma epinephrine concentrations. (*From* Jastak JT, Yagiela JA, Donaldson D. Local anesthesia of the oral cavity. Philadelphia: WB Saunders; 1995; with permission.)

Heart transplants have created a special group of patients who are supersensitive to injected catecholamines. When a heart is transplanted, it is of necessity surgically denervated. The loss of sympathetic nerves to the heart eliminates the adrenergic nerve terminals that both release norepinephrine and take it back up for later reuse (by a transport system known as uptake$_1$) [4]. This reuptake process is also the principal means by which the actions of epinephrine and levonordefrin molecules reaching the cardiac adrenoceptors are terminated [26]. The resulting increased exposure to these drugs magnifies cardiac stimulation in these patients [27]. Though there are no published recommendations regarding vasoconstrictors in these patients, the dentist should be cautious in their use, administering local anesthetic solutions in small divided doses and monitoring the heart for any changes in rate or rhythm.

Pregnancy

Prudence dictates that elective dental procedures be deferred when a patient is pregnant. When delay is not possible, necessary treatment—including the administration of local anesthesia for pain relief—must be provided in an optimally safe manner for both mother and fetus. Occasionally, the use of vasoconstrictors in this regard has been questioned. Potential concerns regarding epinephrine involve the drug's effects on uterine muscle tone and blood flow.

Experimentally, stimulation of α_1-adrenergic receptors causes contraction of uterine muscle strips. But the principal effect of clinically used doses of epinephrine during pregnancy is uterine relaxation during the third trimester, a β_2-adrenoceptor effect. Because it only weakly stimulates α_1 and β_2 adrenoceptors, levonordefrin probably has little effect on uterine tone.

As with many vascular beds, epinephrine can cause vasoconstriction and decrease uterine blood flow. This effect has been examined in pregnant women receiving epidural local anesthesia for labor. Most studies have shown that uterine and umbilical blood flow are not compromised by epinephrine [28–31]. A possible exception includes women whose pregnancies are complicated by hypertension [32]. In this case, epinephrine may increase vascular resistance in the uteroplacental circulation, indicating impaired blood flow. Even so, there is no evidence of increased deleterious effects. Because the use of a vasoconstrictor can reduce the amount of local anesthetic administered and concomitantly reduce fetal drug exposure [31], it has been argued that vasoconstrictors are appropriate when local anesthesia is administered to a pregnant woman [33].

Drug interactions

With the growing variety and number of drugs patients are taking, and the rising use of multiple medications, drug interactions are of increasing concern. The most important and best characterized interactions with vasoconstrictors include the tricyclic antidepressants, nonselective β-adrenergic blocking agents, certain general anesthetics, and cocaine. These and other drug interactions that have been discussed in the dental/medical literature are listed below (Table 4).

Tricyclic antidepressants (TCAs) such as imipramine (Tofranil®), amitriptyline (Elavil®), and doxepin (Sinequan®) are now second-line agents for the treatment of depression as well as for orofacial and other chronic pain disorders. These drugs act on the central and peripheral nervous systems by blocking the reuptake of certain neurotransmitters, most notably norepinephrine and 5-hydroxytryptamine. The affected neurotransmitters are thus free to interact more effectively with their receptors, augmenting their physiologic effects. Epinephrine and levonordefrin are subject to the same uptake process and, therefore, the same potentiation. Significant increases in blood pressure and disturbances of the normal cardiac rhythm may occur [34–36].

The potentiation of epinephrine with TCAs is about threefold, at least early in TCA therapy. The potentiation is six- to eightfold with levonordefrin. It is recommended that levonordefrin not be used with patients on TCAs because of the acute hypertension and cardiac dysrhythmias that might occur after an accidental intravascular injection [36]. Epinephrine-impregnated gingival retraction cord is also contraindicated because of the large amounts of epinephrine available for absorption. If a local anesthetic with epinephrine is to be used, it should have no more than 1:100,000 epinephrine, and the maximum recommended dose should be reduced by one-third [34,36].

β-Adrenergic antagonists (also referred to as β-adrenoceptor blockers or β blockers) are prescribed for numerous conditions: essential hypertension, angina pectoris, myocardial infarction, hyperthyroidism, cardiac dysrhythmias, and disorders with excessive sympathetic nervous system activity. Some β blockers affect β_1 and β_2 receptors similarly; others are selective for β_1 receptors. Both types attenuate epinephrine's stimulation of the heart but only the nonselective forms prevent the ability of epinephrine to stimulate β_2 receptors and dilate skeletal muscle blood vessels. When epinephrine is administered to a patient with nonselective β blockade, unopposed α-adrenergic stimulation may lead to a serious rise in blood pressure and reflex bradycardia [34,36]. Therefore, patients taking nonselective β blockers should receive a minimal initial dose such as one half of a cartridge of local anesthetic with 1:100,000 epinephrine and then be monitored for systemic effects at 5 minutes before additional drug is administered [36] Special care should also be taken to avoid intravascular injection. This interaction is not evident in patients receiving selective β_1 blockers.

Certain general anesthetics are known to potentiate dysrhythmias associated with the administration of vasoconstrictors. The inhalation agent halothane (Fluothane®) has the greatest potential of all currently available inhalation anesthetics to elicit this reaction, and epinephrine should not be administered in single doses over 2 μg/kg when used with halothane [36]. (For a 70-kg [154-lb] man, 2 μg/kg would equal 14 mL of a 1:100,000 epinephrine solution.) The intravenous anesthetic thiopental (Pentothal®) is likewise capable of enhancing the dysrhythmic activity of adrenergic drugs. Thiopental may be used as an induction agent, and when given concomitantly with halothane the recommended maximum dose of epinephrine is reduced to 1 μg/kg [36]. Gingival retraction cord containing epinephrine is best avoided in all patients receiving general anesthesia.

Cocaine and epinephrine possess a potentially lethal interaction. Cocaine is occasionally applied as a topical anesthetic for mucosal membranes; however, its most prominent use is illicit consumption. Cocaine is a stimulant that blocks the reuptake of norepinephrine, dopamine, and 5-hydroxytryptamine at presynaptic nerve terminals. This action also includes epinephrine and levonordefrin used in local anesthesia. Serious adrenergic stimulation leading to hypertension, myocardial infarction, and even sudden death may ensue in patients actively abusing cocaine [37]. Therefore, patients who are under the influence of cocaine should have elective dental treatment postponed for at least 24 hours after the last drug exposure.

A number of the interactions listed below (see Table 4) are poorly documented clinically or occur in situations not likely to be encountered in dental practice. The monoamine oxidase inhibitors (MAOIs) illustrate a widely mentioned interaction that actually has little clinical relevance for adrenergic vasoconstrictors used in dentistry. The MAOIs include the antidepressants phenelzine (Nardil®) and tranylcypromine (Parnate®), the antiparkinson drug selegiline (Eldepryl®) and the antimicrobial agents

Table 4
Drug interactions involving catecholamine vasoconstrictors

Drug class	Examples	Mechanism	Effect	Recommendation
Tricyclic antidepressants and related drugs	Amitriptyline (Elavil®), doxepin (Sinequan®), imipramine (Tofranil®), maprotiline (Ludiomil®)	TCAs block the uptake of catecholamines by sympathetic nerve terminals, increasing their actions	Potentiation of cardiovascular effects	Use epinephrine cautiously, avoid levonordefrin and gingival retraction cord with epinephrine
Nonselective β-adrenergic blockers	Nadolol (Corgard®), propranolol (Inderal®)	Unopposed α-adrenergic stimulation of catecholamines	Hypertension and reflex bradycardia	Use epinephrine and levonordefrin cautiously; avoid gingival retraction cord with epinephrine
Volatile general anesthetics	Desflurane (Suprane®), enflurane (Ethrane®), halothane (Fluothane®)	Potentiation of the dysrhythmic potential of catecholamines	Ventricular dysrhythmias	Use epinephrine and levonordefrin cautiously after informing anesthesiologist; avoid gingival retraction cord with epinephrine
Intravenous general anesthetics	Thiopental (Pentothal®)	Potentiation of the dysrhythmic potential of catecholamines	Ventricular dysrhythmias	Use epinephrine and levonordefrin cautiously after informing anesthesiologist; avoid gingival retraction cord with epinephrine
Recreational drugs	Cocaine	Cocaine potentiates sympathetic nervous system activity and blocks the uptake of catecholamines by sympathetic nerve terminals, increasing their actions	Hypertension, myocardial infarction, ventricular dysrhythmias	Have patient abstain from cocaine for 48 hours before treatment; avoid catecholamines if emergency dental treatment necessary
COMT inhibitors	Entacapone (Comtan®), tolcapone (Tasmar®),	Metabolism of catecholamines by COMT is inhibited, increasing their actions	Potential of cardiovascular effects	Use epinephrine and levonordefrin cautiously; avoid gingival retraction cord with epinephrine
Antiadrenergic agents	Guanadrel (Hylorel®), guanethidine (Ismeline®), methyldopa (Aldomet®)	Uptake of catecholamines is inhibited and/or target tissue responsiveness is increased	Possible potentiation of cardiovascular effects	Use epinephrine and levonordefrin cautiously; avoid gingival retraction cord with epinephrine

Nonselective α-adrenergic blockers	Chlorpromazine (Thorazine®), clozapine (Clozaril®), haloperidol (Haldol®), olanzapine (Zyprexa®)	Unopposed β2-adrenergic stimulation of catecholamines	No interaction with normal doses of interacting drugs; hypotension with large doses	No special precautions in ambulatory patients; avoid epinephrine when treating hypotensive emergencies
Digitalis glycosides	Digoxin (Lanoxin®)	Additive dysrhythmogenic effects	Potentially dangerous dysrhythmias with large doses of vasoconstrictor	Use epinephrine and levonordefrin cautiously; avoid gingival retraction cord with epinephrine
Thyroid hormones	Desiccated thyroid (Armour Thyroid®), levothyroxine (Synthroid®), liothyronine (Cytomel®)	Additive dysrhythmogenic effects	Potentially dangerous dysrhythmias with large doses	No special precautions in euthyroid patients; use epinephrine and levonordefrin cautiously and avoid gingival retraction cord with epinephrine in hyperthyroid patients
MAO inhibitors	Furazolidone (Furoxone®), linezolid (Zyvox®), phenelzine (Nardil®), selegiline (Eldepryl®), tranylcypromine (Parnate®)	Exogenously administered catecholamines are not inactivated by monoamine oxidase	No interaction	None

COMT, catecholamine-O-methyltransferase; MAO, monoamine oxidase; TCAs, tricyclic antidepressants.

furazolidone (Furoxone®) and linezolid (Zyvox®). The package insert for local anesthetics with vasoconstrictors lists MAOIs as interacting drugs. It was once thought that this interaction might be significant because MAOIs block the metabolism of some adrenergic drugs as well as the intraneuronal breakdown of norepinephrine, increasing the pool of neurotransmitter that can be released by indirect-acting adrenergic drugs. A MAOI drug interaction is significant with such drugs as dextroamphetamine, used to treat narcolepsy, and pseudoephedrine found in nasal decongestants. A MAOI interaction is not clinically significant, however, with epinephrine or levonordefrin as used in dentistry [34–36]. These direct-acting, exogenously administered catecholamines are primarily inactivated by the enzyme catechol-O-methytransferase (COMT).

Two drugs, tolcapone (Tasmar®) and entacapone (Comtan®), have been recently introduced that inhibit COMT. These medications are used in the management of Parkinson's disease by helping to prevent the breakdown of levodopa, the principal therapeutic agent used for this disorder. Because COMT is directly involved in the metabolism of epinephrine and levonordefrin, care should be taken when using local anesthetics with vasoconstrictors in patients taking these medications. There are little data on the clinical significance of this interaction, possibly because of the short time that the drugs have been on the market, but it is recommended that no more than the equivalent of one cartridge of lidocaine with 1:100,000 epinephrine be administered initially and that the patient's heart rate and blood pressure be checked 5 minutes afterward before giving more local anesthetic [38].

Sulfite intolerance

Numerous reports exist of alleged allergic reactions to local anesthetics. The majority of true allergic reactions to amide local anesthetic solutions are probably responses to the methyparaben preservative used in multidose vials. Reactions have also been attributed to sulfites, most notably, sodium metabisulfite.

Sulfites are found naturally in many common foods and beverages [39]. Sulfites are also added to prevent or delay undesirable changes in the color, taste, or texture of such edibles. Wine, for example, contains about 10 mg/oz sulfites [39]. Sulfites are used in local anesthetic solutions as antioxidants to prevent the breakdown of the vasoconstrictor components. Local anesthetics with vasoconstrictors can contain as much as 2 mg/mL of sulfite salts [40].

Allergic-like reactions to sulfites are most commonly seen in asthmatic adults who react to inhaled or ingested sulfites through a nonimmunologic pathway. These individuals are not particularly sensitive to small amounts of injected sulfites. In fact, documented anaphylactic reactions to sulfites, which would be expected to be more intense with an injected allergen, are quite rare.

Although most patients who describe themselves as being sulfite-sensitive can receive intraoral injections of sulfite-containing solutions safely, whenever a patient reports a history of "allergy" to a local anesthetic, the treating dentist must include sulfite intolerance in the differential diagnosis. Local anesthetics with adrenergic vasoconstrictors are absolutely contra-indicated in the rare patient with a true sulfite allergy.

References

[1] Cassidy JP, Phero JC, Grau WH. Epinephrine: systemic effects and varying concentrations in local anesthesia. Anesth Prog 1986;33(6):289–97.

[2] Jastak JT, Yagiela JA, Donaldson D. Local anesthesia of the oral cavity. Philadelphia: WB Saunders; 1995. p. 61–85.

[3] Malamed SF. Handbook of local anesthesia. 4th edition. St. Louis: Mosby–Year Book; 1997. p. 37–48.

[4] Åberg G. Studies on the duration of local anesthesia: a possible mechanism for the prolonging effect of "vasoconstrictors" on the duration of infiltration anesthesia. Int J Oral Surg 1980;9(2):144–7.

[5] Hersh EV, Hermann DG, Lamp CJ, et al. Assessing the duration of mandibular soft tissue anesthesia. J Am Dent Assoc 1995;126(11):1531–6.

[6] Trieger N, Gillen GH. Bupivacaine anesthesia and post-operative analgesia in oral surgery. Anesth Prog 1979;26(1):20–3.

[7] Hecht A, App GR. Blood volume lost during gingivectomy using two different anesthetic techniques. J Periodontol 1974;45(1):9–12.

[8] Sveen K. Effect of the addition of a vasoconstrictor to local anesthetic solution on operative and postoperative bleeding, analgesia and wound healing. Int J Oral Surg 1979;8(4):301–6.

[9] Buckley JA, Ciancio SG, McMullen JA. Efficacy of epinephrine concentration in local anesthesia during periodontal surgery. J Periodontol 1984;55(11):653–7.

[10] Ueda W, Hirakawa M, Mori K. Acceleration of epinephrine absorption by lidocaine. Anesthesiology 1985;63(6):717–20.

[11] Brand HS, Abraham-Inpijn L. Cardiovascular responses induced by dental treatment. Eur J Oral Sci 1996;104(3):245–52.

[12] Pallasch TJ. Vasoconstrictors and the heart. J Calif Dent Assoc 1998;26(9):668–73.

[13] Glover J. Vasoconstrictors in dental anæsthetics: contra-indication—fact or fallacy? Aust Dent J 1968;13(1):65–9.

[14] Cannell H, Walters H, Beckett AH, Saunders A. Circulating levels of lignocaine after peri-oral injections. Br Dent J 1975;138(3):87–93.

[15] Goebel WM, Allen GD, Randall F. Comparative circulating serum levels of mepivacaine with levo-nordefrin and lidocaine with epinephrine. Anesth Prog 1979;26(4):93–7.

[16] Goebel WM, Allen GD, Randall F. Comparative circulating serum levels of 2 per cent mepivacaine and 2 per cent lignocaine. Br Dent J 1980;148(11–12):261–4.

[17] Åström A, Persson NH, Örtengren B. The effects of adrenaline on the toxicities and absorptions of L 67 (Citanest ®) and some other local anaesthetics studied in mice and rabbits. Acta Pharmacol Toxicol 1964;21(2):161–71.

[18] Avant WE, Weatherby JH. Effects of epinephrine on toxicities of several local anesthetic agents. Proc Soc Exp Biol Med 1960;103(2):353–6.

[19] Yagiela JA. Intravascular lidocaine toxicity: influence of epinephrine and route of administration. Anesth Prog 1985;33(2):57–61.

[20] Yagiela JA. Vasoconstrictors: their role in local anesthetic toxicity. Int J Oral Biol 1999;24(4):143–54.

[21] Pérusse R, Goulet J-P, Turcotte J-Y. Contraindications to vasoconstrictors in dentistry: part I. Cardiovascular diseases. Oral Surg Oral Med Oral Pathol 1992;74(5):679–86.

[22] Hirota Y, Sugiyama K, Joh S, et al. An echocardiographic study of patients with cardiovascular disease during dental treatment using local anesthesia. J Oral Maxillofac Surg 1986;44(2):116–21.

[23] New York Heart Association. Use of epinephrine in connection with procaine in dental procedures: report of the Special Committee of the New York Heart Association, Inc., on the Use of Epinephrine in Connection with Procaine in Dental Procedures. J Am Dent Assoc 1955;50(1):108.

[24] Management of dental problems in patients with cardiovascular disease: report of a working conference jointly sponsored by the American Dental Association and American Heart Association. J Am Dent Assoc 1964;68:334–42.

[25] Kaplan EL, editor. Cardiovascular disease in dental practice. Dallas (TX): American Heart Association; 1986.

[26] Gilbert EM, Eiswirth CC, Mealey PC, et al. β-Adrenergic supersensitivity of the transplanted human heart is presynaptic in origin. Circulation 1989;79(2):344–9.

[27] Meechan JG, Cole B, Welbury RR. The influence of two different dental local anaesthetic solutions on the haemodynamic responses of children undergoing restorative dentistry: a randomised, single-blind, split-mouth study. Br Dent J 2001;190(9):502–4.

[28] Alahuhta S, Räsänen J, Jouppila P, et al. Effects of extradural bupivacaine with adrenaline for Caesarean section on uteroplacental and fetal circulation. Br J Anaesth 1991;67(6): 678–82.

[29] Morrow RJ, Rolbin SH, Ritchie JWK, et al. Epidural anaesthesia and blood flow velocity in mother and fetus. Can J Anaesth 1989;36(5):519–22.

[30] Okutomi T, Amano K, Morishima HO. Effect of standard diluted epinephrine infusion on epidural anesthesia in labor. Reg Anesth Pain Med 2000;25(5):529–34.

[31] Okutomi T, Mochizuki J, Amano K, et al. Effect of epidural epinephrine infusion with bupivacaine on labor pain and mother-fetus outcomes in humans. Reg Anesth Pain Med 2000;25(3):228–34.

[32] Alahuhta S, Räsänen J, Jouppila P, et al. Uteroplacental and fetal circulation during extradural bupivacaine-adrenaline and bupivacaine for Caesarean section in hypertensive pregnancies with chronic fetal asphyxia. Br J Anaesth 1993;71(3):348–53.

[33] Haas DA, Pynn BR, Sands TD. Drug use for the pregnant or lactating patient. Gen Dent 2000;48(1):54–60.

[34] Goulet J-P, Pérusse R, Turcotte J-Y. Contraindications to vasoconstrictors in dentistry: part III, Pharmacologic interactions. Oral Surg Oral Med Oral Pathol 1992;74(5):692–7.

[35] Jastak JT, Yagiela JA. Vasoconstrictors and local anesthesia: a review and rationale for use. J Am Dent Assoc 1983;107(4):623–30.

[36] Yagiela JA. Adverse drug interactions in dental practice: interactions associated with vasoconstrictors. Part V of a series. J Am Dent Assoc 1999;130(5):701–9.

[37] Pallasch TJ, McCarthy FM, Jastak JT. Cocaine and sudden cardiac death. J Oral Maxillofac Surg 1989;47(11):1188–91.

[38] Rosenberg M, Yagiela J. Drug interactions: COMT inhibitors. J Mass Dent Soc 2001; 50(2):44–6.

[39] Blackmore JW. Local anesthetics and sulphite sensitivity. J Can Dent Assoc 1988;54(5): 349–52.

[40] Schwartz HJ, Gilbert IA, Lenner KA, et al. Metabisulfite sensitivity and local dental anesthesia. Ann Allergy 1989;62(2):83–6.

THE DENTAL
CLINICS OF
NORTH
AMERICA

Dent Clin N Am 46 (2002) 747–757

Adverse drug reactions to local anesthesia

Richard L. Finder, DMD, MS[a,b],
Paul A. Moore, DMD, PhD, MPH[c,*]

[a]Department of Physiology and Pharmacology, School of Dental Medicine,
University of Pittsburgh, 3501 Terrace Street, Pittsburgh, PA 15261, USA
[b]Ambulatory Anesthesia Associates, 2 Parkway Center, Suite G-1,
Pittsburgh, PA 15220, USA
[c]Department of Dental Public Health, University of Pittsburgh School of Dental Medicine,
552 Salk Hall, 3501 Terrace Street, Pittsburgh, PA 15261, USA

A dentist's ability to safely administer regional anesthesia is essential for dental practice. Local anesthetic solutions used in the United States for dental anesthesia are formulated with several components. The contents of a standard local anesthetic cartridge may include an amide or ester local anesthetic drug, an adrenergic vasoconstrictor, and an antioxidant. In susceptible patients, any of these components may induce systemic, dose-dependent adverse reactions. Although extremely rare, allergic reactions may also occur. Signs and symptoms of the various adverse reactions associated with local anesthetics are quite distinctive, permitting rapid diagnosis and treatment (see box below). Serious reactions are extremely infrequent and, when treated properly, are unlikely to result in significant morbidity or mortality.

Local anesthesia toxicity

When the local anesthetic contained in a dental cartridge diffuses away from the site of injection, it is absorbed into the systemic circulation where it is metabolized and excreted. The doses of a local anesthetic used in dentistry are usually minimal, and systemic effects are therefore uncommon. However, if an inadvertent vascular injection occurs or when repeated injections are administered, blood levels of a local anesthetic may become elevated.

Signs and symptoms

Initially, excitatory reactions to local anesthetic overdose are seen such as tremors, muscle twitching, shivering, and clonic-tonic convulsions [1–3].

---

* Corresponding author.
E-mail address: pam7@pitt.edu (P.A. Moore).

Diagnosis of local anesthesia reactions

Local anesthesia toxicity

Initial symptoms include tremors, muscle twitching, and convulsions. Following the initial phase, respiratory depression, lethargy, and loss of consciousness are possible. Cardiovascular depression may induce hypotension at extremely high blood concentrations. Hypoxia secondary to respiratory depression can rapidly produce the most serious outcomes including cardiovascular collapse, brain damage, and death.

Vasoconstrictor reactions

Initial signs of the sympathetic nervous system stimulation include palpitations, increased heart rate, and elevated blood pressure. Anxiety, nervousness, and fear are often associated with the palpitations. With severe overdose, arrhythmia, stroke, and myocardial infarction are possible.

Methemoglobinemia

Because methemoglobinemia is caused by metabolites of prilocaine, symptoms frequently do not occur for 1–3 hours following treatment. Methemoglobinemia also has been reported following benzocaine and other local anesthetics. Cyanosis without signs of respiratory distress may be apparent when methemoglobin levels reaches 10–20%. Vomiting and headache have been described. At higher blood concentrations of methemoglobin, dyspnea, seizures, stupor, coma, and death are possible.

Allergic reactions to local anesthetics

Mild manifestations of allergy to systemic drugs include urticaria, erythema, and intense itching. More severe reactions may include angioedema and respiratory distress. Although extremely unlikely, one should be prepared for the life-threatening anaphylactic responses including dyspnea, hypotension, and loss of consciousness.

Sulfite antioxidant reactions

Asthma-like signs of taychypnea, wheezing, bronchospasm, dyspnea, tachycardia, dizziness, and weakness have been reported, usually after exposure to foods (salads, shellfish, wines) containing sulfite antioxidants. Severe flushing, generalized urticaria, angioedema, tingling, pruritis, rhinitis, conjunctivis, dysphagia, nausea, and diarrhea have also been reported.

These initial excitatory reactions are thought to be disinhibition phenomena resulting from selective blockade of small inhibitory neurons within the limbic system of the central nervous system (CNS). Whether this initial excitatory reaction is seen or not, a generalized CNS depression with symptoms of sedation, drowsiness, lethargy, and life-threatening respiratory depression follow as blood levels continue to rise [4,5]. With extremely high toxic doses, myocardial excitability and conductivity may also be depressed, particularly with the highly lipid-soluble long-acting local anesthetics etidocaine and bupivacaine. Cardiac toxicity to local anesthetic overdose is most often manifested as ectopic cardiac rhythms and bradycardia. With extreme local anesthetic overdose, cardiac contractility is depressed and peripheral vasodilation occurs, leading to significant hypotension.

Prevention

Compliance with local anesthetic dosing guidelines is the first and most important strategy for preventing this adverse event. Dosing calculations and systemic reactions to local anesthetics are dependent on body weight. True dose-dependent toxicity reactions to local anesthetics are most frequently reported in pediatric patients. Children may be at greater risk of toxicity reactions because their lower body weight does not represent a proportionate decrease in orofacial anatomy. Because the mandible and maxilla of a 50-lb child are not one third the size of an adult (150 lbs), there is an apparent need to use relatively larger volumes when inducing local anesthesia in pediatric dental patients. The consequence of this disparity is that local anesthetic toxicity reactions occur more frequently in children. Additionally, systemic drug interactions involving local anesthetics and other CNS depressant drugs are more likely to occur in children [2,6].

The local anesthetic formulation of 3% mepivacaine plain appears to be associated with a disproportionate number of local anesthetic toxicity reports [6–9]. This may be caused by the absence of a vasoconstrictor, thereby allowing more rapid systemic absorption of the anesthetic. Additionally, the higher concentration used in its anesthetic formulation (3%) may result in the administration of larger relative doses. Pharmacokinetic studies by Goebel et al have demonstrated that peak anesthetic blood levels of 3% mepivacaine occur more rapidly and exceed that of an equal volume of 2% lidocaine with 1:100,000 epinephrine by approximately threefold following maxillary infiltration injections [10,11].

The 3% mepivacaine formulation is often chosen for children because it is considered by some to have a shorter duration of soft tissue anesthesia, therefore limiting severe lip biting and oral trauma seen in children following dental local anesthesia. The results of a recent double-blind randomized trial has found, however, that onset time, peak effects, and duration of soft tissue anesthesia following mandibular block injections with 2% lidocaine 1:100,000 epinephrine, 3% mepivacaine plain, or 4% prilocaine plain were very similar [12]. The selection of anesthetic formulations that do not contain a vasoconstrictor, such as 3% mepivacaine, may not be a significant therapeutic advantage when anesthetizing children.

The maximum volume of 3% mepivacaine plain for anesthetic injection (7 cartridges for a 150-lb adult) is the most restrictive of any local anesthetic used in dentistry. In comparison, the maximum volume for 2% lidocaine with epinephrine (14 cartridges for a 70 kg adult) permits the greatest volume for safe anesthesia injection. With children, selection of 2% lidocaine with 1:100,000 epinephrine is the least likely to cause toxicity reactions if multiple injections are required [13].

The calculation of maximum recommended doses (MRDs) for children receiving local anesthetics is complicated by the conflicting published dosage recommendations found in the literature and the various units involved in the determination (mg, %, cc, ml, kg, lb, cartridges). The MRDs for dental local anesthetics recently published in the American Dental Association (ADA) Guide to Dental Therapeutics is possibly the most current authoritative source [14]. These values are summarized in Table 1. It should be noted that these recommendations for lidocaine with epinephrine permit the largest volume of anesthetic, and for mepivacaine permit the smallest volume of anesthetic. Additionally, because of our desire to prevent oral trauma following dental anesthesia, the long-acting local anesthetics are generally not indicated for young children [15].

A simplified alternative for calculating maximum safe doses of local anesthesia has been to establish a conservative recommendation that can be applied to all anesthetic formulations used in dentistry. This recommendation, "The Rule of 25," states that a dentist may safely use 1 cartridge of any marketed local anesthetic for every 25 lbs of patient weight: ie, 3 cartridges for a 75-lb patient, 6 cartridges in a 150-lb patient [13].

Practical management

Tonic-clonic convulsions are the most common manifestation of a true overdose situation. Fortunately, local anesthetic-induced convulsions are usually transient. Following a convulsive episode, loss of consciousness and severe, prolonged respiratory depression is likely. Immediate treatment of this emergency should address both the convulsions and the potential respiratory depression. One must monitor vital signs (particularly respiratory adequacy), protect the patient from injury, place the patient in supine position, and maintain the airway. If the patient is unconscious, positive pressure oxygen is essential. Although rarely required, intravenous diazepam 5–10 mg is the definitive treatment if convulsions persist.

Vasoconstrictor reactions

With the possible exception of mepivacaine (Carbocaine®, Polocaine®) and prilocaine (Citanest®), most local anesthetics induce some degree of

Table 1
Dosage guidelines for local anesthetics[a]

| | Max rec dose | | | mg/ cartridge | Max # cartridges | |
Anesthetic agent	dose	mg/lb	Conc		150-lb adult	50-lb child
Lidocaine						
2% with epinephrine	500 mg	3.3 mg/lb	20 mg/ml	36 mg	14	5
2% plain	300 mg	2.0 mg/lb	20 mg/ml	36 mg	8	3
Mepivacaine						
3% plain	400 mg	2.6 mg/lb	30 mg/ml	54 mg	7	2
2% with levonordefrin	400 mg	2.6 mg/lb	20 mg/ml	36 mg	11	4
Prilocaine						
4% plain or epi	600 mg	4.0 mg/lb	40 mg/ml	72 mg	8	3
Articaine[b]						
4% with epinephrine	500 mg	3.3 mg/lb	40 mg/ml	68 mg[c]	7	2
Bupivacaine						
0.5% with epinephrine	90 mg	0.6 mg/lb	5 mg/ml	9 mg	10	_[d]
Etidocaine						
1.5% with epinephrine	400 mg	2.6 mg/lb	15 mg/ml	27 mg	15	_[d]

[a] *Data from* Yagiela J, Malamed SF. Injectable and topical local anesthetics. In: Ciancio SG, editor. ADA guide to dental therapeutics. Chicago: ADA Publishing Co; 1998, and manufacturer's product information; with permission.

[b] Cartridges are packaged with 1.8 ml except articaine which is available as 1.7 ml.

[c] Some manufacturers uses a lower dosage recommendation for articaine (2.3 mg/lb) with children 4–12 years of age.

[d] The long-acting local anesthetics bupivacaine and etidocaine are not recommended for children younger than 12 years of age.

vasodilation at the site of injection [16]. To limit systemic uptake and to prolong the duration of the anesthesia, vasoconstrictors are often added to local anesthetic formulations. A concentration as low as 1:200,000 epinephrine (0.005 mg/mL) improves the onset, profundity, and duration of regional anesthesia.

The vasoconstricting agents most commonly used in dental local anesthetic formulations, epinephrine and levonordefrin, have catecholamine structures and act by stimulating postsynaptic receptors of the sympathetic nervous system. Vasoconstriction at the site of injection is the therapeutic goal for adding adrenergic vasoconstrictors to local anesthetic solutions. Systemic epinephrine and levonordefrin have both alpha and beta adrenergic-stimulating properties, thereby increasing cardiac heart rate and contraction, as well as inducing vasoconstriction in skin and vasodilation in muscle tissue.

Signs and symptoms

Following injection of one or two cartridges of a dental local anesthetic containing epinephrine, normal circulating levels of epinephrine may increase two or threefold [17]. This additional exogenous epinephrine is generally well tolerated in healthy adults. Reactions associated with the vasoconstrictor in a local anesthetic solution are usually seen as mild stimulation of the cardio-vascular system; the resulting rises in heart rate and blood pressure are usu-ally transient. Of greater concern, particularly with a massive adrenergic vasoconstrictor overdose, are cardiac dysrhythmias including premature ventricular contractions and ventricular fibrillation. When considering a patient's tolerance to cardiovascular stimulation, there is little to indicate that epinephrine 1:100,000 or levonordefrin 1:20,000 differ substantially.

Prevention

Slow injections and careful aspiration will prevent rapid systemic absorp-tion of epinephrine and levonordefrin. A patient's health history that indicates significant cardiovascular impairment may indicate limiting the use of vaso-constrictors. Although rarely contraindicated, a common recommendation, when there is a medical history that suggests a need for caution, is to limit the dose of epinephrine to 0.018–0.036 mg, the amount of epinephrine contained in one to two cartridges of 2% lidocaine with 100,000 epinephrine [18].

Additionally, practitioners must be alert to drug-patient interactions when using local anesthetics containing the vasoconstrictors epinephrine and levonordefrin. Vasoconstrictors should be used with caution with pa-tients currently taking nonselective beta-adrenoreceptor blockers, tricyclic antidepressants, cocaine, and alpha-adrenergic blockers [19]. Patients taking nonselective beta-adrenergic antagonists such as propranolol may experi-ence exaggerated systemic vasoconstrictive responses to epinephrine or lev-onordefrin [20]. The tricyclic antidepressants may also enhance the systemic adrenergic response. Cocaine and the halogenated general anesthetics, most notably halothane, may increase the sensitivity of the heart to life-threaten-ing arrhythmias following the use of adrenergic vasoconstrictors. These interactions are clinically relevant and potentially life-threatening [19]. Other drugs that may adversely interact with adrenergic vasoconstrictors, such as alpha adrenergic blockers (ie, chlorpromazine), adrenergic neuronal blockers (ie, guanadrel), local anesthetics, thyroid hormones, and mono-amine oxidase inhibitors are poorly documented and are probably of little clinical significance when dose guidelines are followed. These reactions are addressed more comprehensively in Yageila's article, "Vasoconstrictors: indications and contraindications."

Practical management

If a reaction does result from local anesthetic administration, treatment recommendations include monitoring vital signs, explaining to the patient the cause of the symptoms, and assuring the patient that the response will last only a few minutes. If a significant rise in blood pressure is noted, defin-itive drug treatment in a dental office is sublingual nitroglycerin and imme-diate transport to the local hospital emergency room.

Methemoglobinemia

Methemoglobinemia is a unique dose-dependent reaction reported to occur following the administration of nitrates, aniline dyes, and some amide-containing medications. When administered in excessive doses, the dental anesthetics prilocaine and benzocaine (and rarely lidocaine and articaine) may also induce methemoglobinemia. These local anesthetics, as well as nitrogylcerin and various nitrite preparations and the antimicrobials dapsone and the sulfonamide antibiotics (such as sulfamethoxazole and sulfasoxazole), can cause the oxidation of the iron atom within hemoglobin, producing methemoglobin.

Signs and symptoms

With toxicity, clinical signs of cyanosis are initially observed as blood levels of methemoglobin reach 10–20%. Dyspnea and tachycardia are observed as methemoglobin levels reach 35–40%. Reports of methemoglobinemia following administration of prilocaine and benzocaine are most often associated with large doses. Because this reaction is associated with prilocaine's metabolite toluidine, symptoms often develop after the patient has left the dental office. This serious reaction has been repeatedly documented following dental anesthesia using prilocaine, although fatalities have not been reported [21,22]. Methemoglobinemia following the topical administration of EMLA, a Eutectic Mixture of Prilocaine and Lidocaine, has occurred in infants [23].

Prevention

Risk factors for this reaction include extremes of age, anemia, respiratory disease, hereditary methemoglobinemia, deficiencies in glucose-6-phosphate dehydrogenase and methemoglobin reductase, and possibly combinations of oxidant drugs [1,24]. It is recommended that the total dose of prilocaine and other local anesthetics be calculated carefully and that weight-based MRDs not be exceeded.

Practical management

Treatment strategies are usually symptomatic. This drug reaction reverses itself within a few hours in healthy patients, as the drug and/or its metabolites are eliminated. In general, if the patient is not in distress, treatment recommendations include: monitoring cardiovascular and respiratory function, administering 100% oxygen via facemask, and transportation to the local emergency room. If cyanosis, hypoxia, and respiratory distress are clinically significant, intravenous methylene blue (1–2 mg/kg), which rapidly reverts the methemoglobin to hemoglobin, is the definitive treatment.

Allergic reactions to local anesthetics

Although extremely rare, allergic reactions to local anesthetics may occur. True allergy has been reported most often for ester local anesthetics such as procaine and tetracaine. Fortunately, the most common agents used in dentistry are the amide anesthetics that possess very limited ability to induce hypersensitivity reactions [25].

Additionally, the removal of methylparaben, a preservative additive, from dental local anesthetic formulations in the 1980s, has also diminished reports of allergic reactions in dentistry [26]. Since then, serious allergic reactions following local anesthesia administration in dentistry are almost never reported. Although a practitioner should be prepared to treat local anesthetic hypersensitivity reactions, most suspected reactions are psychogenic. Experience reported by allergy clinics have suggested that most patients referred for local anesthetic allergenicity testing have been misdiagnosed [27,28]. Comprehending a patient's anxiety and fear of dental injections may provide useful information for recognizing psychogenic reactions.

Signs and symptoms

Although patients often report allergy to local anesthetics, confirmed responses of true allergy are extremely rare. Reactions considered to indicate true allergy include cutaneous responses such as rash and urticaria, as well as systemic anaphylactoid responses such as dyspnea and hypotension.

Prevention

Taking a complete drug history and avoiding medications listed under allergies can prevent most of these reactions. Because alternatives to local anesthetics, such as diphenydramine injection, deep sedation, and general anesthesia, are not ideal, a referral for allergy testing to confirm the diagnosis is recommended. Results of allergy testing will most often rule out true allergy or will identify a specific local anesthetic agent that can be used for dental anesthesia.

Practical management

Allergic reactions to injected medications range from mild to severe. Mild skin responses are managed with an antihistamine such as diphenhydramine 25–50 mg administered either orally or intramuscularly. Frequently, a patient having an allergic reaction for the first time will be extremely anxious. A rapid rate of onset of an allergic drug reaction should alert practitioners to a possible anaphylactoid response. If dyspnea, nausea, vomiting, hypotension, or other acute signs of anaphylaxis occur, immediate treatment is required. Recommended treatment includes basic life support, intramuscular or subcutaneous epinephrine 0.3–0.5 mg, summoning medical assistance, and transportation to the local hospital emergency room. Additional therapy including antihistamines and corticosteroids may be required subsequent to the acute therapy.

Sulfite antioxidant reactions

Concern has recently developed for possible dose-dependent reactions to the antioxidant sulfites used in the local anesthetic formulations containing epinephrine or levonordefrin [29]. Sulfites are included in local anesthetic solutions to prevent nonenzymatic oxidation of the catecholamine vasoconstrictors, thereby prolonging the shelf life of these formulations. Local anesthetic solutions that do not include vasoconstrictors, such as 3% mepivacaine and 4% prilocaine, do not include antioxidants in their formulations. Sulfite antioxidants (sulfur dioxide, sulfites, bisulfites, and metabisulfites) have been found to sensitize some asthmatic patients when they are exposed to rather large amounts of these preservatives. Large doses, such as those previously used in restaurant salad bars and homemade wines, had been linked to six deaths in 1984 [30]. Five percent of the 9 million asthmatic patients in the United States may be sulfite-sensitive [31].

Signs and symptoms

Reactions of urticaria, angioedema, bronchospasm, and anaphylactic shock have been reported [22]. The most common reactions are wheezing and bronchospasm. Other symptoms of sulfite sensitivity include tachypnea, dizziness, nausea, and weakness [32].

Prevention

Adverse reaction to sulfites occurs most frequently in patients with a history of atopic allergy or asthma. History of asthma, particularly if sulfite sensitivity is noted, may be important in selecting an anesthetic agent. Although some concern and caution is justified when using local anesthetics containing vasoconstrictors and sulfites, a documented reaction in dental practice has not been published, probably because the amount of this antioxidant sulfite in a dental formulation is too small to stimulate a significant life-threatening reaction.

Practical management

Reactions usually occur within 30 minutes of oral ingestion. Severe respiratory distress should be treated with a beta-agonist inhaler if possible. Anaphylactoid reactions should be treated immediately with intramuscular or subcutaneous epinephrine (0.3–0.5 mg).

References

[1] Moore PA. Adverse drug interactions in dental practice: interactions associated with local anesthetics, sedatives and anxiolytics. Part IV of a series. J Am Dent Assoc 1999;130: 541–54.

[2] Moore PA, Goodson JM. Risk appraisal of narcotic sedation for children. Anesth Prog 1985;32:129–39.

[3] Reynolds F. Adverse effects of local anesthetics. Br J Anaesth 1987;59:78–95.

[4] Covino BG, Vassallo HG. Local anesthetics: mechanisms of action and clinical use. New York: Grune & Stratton, Inc; 1976.

[5] Liu PL, Feldman HS, Giasi R, et al. Comparative CNS toxicity of lidocaine, etidocaine, bupivacaine, and tetracaine in awake dogs following rapid intravenous administration. Anesth Analg 1983;62:375–9.

[6] Goodson JM, Moore PA. Life-threatening reactions following pedodontic sedation: an assessment of narcotic, local anesthetic and antiemetic drug interaction. J Am Dent Assoc 1983;107:239–45.

[7] Hersh EV, Helpin ML, Evans OB. Local anesthetic mortality: report of case. J Dent Child 1991;58:489–91.

[8] Moore PA. Prevention of local anesthesia toxicity. J Am Dent Assoc 1992;123:60–4.

[9] Virts BE. Local anesthesia toxicity review. Ped Dent 1999;21:375.

[10] Goebel WM, Allen G, Randall F. Circulating serum levels of mepivacaine after dental injection. Anesth Prog 1978;25:52–6.

[11] Goebel WM, Allen G, Randall F. The effect of commercial vasoconstrictor preparations on the circulating venous serum level of mepivacaine and lidocaine. J Oral Med 1980;35: 91–6.

[12] Hersh EV, Hermann DG, Lamp CJ, et al. Assessing the duration of mandibular soft tissue anesthesia. J Am Dent Assoc 1995;126:1531–6.

[13] Moore PA. Manual of local anesthesia in dentistry. 4th edition. Rochester (NY): Eastman-Kodak Co; 1996.

[14] Yagiela J, Malamed SF. Injectable and topical local anesthetics. In: Ciancio SG, editor. ADA guide to dental therapeutics. Chicago: ADA Publishing Co; 1998.

[15] Moore PA. Long-acting local anesthetics: a review of clinical efficacy in dentistry. Compend Cont Dent Ed 1990;11:22–30.

[16] Lindorf HH. Investigation of the vascular effect of newer local anesthetics and vaso-constrictors. Oral Surg 1979;48:292–7.

[17] Yagiela JA. Local anesthetics. In: Dionne RA, Phero JC, editors. Management of pain and anxiety in dental practice. New York: Elsevier; 1991.

[18] Little JW, Falace DA. Dental management of the medically compromised patient. 4th edition. St. Louis: Mosby; 1993. p. 228.

[19] Yagiela JA. Adverse drug interactions in dental practice: interactions associated with vasoconstrictors. Part V of a series. J Am Dent Assoc 1999;130:701–9.

[20] Mito RS, Yagiela JA. Hypertensive response to levonordefrin in a patient receiving pro-pranolol: report of case. J Am Dent Assoc 1988;116:280–1.

[21] Epidemiologic notes and reports. Prilocaine-induced methemoglobinemia-Wisconsin, 1993. Morbidity & Mortality Weekly Report 1994;43(35):655–7.

[22] Jakobson B, Nilsson A. Methemoglobinemia associated with a prilocaine-lidocaine cream and trimetoprim-sulphamethoxazole. A case report. Acta Anaesthesiol Scand 1985;29(4):453–5.

[23] Kumar AR, Dunn N, Naqvi M. Methemoglobinemia associated with a prilocaine-lidocaine cream. Clin Pediatrics 1997;36(4):239–40.

[24] Wilburn-Goo D, Lloyd LM. When patients become cyanotic: acquired methemoglobine-mia. J Am Dent Assoc 1999;130:826–31.

[25] Seng GF, Kraus K, Cartridge G, et al. Confirmed allergic reactions to amide local anes-thetics. Gen Dent 1996;44:52–4.

[26] Larson CE. Methylparaben-an overlooked cause of local anesthetic hypersensitivity. Anesth Prog 1977;24:72–4.

[27] deSharo RD, Nelson HS. An approach to the patient with a history of local anesthetic hypersensitivity: experience with 90 patients. J Allergy Clin Immunol 1979;63:387–94.

[28] Incaudo G, Schatz M, Patterson R, et al. Administration of local anesthetics to patients with a history of prior adverse reactions. J Allergy Clin Immunol 1978;61:339–45.

[29] Seng GF, Gay BJ. Dangers of sulfites in dental local anesthetic solutions: warning and recommendations. J Am Dent Assoc 1986;113:769–70.

[30] New sulfite regulations. FDA Drug Bull 1986;16:17–8.

[31] Bush RK, Taylor SL, Holden K, et al. Prevelance of sensitivity to sulfiting agents in asthmatic patients. Am J Med 1986;81:816–20.

[32] Schwartz HJ. Sensitivity to ingested metabisulfite: variations in clinical presentation. J Allergy Clin Immunol 1983;71(5):487–9.

THE DENTAL
CLINICS OF
NORTH
AMERICA

Dent Clin N Am 46 (2002) 759–766

Effective topical anesthetic agents and techniques

John G. Meechan, BSc, BDS, FDSRCPS, PhD

*Department of Oral and Maxillofacial Surgery, The Dental School, Framlington Place,
Newcastle upon Tyne, England NE2 4BW, United Kingdom*

Anxiety is still a barrier to dental attendance [1]. Fear of pain is one reason a patient may be apprehensive about dental treatment. That the most common form of pain control in dentistry, namely local anesthesia, can itself produce anxiety [2] is unfortunate. There are several factors that influence dental injection pain. A variety of techniques are used to overcome this discomfort. These include suggestion [3], alteration of factors related to the injected solution such as pH and temperature [4,5], and a reduced speed of injection. Another method is to prepare the surface tissues before needle penetration. Methods of surface anesthesia include refrigeration [6], transcutaneous electronic nerve stimulation [7], and topical anesthesia. Topical anesthesia relies on the pharmacologic effect of anesthetics when applied to surface tissue. In addition to its use as a means of reducing injection discomfort, topical anesthetics may be used alone or as components of proprietary preparations used as symptomatic treatments for painful oral mucosal lesions such as ulcers [8]. Topical anesthesia also has been used as the sole means of anesthesia for intraoral soft tissue surgery [9,10] and extraction of teeth [11,12]. One of the "holy grails" in dentistry is the achievement of pulpal anesthesia by topical application of an anesthetic, and although this is not yet a reliable technique, this objective has been pursued [13].

Topical anesthetics are available in several formulations in North America. They are supplied in the forms of aerosols, ointments, gels, lozenges, tablets, pastes, powders, solutions, and impregnated patches (Fig. 1). Specialized application systems, such as incorporation into liposomes [14,15] or delivery by iontophoresis [11], also have been investigated.

This article is concerned with the use of topical anesthetics before the injection of local anesthetics in dentistry. The first important question to ask in relation to topical anesthetics is, are they effective? Preparation of the

E-mail address: J.G.Meechan@ncl.ac.uk (J.G. Meechan).

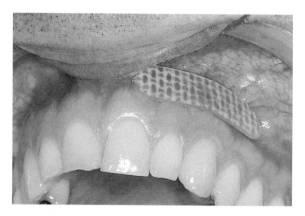

Fig. 1. Topical anesthesia is effective in masking injection discomfort when applied to the maxillary buccal fold. The time of application influences efficacy, however. A lidocaine-impregnated patch has been applied in this case.

surface tissues could reduce discomfort by two mechanisms. There may be an advantageous effect psychologically and there may be a pharmacologic action. In dental practice, any benefit is important and thus the psychologic impact of topical anesthetics should not be disregarded. Martin et al [16] have shown that subjects who are informed they are to receive a topical anesthetic for comfort anticipate less injection pain than those not offered such counseling. This may decrease apprehension [16]. If there is no pharmacologic effect, however, why use an anesthetic agent? If there is a pharmacologic effect, then the use of an anesthetic is sensible. It is possible to separate psychologic and pharmacologic effects in well designed clinical trials and this article considers this aspect.

What is the evidence that topical anesthetics are effective?

There are several published studies that have investigated the pharmacologic effect of intraoral topical anesthetics and the results are conflicting. Reasons for variation in results are caused by different methodology, such as the use of a variety of agents, differing sites of test, and various types of test stimuli. To reduce confounding factors, the studies referred to in this section are limited to those that have compared topical anesthetics with placebo before either needle penetration of oral mucosa or intraoral injection. In addition, as several factors such as bias and the order of injection [16] can influence the results, only randomized, double-blind studies have been included.

Hersh et al [17] investigated the efficacy of patches containing 10% (23 mg) or 20% (46.5 mg) lidocaine (Dentipatch) when applied for 15 minutes just apical to the mucogingival junction in the maxillary and mandibular premolar region. The test stimulus was insertion of a 25-gauge needle to the point of bony contact. Efficacy was tested at several time points following application of the patch. These investigators found that neither patch differed from placebo 2.5 minutes after maxillary application. Both patches achieved an analgesic effect at 5 minutes, however, and this lasted for 15 minutes. With the 20% patch there was still an analgesic effect at 45 minutes. These workers considered the duration of anesthesia to be 10 minutes for the 23-mg patch and at least 40 minutes for the 46.5-mg patch in the maxilla. In the mandible, the 46.5-mg patch achieved an effect at 2.5 minutes and the 23-mg patch at 5 minutes. An analgesic effect in the mandible was still present at the 45-minute test. There was a clear dose response in the mandible.

Holst and Evers [18] compared 5% lidocaine with placebo and found that in the lower buccal fold a 2-minute application produced an analgesic effect when the test stimulus was insertion of a 30-gauge needle to a depth of approximately 2 mm.

Rosivack et al [19] compared the 3-minute application of 20% benzocaine and 5% lidocaine with placebo in reducing the discomfort of 27-gauge needle penetration in the maxillary buccal sulcus. Both topical agents reduced discomfort compared with placebo.

Carrell et al [20] reported that topical anesthetics containing 5% lidocaine reduced the incidence of crying in children during local anesthesia compared with the application of placebo.

Svensson and Petersen [21] investigated insertion of a 27-gauge needle in palatal mucosa and noted that a 5-minute application of eutectic mixture of local anesthetics (EMLA) (a 5% eutectic mixture of lidocaine and prilocaine) reduced discomfort compared with placebo.

Vickers and Punnia Moorthy [22] compared three different topical agents to placebo after a 2-minute application in the maxillary buccal sulcus. EMLA cream, 5% lidocaine, and the combination of 15% benzocaine with 1.7% amethocaine were all better than placebo at reducing the discomfort of 27-gauge needle penetration.

Unlike the other studies described that looked at only needle penetration, Hutchins et al [23] studied the effect of a 1-minute application of 20% benzocaine compared with placebo before local anesthetic injections by way of a 27-gauge needle. They found that in the maxillary buccal fold, the topical anesthetic was more effective than placebo in reducing injection discomfort; however, in the palatal mucosa there was no difference between active and placebo treatments.

All of the investigations considered earlier demonstrated a positive result in at least one aspect studied. Not all randomized, double-blind, placebo-controlled trials have reported differences between topical anesthetics and placebo, however. Gill and Orr [24] compared three topical anesthetics (5% lidocaine, 22% benzocaine, 2% amethocaine with 18% benzocaine) with placebo. They used a 30-second application on palatal mucosa and stimulated the mucosa with penetration of a 25-gauge needle. They found no difference in injection discomfort between treatments.

Kincheloe et al [25] compared the 3-minute application of an unnamed topical anesthetic at various sites intraorally and found no benefit in relation to placebo.

In summary, there is evidence from several double-blind, placebo-controlled trials [17–19,21,22,23,26] that topical anesthetics have a pharmacologic effect.

Factors governing the efficacy of topical anesthetics

The studies mentioned earlier demonstrated mixed results. In addition to variations caused by different test stimuli in trials [17], other factors that influence the efficacy of topical anesthetics include:

- The agent used
- Duration of application
- Site of application

These factors are discussed later.

Topical anesthetic agents

Is there any evidence that the anesthetic used is important in relation to efficacy? Several studies have investigated this question. Two aspects are relevant here: the concentration used and the anesthetic agent itself.

It was mentioned earlier that different delivery vehicles are used to administer topical anesthetics. Different formulations of the same drug need different concentrations to achieve a similar effect, for example sprays require a higher concentration than patches [27]. Animal studies have shown that the rate of transfer of anesthetics applied topically is concentration-dependent [28]. Hersh et al [17] showed a dose response in humans with a patch containing 46.5 mg lidocaine being more effective than one that contained 23 mg when applied topically in the mouth. Thus, the concentration is important.

A variety of agents are used as anesthetics; local anesthetics of the ester and the amide groups may be used. This is important in relation to allergic reactions. Most injectable local anesthetic agents such as lidocaine, prilocaine, and bupivacaine are amides that have a low incidence of producing allergies. Ester anesthetics, however, such as benzocaine and tetracaine (amethocaine) are included in topical preparations in North America and this group has a higher incidence of allergy. The studies mentioned earlier [17–19,21,22,23,26] have shown lidocaine (alone and in combination with prilocaine) and benzocaine (alone and in combination with amethocaine) exert an effect when applied topically to oral mucosa.

Two double-blind investigations have shown an increase in efficacy when lidocaine is used in combination with prilocaine in the eutectic mixture EMLA. Holst and Evers [18] have shown that a 5-minute application of

EMLA to the palate decreases discomfort of needle penetration compared with 5% lidocaine. Similarly, Meechan and Thomason [29] reported that a 5-minute application of EMLA was more effective than a similar regimen using 5% lidocaine in reducing the discomfort of intraligamentary injections.

Thus there is evidence that the choice of material influences the efficacy of topical anesthesia. Not all studies have reported variation between agents, however, as Rosivack et al [19] found no difference in the 3-minute application of 5% lidocaine and 20% benzocaine in the maxillary buccal sulcus.

Site

Local anesthetic injections are administered at different intraoral sites. The placement of topical anesthetics can therefore vary. The duration of the effect of applied topical anesthetics varies in different areas of the mouth [30]. Factors relating to site that might influence efficacy are keratinized versus non-keratinized mucosa, for example maxillary buccal sulcus (see Fig. 1) versus palatal mucosa (Fig. 2). In addition, eliminating the discomfort at a site that is going to receive a superficial infiltration injection may be easier than masking the pain of a deep regional block injection. Even the effectiveness of topical anesthetics in reducing infiltration pain varies between sites. Hersh et al [17] showed that a 2.5-minute application of a 46.5-mg lidocaine patch was successful in eliminating needle penetration discomfort in the mandibular buccal fold but not in the maxillary buccal sulcus.

Holst and Evers [18] noted that a 2-minute application of 5% lidocaine to the mandibular buccal fold was effective in reducing the pain of needle insertion; however, this regimen was no better than placebo on the palate. Similarly, Hutchins et al [23] found that although effective in the buccal fold, a 1-minute application of 20% benzocaine was no better than placebo in the palate.

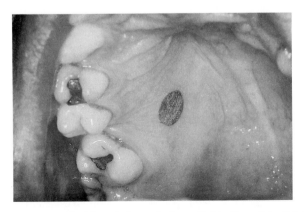

Fig. 2. A patch impregnated with topical anesthetic applied to the palate. Palatal mucosa is more resistant to the effects of topical anesthetics compared with the buccal fold.

The only material that has been shown to reduce palatal injection pain in double-blind, randomized studies is EMLA. Other trials [31], however, have suggested that this material is no better than 20% benzocaine when used to mask palatal injection pain in children.

The author is unaware of any double-blind studies on the efficacy of topical anesthetics before deep regional block injections (Fig. 3). One study [32] that investigated the effects of needle penetration in the pterygotemporal depression to mimic block anesthesia showed no difference in insertion pain following application of 20% benzocaine or placebo for 4 minutes. Another single-blind study [7] comparing the 2-minute application of 20% benzocaine with no topical treatment before the injection of inferior alveolar nerve blocks reported no difference in injection discomfort between treatments. Thus there is no evidence to support the use of topical anesthetics before inferior alveolar nerve block injections.

Duration of application

Most local anesthetic injections do not have an immediate effect. It is common practice to allow a few minutes to elapse before beginning a procedure on a tooth that has been anesthetized. The same rule applies to topical application of a local anesthetic. Not surprisingly, the depth of penetration of the applied agent is governed by the duration of application [26].

One double-blind trial [23] has shown an application time of 1 minute to achieve success in the maxillary buccal fold with 20% benzocaine. On the contrary, another investigation [17] has shown a 2.5-minute application of a 23-mg lidocaine patch at that site was no better than placebo. In the latter study, however, an effect was apparent at 5 minutes. Yet another trial [25]

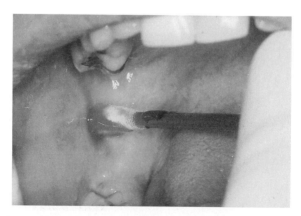

Fig. 3. There is no evidence that topical anesthesia masks the discomfort of inferior alveolar nerve block injections. Here, 20% benzocaine gel is being applied to the needle insertion point before administration of an inferior alveolar nerve block.

has shown that a 3-minute application of an unnamed topical was ineffective. Holst and Evers [18] noted that an application time of 5 minutes increased the efficacy of 5% lidocaine compared with a 2-minute application.

Summary

What conclusions can be drawn concerning intraoral topical anesthesia? First, a variety of agents have been shown to have a pharmacologic effect. When used as a single agent, lidocaine is effective at concentrations between 5% and 20%. There is evidence of a dose response with lidocaine [17]. The combination of 2.5% lidocaine and 2.5% prilocaine has been shown to be a reliable agent; however, at the time of writing, this mixture is not licensed for intraoral use. Benzocaine is effective when used alone at a concentration of 20% and when combined at a dose of 15% with 1.7% amethocaine.

Second, a crucial factor governing effectiveness is the time of application. One study cited in this paper [23] has shown an effect occurring in the maxillary buccal sulcus after a 1-minute application. Others [17,25] have shown that a 2- to 3-minute application at the same site is no better than placebo. The differences in these studies may be caused by the use of different test stimuli, such as the gauge of the needle used and the depth of insertion. When applied for 5 minutes, it seems that success is guaranteed when used in the buccal fold of either jaw.

Finally, the site of application is important. Palatal mucosa is more resistant to the effects of topical anesthetics than other intraoral sites investigated. There is no evidence that topical anesthetics have any value in reducing the discomfort of deep regional block administrations such as inferior alveolar nerve block injections.

References

[1] Nuttall NM, Bradnock G, White D, et al. Dental attendance in 1998 and implications for the future. Br Dent J 2001;190(4):177–82.

[2] Fiset L, Milgrom P, Weinstein P, et al. Psychophysiological responses to dental injections. J Am Dent Assoc 1985;111:578–83.

[3] Pollack S. Pain control by suggestion. J Oral Med 1966;21(2):89–95.

[4] Courtney D, Agrawal S, Revington PJ. Local anaesthesia: to warm or alter the pH? A survey of current practice. J R Coll Surg Edinb 1999;44:167–71.

[5] Oikarinen VJ, Ylipaavalnpemi P, Evers H. Pain and temperature sensations related to local analgesia. Int J Oral Surg 1975;4:151–56.

[6] Harbert H. Topical ice: a precursor to palatal injections. J Endodont 1989;15(1):27–8.

[7] Meechan JG, Gowans AJ, Welbury RR. The use of patient-controlled transcutaneous electronic nerve stimulation (TENS) to decrease the discomfort of regional anaesthesia in dentistry: a randomised controlled clinical trial. J Dent 1998;26:417–20.

[8] Yankell SL, Welsh CA, Cohen DW. Evaluation of benzydamine HCl in patients with aphthous ulcers. Comp Cont Educ Dent 1981;2(1):14–6.

[9] Meechan JG. The use of EMLA for an intra-oral biopsy in a needle phobic: a case report. Anesth Prog 2001;48:32–4.

[10] Roller NW, Ship II. Lidocaine topical film strip for oral mucosal biopsies. J Oral Med 1975;30:55–8.
[11] Gangarosa LP. Iontophoresis for surface local anaesthesia. J Am Dent Assoc 1974;88: 125–8.
[12] Taware CP, Mazumdar S, Pendharkar M, et al. A bioadhesive delivery system as an alternative to infiltration anaesthesia. Oral Surg Oral Med Oral Path 1997;84:609–15.
[13] Vickers ER, Punnia Moorthy A. Pulpal anesthesia from an application of a eutectic topical anesthetic. Quintessence Int 1993;24:547–51.
[14] Lener EV, Bucalo BD, Kist LDA, et al. Topical anesthetic agents in dermatologic surgery. A review. Dermatol Surg 1997;23:673–83.
[15] Zed CM, Epstein J, Donaldson D. Topical liposome encapsulated tetracaine versus benzocaine: a clinical investigation [abstract 1840]. J Dent Res 1996;75:247.
[16] Martin MD, Ramsay DS, Whitney C, et al. Topical anesthesia: differentiating the pharmacological and psychological contributions to efficacy. Anesth Prog 1994;41:40–7.
[17] Hersh EV, Houpt MI, Cooper SA, et al. Analgesic efficacy and safety of an intra-oral lidocaine patch. J Am Dent Assoc 1996;127:1626–34.
[18] Holst A, Evers H. Experimental studies of new topical anaesthetics on the oral mucosa. Swed Dent J 1985;9:185–91.
[19] Rosivack RG, Koenigsberg SR, Maxwell KC. An analysis of the effectiveness of two topical anaesthetics. Anesth Prog 1990;37:290–2.
[20] Carrel R, Friedman L, Binns WH. Laboratory and clinical evaluation of a new topical anesthetic. Anesth Prog 1974;21:126–31.
[21] Svensson P, Petersen JK. Anesthetic effect of EMLA occluded with orahesive oral bandages on oral mucosa. A placebo-controlled study. Anesth Prog 1992;39:79–82.
[22] Vickers ER, Punnia Moorthy A. A clinical evaluation of three topical anaesthetic agents. Aust Dent J 1992;37:266–70.
[23] Gill CJ, Orr DL. A double blind crossover comparison of topical anesthetics. J Am Dent Assoc 1979;98:213–4.
[24] Kincheloe JE, Mealiea WL, Mattison GD, et al. Psychophysical measurement on pain perception after administration of a topical anesthetic. Quintessence Int 1991;22:311–5.
[25] Bjerring P, Arendt-Nielsen L. Depth and duration of skin analgesia to needle insertion after topical application of EMLA cream. Br J Anaesth 1990;64:173–7.
[26] Hutchins HS, Young FA, Lackland DL, et al. The effectiveness of topical anesthesia and vibration in alleviating the pain of oral injections. Anesth Prog 1997;44:87–9.
[27] Giddon DB, Quadland M, Rachwall PC, et al. Development of a method for comparing topical anesthetics in different application and dosage forms. J Oral Ther Pharm 1968; 4:270–4.
[28] Bergman S, Kane D, Siegal IA, et al. In vitro and in situ transfer of local anaesthetics across the oral mucosa. Arch Oral Biol 1969;14:35–43.
[29] Meechan JG, Thomason JM. A comparison of two topical anesthetics on the discomfort of intraligamentary injections: a double-blind split mouth volunteer clinical trial. Oral Surg Oral Med Oral Path 1999;87:362–5.
[30] Adriani J, Zepernick R, Arens J, et al. The comparative potency and effectiveness of topical anesthetics in man. Clin Pharmacol Ther 1963;5:49–62.
[31] Primosch RE, Rolland-Asensi G. Comparison of topical EMLA 5% oral adhesive to benzocaine 20% on the pain experienced during palatal anesthetic infiltration in children. Ped Dent 2001;23(1):11–4.
[32] Nakanishi O, Haas D, Ishikawa T, et al. Efficacy of mandibular topical anesthesia varies with the site of administration. Anesth Prog 1996;43:14–19.

Conscious sedation for dentistry: risk management and patient selection

Douglass L. Jackson, DMD, MS, PhD[a,*],
Barton S. Johnson, DDS, MS[b]

[a]*Department of Oral Medicine, University of Washington School of Dentistry,
B412 Health Sciences Building, Seattle, WA 98195, USA*
[b]*Departments of Restorative Dentistry and Hospital Dentistry, University of Washington
School of Dentistry, Seattle, WA 98195, USA*

Despite the many advances in pain control that have expanded our abilities to perform a wide range of dental treatment in a pain-free environment, many adult dental patients still have a great deal of fear about treatment-evoked pain. Discussions about conscious sedation, and possibly general anesthesia, seem to be appropriate in developing treatment plans for this population of fearful patients. Are there other adult populations that also may benefit from sedation during dental treatment? For example, what about the developmentally disabled adult who is unable to cooperate with the dental treatment team, thus decreasing the efficiency and safety of delivering dental treatment? Or what about the adult with a medical history of angina that can be precipitated by moderately stressful events like intraoral injections of local anesthesia? These two examples should suggest that there are other patient populations that would also benefit from sedation during dental treatment.

Given the unpleasant nature of many dental procedures, one could argue that sedation is used too little in the practice of dentistry. In contrast, many disciplines of medicine use some sort of sedation when performing procedures that can be considered simple and less stressful when compared with many dental procedures. There are clearly several situations in which local anesthesia alone may be insufficient to deliver dental treatment. In some cases the use of parenteral sedation (ie, intramuscular and intravascular) or general anesthesia may be among the pharmacologic methods for consideration as treatment adjuncts. Advanced clinical training and licensing is

---

* Corresponding author.
E-mail address: jacksond@u.washington.edu (D.L. Jackson).

required to deliver parenteral sedation and general anesthesia, however. Additionally, some parenteral sedation techniques and general anesthesia depress the patient's level of consciousness to a point at which several significant risks arise that need to be considered. We would like to suggest that nitrous oxide/oxygen (N_2O/O_2) inhalational sedation and enteral (oral) sedation with a single pharmacologic agent are two additional conscious sedation techniques that can be used by most dental practitioners with reasonable success. Unlike parenteral sedation and general anesthesia, the amount of advanced training required to administer N_2O/O_2 inhalational sedation and enteral sedation with a single pharmacologic agent is considerably less, and the margin of safety is much greater.

The goal of this article is to review the many aspects of risk management that need to be considered when using N_2O/O_2 inhalational sedation and enteral sedation in adults and children. Understanding the regulations and guidelines that need to be followed when delivering conscious sedation greatly increases the margin of safety. This article reviews the definitions and guidelines for delivering conscious sedation, establishes the criteria for selecting appropriate patients, and discusses the many aspects of clinical preparedness. These risk management discussions are applicable to the following two articles in which N_2O/O_2 inhalational sedation and enteral sedation in adults and children is discussed, and the remaining article in this section that reviews emergency drugs and their use in dental situations.

Definitions

The anxiety evoked by dental treatment can be successfully controlled by slightly depressing the level of consciousness in many patients. For these patients, the use of conscious sedation may be appropriate. Before engaging in a comprehensive review of N_2O/O_2 and enteral sedation for any dental patients, however, it is important to be familiar with some definitions that establish the guidelines for keeping sedation safe. The House of Delegates of the American Dental Association (ADA) has adopted a policy statement and guidelines for the use of sedation and general anesthesia in dentistry [1]. Although the ADA's guidelines provide a reasonable foundation for defining the scope of anxiety and pain control in the practice of dentistry, most states also have published a modification of these guidelines to meet their individual needs. The guidelines of most states are similar to those adopted by the ADA, but we recommend that all dentists review the exact guidelines they are expected to follow.

The ADA's House of Delegates has provided definitions for sedation and general anesthesia (see box below). The House of Delegates defines *conscious sedation* as "a minimally depressed level of consciousness that retains the patient's ability to independently and continuously maintain an airway and respond appropriately to physical stimulation or verbal command and

Definitions of sedation and general anesthesia

Conscious sedation

A minimally depressed level of consciousness that retains the patient's ability to independently and continuously maintain an airway and respond appropriately to physical stimulation or verbal command and that is produced by a pharmacologic or nonpharmacologic method or a combination thereof.

Deep sedation

An induced state of depressed consciousness accompanied by partial loss of protective reflexes, including the inability to continually maintain an airway independently and/or to respond purposefully to physical stimulation or verbal command, and that is produced by a pharmacologic or nonpharmacologic method or a combination thereof.

General anesthesia

An induced state of unconsciousness accompanied by partial or complete loss of protective reflexes, including the inability to continually maintain an airway independently and respond purposefully to physical stimulation or verbal command, and that is produced by a pharmacologic or nonpharmacologic method or a combination thereof.

ADA Policy Statement on Use of Conscious Sedation, Deep Sedation and General Anesthesia in Dentistry; as adopted by the American Dental Association House of Delegates, October 2000.

that is produced by a pharmacological or non-pharmacological method or a combination thereof" [1]. The drugs and techniques that are acceptable for producing conscious sedation should have a reasonably large therapeutic index, making it unlikely that the patient will lose consciousness [1]. Depressing the level of consciousness to the point at which the patient's only response is a reflex withdrawal from painful stimulation is well outside of the range of conscious sedation and is to be avoided. Conscious sedation is NOT to be used as a way to reduce pain during dental treatment! Local anesthesia is still required as the principle means for eliminating the sensation of orofacial pain during treatment. Conscious sedation may make the process of local anesthetic administration much more acceptable to the patient, however.

In contrast, the ADA defines *deep sedation* as "an induced state of depressed consciousness accompanied by partial loss of protective reflexes, including the inability to continually maintain an airway independently and/ or to respond purposefully to physical stimulation *or* verbal command..." [1]. Deep sedation is similar to *general anesthesia*, with the only difference being that a state of unconsciousness is induced with general anesthesia.

It should be clear from these definitions that maintaining a certain level of responsiveness in which the patient is capable of responding appropriately to stimuli is an important safety consideration in conscious sedation. As long as the patient maintains this level of consciousness there is a high degree of safety with any chosen sedation technique. Once protective reflexes become compromised, especially the ability to maintain and clear one's airway, the person providing the sedation assumes a greater responsibility for the patient's well-being and must have the appropriate training and certifications to do so.

Patient selection and preparation

Physical assessment

An important step in determining whether any patient is a candidate for conscious sedation of any type is to have a thorough and current written medical history. This comprehensive medical history should include a review of the major physiologic systems (ie, cardiovascular, respiratory, central nervous, endocrine, hepatic, and renal). Particularly close attention should be given to the central nervous, respiratory, and cardiovascular systems because the actions of sedative agents and the physiologic responses to stress may have profound effects on these three specific systems. Information about the hepatic and renal systems provides valuable information about the patient's ability to effectively metabolize and eliminate certain medications that require these organ systems for their deactivation. Careful assessment of the central nervous system function alerts the dentist to disease processes (eg, seizure disorder) or medical therapies that may have an impact on the selection and dosage of sedative agents (eg, depression). Finally, the medical history must include a current list of all prescription and over-the-counter medications (including "herbal," "alternative," or "complimentary" medications) that are taken by the patient, and any drug allergies and unpleasant side effects. It is prudent to extend the inquiry about medications to include any that may have been discontinued within the last 6 months.

Most clinicians ask their patients or the patient's guardian to complete a written health questionnaire. The completed questionnaire should be reviewed with the patient to verify specific responses, obtain more in-depth information, and make sure that all the questions were understood by the person completing it. The medical history should be updated at a minimum of every 6 months. It also is wise to inquire at each appointment whether there have been any changes to the history since the last visit.

A basic physical inspection of the patient also provides valuable information that may be useful in making determinations about whether conscious sedation can be used safely. Besides looking for obvious physical signs that are suggestive of systemic conditions (eg, shortness of breath in response to minimal physical exertion, distended jugular veins when seated, the scent of acetone on the breath), observe the patient for signs of fear (eg, sweaty palms, nervous tremor in the voice). Included in this initial physical assessment of the patient are their baseline vital signs, consisting of blood pressure, heart rate, respiratory rate, and temperature. Because the dosages of some sedative medications depend on the patient's weight, information about their height and weight should also be recorded. Besides measuring and recording vital signs at the initial screening appointment, it is recommended that the vital signs be measured and recorded immediately before administering any sedatives or local anesthetics.

If one has any concerns or questions about a patient's responses to the medical history questionnaire or one's physical findings during the patient inspection, consideration should be given to consulting their physician. One should be specific in the request to the physician. Most importantly, one should be sure to include the nature of any abnormal or questionable findings from the assessment, specifics about the proposed procedure, and information about the patient's anticipated response and ability to tolerate the proposed procedure. Be sure to ask for a written confirmation of this consultation to complete documentation.

A useful method of assessing the level of risk involved in treating a patient is to assign a physical status classification to the patient. A classification scheme that is easy to use has been developed by the American Society of Anesthesiologists (ASA) [2]. This classification scheme is presented in the following box (American Society of Anesthesiologists, 1963). As the patient's classification number increases, so does the inherent risk for evoking unwanted medical complications during dental treatment. ASA I and II patients are the most appropriate to receive conscious sedation for dental appointments. The general health of ASA I and II patients is reasonably good, and there is minimal likelihood that the physiologic stressors of the dental procedure, local anesthetics, or the sedative will precipitate a significant medical complication. In contrast, more severe, life-threatening systemic disease dictates that a patient receives an ASA classification greater than II. An ASA status greater than II indicates the likelihood of a high level of risk when treating these patients in normal situations without taking appropriate precautions. In some situations, the use of sedation may be appropriate in this more seriously compromised patient population as a way of reducing the physiologic stress the dental procedure may produce. Providing sedative medications during dental treatments with some of these compromised patients (eg, ASA III) is not advised without first consulting the patient's primary physician. Serious consideration should be given to having someone with more training in

---

Physical status classification for patients as defined by the American Society of Anesthesiologists (ASA)

ASA I: A normal healthy patient

ASA II: A patient with mild systemic disease (eg, well-controlled hypertension)

ASA III: A patient with severe systemic disease (eg, congestive heart failure)

ASAIV: A patient with severe systemic disease that is a constant threat to life (eg, unstable angina)

ASA V: A moribund patient who is not expected to survive without the operation

ASA VI: A declared brain-dead patient whose organs are being removed for donor purposes

(E: Emergency operation of any variety; used to modify one of the above classifications [ie, ASA II-E])

Adapted from American Society of Anesthesiologists. New classification of physical status. Anesthesiology 1963;24:111; with permission.

---

sedation techniques and treating medically compromised patients deliver the sedation to these patients in the most appropriate clinical setting.

Once these topics have been considered, informed treatment decisions can be made that minimize the level of risk. Dental treatments are elective procedures in most situations. Therefore, one should not initiate treatment if one's physical assessment results in uncertainty about the health status of the patient.

Psychologic assessment

Fear of dental treatment is an indication that some form of sedation may need to be considered and discussed with the patient. Fearful dental patients can identify several dental instruments and procedures that contribute to their dislike of dentistry. Dental treatments that involve the use of syringes to deliver local anesthetic solutions intraorally and rotary handpieces to prepare hard tissues are consistently cited as producing fear during dental treatment [3–7]. Although these and other physical stimuli inherent to dentistry are capable of producing the psychologic response of fear, they also evoke many physiologic consequences. Increases in the heart rate and blood pressure are among the physiologic changes that accompany dental fear during treatment situations, and indicate profound activation of the sympathetic nervous system. Extreme elevations of these specific vital signs are not well tolerated by some patient populations (eg, persons with angina), and need to be avoided. The best way to prevent these undesirable physiologic changes is to identify what evokes them and take actions to eliminate or reduce their occurrence before initiating treatment.

The patient's behavior may provide clues that the patient is fearful. Behaviors such as not seeking dental care on a regular basis, frequently canceling dental appointments, and arriving late are subtle clues that dental fear is present. Tightly gripping the arms of the dental chair and the asking of numerous questions immediately before a procedure are examples of more overt demonstration of dental fear. Asking the patient or their caregiver about their possible fear of dental treatment is appropriate in these situations. Unfortunately, many patients are embarrassed about their dental fear and are uncomfortable talking about it with their dentist. Once the patient feels comfortable talking with the dental team and is sure that they will not be ridiculed or have negative judgments made about them secondary to their dental fear, the dentist can start to explore treatment options that may minimize the unpleasantness of the situation. Each patient is their own "gold standard" about how dentistry affects them. Questions about the patient's use of dental services (eg, how long since the last visit to the dentist) and their concerns about dental treatment may begin a dialogue that makes the dentist more aware of the treatment challenges that may be ahead.

Standardized questionnaires also can determine the level of fear that dental situations evoke in patients. The Dental Anxiety Scale [8] is among the most widely used instruments to determine how fearful patients are about dental treatment (see box). This particular questionnaire is short and can be completed in a few minutes by most adults. Points are assigned to the patient's choices, ranging from one point for selecting choice (a) through five points for selecting (e). Total scores range between 4 and 20, with scores in the range of 13 or greater being suggestive of at least a moderate degree of dental fear [9].

Patient preparation

After completing the physical and psychologic assessments of the patient, it is time to prepare the patient for the upcoming sedation appointment. This includes providing information about the delivery of the sedative agents, discussing what to realistically expect, answering any questions, and obtaining consent. One of the most important considerations that has an impact on the success of the sedation is being assured that the patient is well informed and has the correct set of expectations. Too often patients have the impression that they will be "knocked out" (ie, asleep) for the appointment. It is important that the patient have an understanding of what is meant by conscious sedation. The ability of inhalational and oral sedation methods to provide relaxation is an important attribute to emphasize when discussing treatment options with the patient. When one is considering using a sedative that produces amnesia, the more skeptical patient may be more willing to

Dental anxiety scale

Questions

1. If you had to go to the dentist tomorrow, how would you feel about it?
   a. I would look forward to it as a reasonably enjoyable experience
   b. I would not care one way or the other
   c. I would be a little uneasy about it
   d. I would be afraid that it would be unpleasant and painful
   e. I would be very frightened of what the dentist might do
2. When you are waiting in the dentist's office for your turn in the chair, how do you feel?
   a. Relaxed
   b. A little uneasy
   c. Tense
   d. Anxious
   e. So anxious that I sometimes break out in a sweat or almost feel physically sick
3. When you are in the dentist's chair waiting while he gets his drill ready to begin working on your teeth, how do you feel?
   a. Relaxed
   b. A little uneasy
   c. Tense
   d. Anxious
   e. So anxious that I sometimes break out in a sweat or almost feel physically sick
4. You are in the dentist's chair to have your teeth cleaned. While you are waiting and the dentist is getting out the instruments that he will use to scrape your teeth around the gums, how do you feel?
   a. Relaxed
   b. A little uneasy
   c. Tense
   d. Anxious
   e. So anxious that I sometimes break out in a sweat or almost feel physically sick

From Corah NL. Development of a dental anxiety scale. J Dent Res 1969;48:596; with permission.

accept the sedation treatment plan. The importance of having the patient able to participate during some aspects of the procedure may need to be emphasized, thus making conscious sedation the most effective manner in which to proceed. Most importantly, the patient needs to recognize that the primary objectives of one's sedation treatment plan are their safety and comfort.

Training requirements

As seen in other articles in this issue, there are many wonderfully effective options when it comes to sedating the adult dental patient. A great deal of emphasis has been placed on the use of N_2O/O_2 inhalational sedation and single enteral agent sedations (especially with benzodiazepines).

To administer N_2O/O_2 inhalational sedation either alone or in combination with a single enteral agent, however, a minimal level of training is required. The amount of training required to administer these conscious sedation modalities is under the jurisdiction of each state or region. Regardless of whether any sedation techniques are used in a dental practice, the dentist and all staff involved in patient care need to be certified in the level of Basic Life Support (BLS) commensurate for healthcare providers. BLS recertification is required at least every 2 years because the guidelines are continually updated based on the results of ongoing research in the area of resuscitation. Effective use of some or all of the BLS skills in emergency situations is necessary to keep critical tissues like the brain and heart perfused with oxygenated blood. The most important of the BLS skills to master when sedation is part of the dental practice are assessing and maintaining the patency of the airway and delivering positive pressure ventilation to the patient having respiratory difficulty. Diligence in monitoring the airway, the adequacy of ventilation, and early recognition and corrective measures of airway and ventilation problems are necessary to keep respiration-related complications from becoming more serious.

Besides maintaining current certification in BLS, the ADA suggests that the dentist administering conscious sedation with a single enteral agent, the inhalation of nitrous oxide and oxygen, or a combination of single enteral agent and of nitrous oxide and oxygen meet certain training criteria. First, the dentist should successfully complete to the level of competency didactic and clinical training consistent with Part I and Part III of the ADA's Guidelines for Teaching the Comprehensive Control of Anxiety and Pain in Dentistry. This training is part of the predoctoral dental curriculum of all accredited dental schools in the United States. Postdoctoral training programs in the United States that offer comprehensive training in the areas of conscious sedation with a single enteral agent and the inhalation of nitrous oxide and oxygen may also satisfy the training criteria. Of course, the regulations of each state or geographic region outline the absolute training requirements to provide this type of conscious sedation. For example, the State of Washington requires that the dentist administering conscious sedation with a single enteral agent or N_2O/O_2 have completed a minimum of 14 hours of either predoctoral dental school or postgraduate instruction that includes the pharmacology and physiology of these sedative agents. To prescribe and purchase enteral sedatives, the dentist must also be registered with the Drug Enforcement Administration (DEA) of the United States Department of Justice.

General office preparedness

Medical emergencies occur in the dental setting regardless of whether conscious sedation is part of the practice repertoire. As long as the sedated patient maintains a level of consciousness in which they are able to respond appropriately to verbal commands and physical stimulation and can maintain control over their protective reflexes, the likelihood of serious medical emergencies is minimal. Even though the likelihood of medical emergencies is rare when sedating patients with N_2O/O_2 either alone or in combination with a single enteral agent, a certain level of preparedness is essential. *Dental treatment needs to be suspended at the first sign of a problem.* Remember, the anesthesia permit holder/provider is responsible for the anesthetic management, adequacy of the facility, and the treatment of emergencies associated with the administration of enteral or combination inhalation-enteral conscious sedation.

As mentioned earlier in the section on training requirements, maintaining current certification in BLS is a requirement for the person administering the sedation, and is highly recommended for all members of the staff that participate in patient care. The responsible administration of sedative agents and monitoring of the sedated patient make it unlikely that cardiopulmonary resuscitation will be necessary. A subset of BLS skills may be necessary in extreme situations, however. For example, in the rare situations in which the patient loses consciousness, positioning the patient's head in a way that keeps the airway patent may become necessary. In extreme situations of depressed consciousness, it also may be necessary to provide positive pressure ventilation with oxygenated air to the lungs until normal respiratory function is restored. Early recognition and treatment of inadequate respiratory function is important in preventing the more serious cardiac complications that begin to appear after prolonged periods of hypoxia.

An emergency kit needs to be readily available when using conscious sedation. An emergency kit can be either bought from a commercial vendor or custom made. Although the commercial kits are a convenient method for compiling and storing all of the drugs and supplies that may be indicated for treating medical emergencies, they tend to be expensive. These kits also tend to contain equipment and drugs that are not indicated in the initial response to an emergency, or one may not be trained in their indications or use (eg, adenosine, laryngoscopes). In contrast, one can make an emergency kit that specifically addresses one's needs and the emergencies one will most likely encounter. The contents of the emergency kit should be in one container that is easily identified and easy to transport. Make sure that the office staff knows where to find the kit and how to use the basic equipment it contains. The contents of a basic emergency kit are listed in the following box. Perhaps the single most important piece of equipment in the emergency kit, especially if one performs sedation, is a device for delivering positive pressure ventilation (eg, bag-valve-mask). Routine inspections of emergency equipment and drugs, including the adequacy of the oxygen supply, should be performed and documented. Don't forget to check the expiration dates on all of the emergency medications during these inspections.

The inclusion of flumazenil (the competitive receptor antagonist for the benzodiazepine drug class) makes the emergency kit used for sedation

---

Contents suggested for a basic dental office emergency kit when using nitrous oxide/oxygen inhalational sedation and enteral sedation

Emergency equipment

- Stethoscope
- Blood pressure cuffs (adult and large adult sizes)
- A mechanism for delivering positive pressure oxygen (eg, self-inflating bag-valve device)
- Clear face masks
- High-volume suction tubing and yankauer suction tips
- Syringes (1-ml tuberculin, 3-ml, 10ml)
- Needles (27-gauge, 20-gauge)
- Dilution fluids (sterile water, 0.9% sodium chloride)
- Alcohol sponges
- Gauze
- Oral and/or nasal airways

Emergency drugs

- Oxygen (at least one portable "E"-sized cylinder with regulator)
- Epinephrine (1:1000 = 1 mg/ml × 3, or an EPI-Pen® × 2)
- Diphenhydramine (Benadryl®, 50 mg/ml)
- Albuterol inhaler (Proventil®)
- Glucose (eg, cake frosting)
- Nitroglycerine (spray or paste)
- Aspirin
- Flumazenil (Romazicon®, benzodiazepine antagonist)

slightly different from the one used in general dental situations. If benzodiazepines are being used to produce sedation, flumazenil needs to be readily available. Although the intravenous route of administration for flumazenil is preferred, especially in the hospital emergency room setting, it can also be administered by way of other routes like sublingual, intramuscular, or rectal [10]. Compared with IV administration, the latency to reverse the complication of profound respiratory depression is slightly longer when using these other routes, requiring a couple of additional minutes. Next to the IV route, the sublingual and IM routes have the next fastest onsets, respectively [10]. Although the outcome of reversing the effects of the benzodiazepine is similar regardless of the route of flumazenil administration, one must be prepared to provide positive pressure ventilation for a slightly longer period of time to adequately oxygenate the patient because of the delay in achieving sufficient blood levels of the antagonist when administered intramuscularly or sublingually.

Having a medical emergency kit readily available is only part of the picture when assessing the preparedness of a dental office that uses sedation. Proper training in the use of the kit's contents is also important. This training should extend beyond the dentist to include other key office personnel that participate directly in patient care (eg, dental assistants and hygienists). In some situations the dentist may not be readily available or able to direct or administer the delivery of emergency care, so others in the office need to be prepared.

Attention also should be given to how the Emergency Medical System (EMS) will be activated if needed. When training office personnel about EMS activation, it is important that they know the telephone number to call (911 in practically all areas in the United States), and how to report the pertinent emergency information. The person activating EMS should be prepared to provide important information that will be asked by the operator regarding the location of the emergency. It is helpful to post the address (including the exact location inside office parks and medical complexes like outpatient clinics) and the phone number of the office on or near each phone to help the person activating the EMS. The person activating EMS may also be responsible for meeting the EMS at the street when they arrive or for reserving an elevator in the building to expedite their arrival at the scene.

Conducting regular emergency drills is a good way of assessing how well the office is prepared to handle medical emergencies, including those emergencies that are related to sedation. These drills serve to reinforce each person's responsibility during the emergency and provide an opportunity to practice the skills. Just like so many other skills, the skills necessary to perform emergency procedures and protocols like positive pressure ventilation and EMS activation can be easily forgotten if not used on a regular basis. Emergency drills should therefore be conducted at a *minimum* of once per year. One of the most important parts of the emergency drill is the critique that follows. Providing each member of the team with feedback about their performance is the only way they will know whether they performed their tasks adequately. It is important to identify tasks they may not have performed satisfactorily, and provide an opportunity for personnel to learn or practice those tasks to proficiency. Don't forget that it is equally important during the critique to acknowledge tasks that were done well. Office personnel should also feel comfortable in performing the tasks they are assigned, and should be given the opportunity to relinquish any tasks that may make them uncomfortable or that they cannot perform.

Summary

There are many safe and effective medications available to the dental practitioner for producing conscious sedation. Given the many sedatives available, all possessing slightly different clinical characteristics and various degrees of risk, careful consideration needs to be given to the objectives of the sedation when deciding which pharmacologic agents to use. Before making plans to sedate dental patients, however, one needs to make sure that several "layers" of risk management are in place to ensure the sedation procedure is as safe as possible.

Included in this risk management plan is a complete understanding of the regulations that define conscious sedation and the training that is required to deliver this state of depressed consciousness. Careful attention also needs to be given to selecting appropriate dental patients for sedation. A thorough understanding of the patient's physical and psychologic status is necessary when making decisions about sedation. Because most dental disease is not life threatening, dental treatment needs tend to be primarily elective in nature. Considering the training requirements for delivering inhalational or enteral conscious sedation with a single agent, it is prudent to limit this type of sedation to the patient population that is healthy (eg, ASA I and II) and psychologically stable as a way of minimizing risk. The amount of additional risk one encounters when sedating more medically compromised patients (ASA III and greater) should suggest that deferring elective dental treatments until the health status improves is prudent. In situations in which an improvement in the patient's health status is not likely, referral to someone with more experience sedating medically compromised patients is strongly recommended. Equally important to the conscious sedation risk management plan is an assurance that the patient understands what is meant by conscious sedation and that their treatment expectations are realistic. Finally, even though conscious sedation is safe when all precautions are followed, being prepared to manage unexpected sedation-related emergencies is necessary.

The principles of risk management covered in this article are applicable to other articles in this issue, in which N_2O/O_2 inhalational sedation and enteral sedation in adults and children are discussed. The remaining article in this section that reviews the prevention of medical emergencies and the pharmacologic agents necessary to treat emergency events that are likely to occur in dental settings further enhances the level of preparedness necessary when administering conscious sedation to adults and children.

References

[1] American Dental Association House of Delegates. Guidelines for the use of conscious sedation, deep sedation and general anesthesia for dentists. Address at: www.ada.org/prof/ed/guidelines/cs-guide.html 2000. Accessed March 26, 2002.

[2] American Society of Anesthesiologists. New classification of physical status. Anesthesiology 1963;24:111.

[3] Bernstein DA, Kleinknecht RA, Alexander LD. Antecedents of dental fear. J Pub Health Dent 1979;39:113–24.

[4] Gale E. Fears of the dental situation. J Dent Res 1972;51:964–6.

[5] Kleinknecht RA, Klepac RK, Alexander LD. Origins and characteristics of fear of dentistry. J Am Dent Assoc 1973;86:842–5.

[6] Milgrom P, Getz T, Weinstein P. Recognizing and treating fears in general practice. Dent Clin N Am 1988;32:657–65.

[7] Milgrom P, Weinstein P, Getz T. Treating fearful dental patients: a patient management handbook. Seattle (WA): Continuing Dental Education, University of Washington; 1995.

[8] Corah NL. Development of a dental anxiety scale. J Dent Res 1969;48:596.

[9] Corah NL, Gale EN, Illig SJ. Assessment of a dental anxiety scale. J Am Dent Assoc 1978;97:816–9.

[10] Heniff MS, Moore GP, Trout A, et al. Comparison of routes of flumazenil administration to reverse midazolam-induced respiratory depression in a canine model. Acad Emerg Med 1997;4:1115–8.

THE DENTAL
CLINICS OF
NORTH
AMERICA

Dent Clin N Am 46 (2002) 781–802

Inhalational and enteral conscious sedation for the adult dental patient

Douglass L. Jackson, DMD, MS, PhD[a],*,
Barton S. Johnson, DDS, MS[b]

[a]Department of Oral Medicine, University of Washington School of Dentistry,
B412 Health Sciences Building, Seattle, WA 98195, USA
[b]Departments of Restorative Dentistry and Hospital Dentistry, University of Washington
School of Dentistry, Seattle, WA 98195, USA

N_2O/O_2 inhalational sedation and enteral sedation are inherently well suited for inducing a level of central nervous system (CNS) depression that is consistent with conscious sedation for a broad population of dental patients. With the appropriate patient population and sufficient training and office preparedness, these two sedation techniques are safe and effective. As discussed elsewhere in this issue, the amount of training necessary to deliver these forms of conscious sedation is considerably less than that required to provide parenteral sedation and general anesthesia. Additionally, both of these forms of sedation have a high level of patient acceptance because the general population perceives minimal discomfort and inconvenience with these techniques. Given the unpleasant nature of many dental procedures, the use of these forms of sedation can make these dental treatment experiences more pleasant for the patient and the dental care providers.

Nitrous oxide is the only inhalational agent that is practical for producing conscious sedation. In contrast to only one inhalational sedative, many enteral sedatives are available, with many having applications in the dental treatment setting. The goal of this article is to comprehensively review N_2O/O_2 inhalational sedation and enteral sedation in the context of conscious sedation for adult dental patients. The pharmacologic properties of nitrous oxide and several oral sedatives are reviewed in this article. Additionally, the techniques of inducing sedation with these pharmacologic agents and monitoring the physiologic status of sedated patients are also discussed. The

* Corresponding author.
  E-mail address: jacksond@u.washington.edu (D.L. Jackson).

adaptation of these sedation techniques for the pediatric population of dental patients is covered in another article.

Nitrous oxide/oxygen inhalational sedation

The historical use of nitrous oxide as a clinical anesthetic is founded in the pioneering work of two dentists, Horace Wells and William T.G. Morton. Nitrous oxide remains one of dentistry's most valuable sedatives. Many physical and clinical properties account for the success of nitrous oxide as an inhalational sedative. The coadministration of nitrous oxide and oxygen results in a sedative technique that is safe and highly efficacious in a large population of mildly apprehensive dental patients. Besides producing sedation, nitrous oxide also produces analgesia and mild skeletal muscle relaxation. Although the exact mechanism of action for nitrous oxide's sedative and analgesic properties has been elusive, the CNS activation of opioid-dependent pathways [1], benzodiazepine receptors [2], and the inhibition of excitatory amino acid receptors [3] are among the likely candidates.

Physical properties, pharmacokinetics, and pharmacodynamics

At room temperature and one atmospheric pressure, nitrous oxide is a colorless nonflammable gas. Even though nitrous oxide is nonflammable, it supports combustion [4]. Nitrous oxide has a mild odor and taste that is described as pleasant by most patients. Additionally, this gas is not irritating to the mucosa of the respiratory system. Nitrous oxide is supplied as a liquid in equilibrium with its gas phase (the gaseous portion located above the liquid) in pressurized metal cylinders. The pressure of the equilibrated gas above the liquid in the cylinder is approximately 750 psi. Dispensing any of the gaseous contents from the cylinder results in a rapid vaporization of some of the remaining liquid to replace the lost gas and restore equilibrium. This action continues until there is no more nitrous oxide liquid in the cylinder to vaporize. Therefore, the gas pressure at the top of the cylinder remains at 750 psi until almost all of the liquid vaporizes. Once the liquid form is depleted there is a quick decline in gas pressure and a rapid depletion of the remaining gas in the cylinder. This property of nitrous oxide makes it difficult to determine with great accuracy how much gas remains in a pressurized cylinder. The most accurate (but inconvenient and impractical) way to determine how much nitrous oxide remains is by intermittently weighing each cylinder while it is in service.

Oxygen is always coadministered with nitrous oxide at a minimum concentration of 30% (the importance of coadministering oxygen with nitrous oxide and the accompanying safety considerations are discussed in greater detail a little later). Oxygen is also supplied in pressurized cylinders, having a pressure of approximately 2000 psi when full. In contrast to nitrous oxide, the oxygen in pressurized cylinders is only in the gaseous state. Therefore, the pressure displayed on the gas regulator is an accurate reflection of the amount of gas remaining in the cylinder (ie, 1000 psi means that half of the total gas supply remains).

The CNS depression that results in sedation depends on the concentration of the sedative in specific brain regions and how these concentrations change as the sedative agent attempts to achieve a state of equilibrium with other bodily tissues (eg, muscle, adipose stores). These same properties of sedation apply to the inhalation of nitrous oxide. Nitrous oxide is poorly soluble in blood. Being poorly soluble in blood results in a small percentage of nitrous oxide being removed from the inhaled mixture of gases in the lung's alveoli before a state of equilibrium is reached between the concentration of gas in the arterial blood supply and air in the alveoli. This property of nitrous oxide results in a rapid onset of sedation (induction) and a quick resolution of the sedative effects (emergence) when the gas is turned off.

A key factor that accounts for nitrous oxide's safety in the practice of dentistry is that it is not a potent anesthetic gas. The minimum alveolar concentration (MAC) is a convenient measure for comparing the potency of anesthetic gases. MAC is defined as the alveolar concentration of an anesthetic at which 50% of patients fail to respond to a standard surgical stimulus [5]. The MAC for nitrous oxide is approximately 105%. Because the nitrous oxide concentrations for producing sedation and analgesia in dental settings are typically in the range of 20–50%, reaching a state of CNS depression in which patients are nonresponsive is highly unlikely without the use of a hyperbaric chamber.

The poor solubility of nitrous oxide in blood and its mild potency are two of the characteristics that make N_2O/O_2 sedation well suited for conscious sedation in dentistry. The characteristics of nitrous oxide are ideally suited for titrating within a wide concentration range the amount of this inhaled sedative necessary to achieve a specific level of CNS depression. By communicating with the patient about the clinical signs of sedation they may or may not be experiencing, adjustments in the inhaled concentration can be made during the dental procedure as needed. This allows for changes in the level of sedation as needed (eg, deeper levels of sedation during the injection of local anesthesia versus lighter levels of sedation during the application of fluoride). The poor solubility of nitrous oxide in blood also means that the latency to observe the desired change in CNS depression after manipulating the inhaled concentration of the gas is short.

Because oxygen concentrations of at least 30% are always coadministered with nitrous oxide, adverse events related to hypoxia and tissue ischemia are not likely with this sedation technique. The cardiovascular and respiratory systems are minimally affected by N_2O/O_2 sedation. Nitrous oxide usually produces no clinically significant changes in cardiovascular function. It has weak myocardial depressant effects and mild sympathomimetic effects [6]. The result of these two opposing effects is usually no clinically evident net change in cardiovascular function. Similarly, nitrous oxide has minimal effects on respiratory function. Although nitrous oxide decreases tidal volume slightly, it also increases respiratory rate, producing a minimal net change in normal patients. Patients whose respiratory drive comes from low oxygen tensions in blood (eg, chronic obstructive pulmonary disease, emphysema), however, represent relative contraindication to N_2O/O_2 sedation. It is the concomitant administration of oxygen, not the nitrous oxide, which produces the problem in these patients. The administration of oxygen concentrations in excess of 30% may be sufficient to blunt the respiratory drive that is driven by hypoxia in these patients [7].

Administration technique and recovery

The induction of anesthesia with nitrous oxide is not technically difficult. An inspection of the system that delivers the gases is an important first step before sedating the patient. Making sure all of the necessary equipment is present and in working order facilitates a smooth induction by eliminating unnecessary technical distractions in the presence of the patient. Most importantly, this inspection should include making sure that an adequate supply of oxygen and nitrous oxide is available, that there are no gas leaks in the system, and that the scavenging system is working properly.

Although not suggested in the sedation guidelines in many states, measuring and recording baseline vital signs is highly recommended immediately before administering any sedative agent to a dental patient. This should include blood pressure, heart rate, and respiratory rate. After verifying that the baseline vital signs are within normal limits and that the consent for the anesthetic and the dental procedure has been obtained, it is time to begin the sedation procedure. Administering oxygen at a concentration of 100% is always the initial part of the induction. A total flow rate of 5–7 liters of gas per minute is typical for the average adult. Adequacy of the chosen flow rate can be determined by observing the reservoir bag on the machine delivering gas. If the bag is completely collapsed the gas flow rate needs to be increased. Conversely, if the bag is completely distended the gas flow rate needs to be decreased.

After establishing that the total gas flow rate is adequate and that the patient is comfortable, the titration of nitrous oxide should commence. Recognizing that there is a great deal of inter- and intrapatient variability in the concentration of nitrous oxide that produces sedation, initial titration at approximately 20% nitrous oxide is a prudent starting point. The rate of sedation induction with nitrous oxide depends on the concentration and the rate and depth of respiration. Instructing the patient to inhale and exhale exclusively through their nose at their regular respiratory rate and depth helps speed the induction. Because titration to the desired effect is one of the benefits of this inhalational technique, make sure that the patient is aware of the signs that the gas produces at concentrations relevant to sedation.

Among the signs and sensations of N_2O/O_2 sedation are feelings of relaxation, tingling in the extremities, circumoral numbness, floating or sinking sensations, changes in the perception of auditory stimuli, and bodily warmth. Titration of increasing concentration of nitrous oxide should continue until the patient is comfortable and experiences any set of these signs.

The delivery of dental treatment should begin once the patient reaches a comfortable level of sedation. By titrating the concentration of nitrous oxide, a higher percentage can be administered during more stressful portions of the procedure (50–70%), producing more profound sedation. In contrast, the concentration of nitrous oxide can be reduced to a lower concentration when the level of stress or stimulation is lower (20–40%). The dentist delivering N_2O/O_2 sedation needs to be attentive to the patient and the sensations they are experiencing, because certain symptoms indicate that nitrous oxide concentrations are too great. Among these symptoms are dysphoria, uncontrolled laughter, sweating, nausea, marked lethargy, unresponsiveness, and the inability to follow commands. The concentration of nitrous oxide should be either immediately decreased or discontinued if these symptoms are encountered.

On completion of the dental procedure or the portion of treatment for which N_2O/O_2 sedation was indicated, the flow of nitrous oxide is discontinued and 100% oxygen is delivered at the predetermined gas flow rate for 3–5 minutes. The poor solubility of nitrous oxide in blood also accounts for the rapid resolution of the signs and sensations of nitrous oxide sedation. Within the 3–5 minutes that the patient is breathing 100% oxygen, the signs and sensations of nitrous oxide sedation usually disappear. Engaging the patient in conversation is a good way for assessing their return to baseline.

The practice of delivering 100% oxygen for 3–5 minutes after nitrous oxide is discontinued has been advocated to prevent diffusion hypoxia. Diffusion hypoxia was first described in 1955 [8]. The poor solubility of nitrous oxide that facilitates a rapid induction also facilitates a rapid dissipation of the effect and removal of the gas from the bloodstream once the gas supply is decreased or discontinued. Because the excretion of nitrous oxide is greater than the uptake of nitrogen from room air in the alveoli, a dilution of alveolar oxygen can occur, resulting in hypoxia. The results of clinical studies measuring end-tidal oxygen concentrations and hemoglobin saturation by way of pulse oximetry in normal, healthy patients with normal respiratory rates, however, do not support this hypothesis because hypoxic conditions during recovery were not evident [9–11]. Although brief reductions in oxygen concentrations and hemoglobin saturations occur immediately after discontinuing nitrous oxide administration, levels indicating hypoxia are not evident, especially in populations of dental patients being treated with no other systemic medications. Collectively, these results suggest that diffusion hypoxia is not a significant problem in the dental setting. Even though diffusion hypoxia is not a concern in most dental patients who have received N_2O/O_2 sedation, it remains prudent to administer 100% oxygen to facilitate an uneventful recovery.

Although not suggested in most sedation guidelines, it is also prudent to measure and record the patient's vital signs once the recovery is complete and the patient is about to be dismissed. Unlike any of the other sedation techniques in which a pharmacologic agent is administered, an adult escort is not necessary at the completion of the procedure. Documentation that supports your assessment of the patient's return to baseline and the resolution of sedative effects is important because the patient can be released without an escort after treatment.

On rare occasions one may encounter a patient who requires more than the usual 3–5 minutes to have the signs and sensation of the inhalational sedation disappear. Although this can be disconcerting to the patient and the dentist, continuing to administer 100% oxygen to the patient, monitoring their vital signs, and reassuring them that this is a normal response in some patients is important. This should be continued until the patient recovers sufficiently to be dismissed from the office.

Safety precautions

Besides striving to effectively relieve patient fear, the dentist providing N_2O/O_2 sedation must also make sure that it is delivered safely. The systematic use of a risk management plan that assesses the patient's physical and psychologic health, as described earlier, is only one part of the process that increases the safety of this sedation technique. The analgesia machine that delivers the nitrous oxide and oxygen incorporates several safety features also. The most important of these safety features are the "fail safe" mechanism and color-coding and pin indexing of the compressed gas supply.

The most important safety feature of the analgesia machine ensures that the patient does not become hypoxic secondary to receiving a mixture of gases that does not contain enough oxygen. This "fail safe" mechanism never allows the delivery of nitrous oxide unless there is oxygen flowing through the machine. For example, if the compressed gas cylinder containing oxygen becomes empty during the procedure, the machine automatically shuts off and delivers no nitrous oxide. Similarly, if the dentist forgets to open the compressed gas cylinder containing oxygen, no nitrous oxide flows through the system for delivery to the patient.

Because the metal cylinders that contain compressed gas all look similar, additional safety mechanisms are in place. A couple of methods are used to distinguish the contents of the cylinders, making it unlikely to mistakenly connect a nitrous oxide cylinder to the oxygen portal of the analgesia machine. The simplest method involves the assignment of different colors to the cylinders depending on the gas they contain. All oxygen cylinders in the United States are green, and nitrous oxide cylinders are blue. If practicing outside of the United States, however, one should be aware that this color-coding system is not universal (eg, oxygen cylinders are white in Canada).

An additional method for preventing the inadvertent attachment of cylinders containing nitrous oxide to the oxygen portal of portable analgesia machines is the system of pin indexing. Two small holes have been drilled into the valve stem of each gas cylinder. These two small holes correspond to the location of two small pins that extend slightly from the section of the analgesia machine's yoke where the compressed gas cylinders connect. These pins of the machine fit snugly inside the holes of the cylinder. The location of the two pins (and the corresponding holes in the cylinder's valve stem) is different for each gas, making it impossible for the incorrect cylinder to be attached to the yoke. A modification of the pin index system has been developed for cylinders of compressed gas that are larger than the portable "E" size (centrally plumbed facilities). The thread size of the connectors for the larger cylinders ("D" and "G" sizes) is unique for each gas, making the inadvertent connection of nitrous oxide to oxygen receptacles impossible.

Even though the analgesia machine has several built-in safety features, the diligence of the operator is still the most important factor in assuring that nitrous oxide administration is safe. The most serious of reported complications involves inadvertent hypoxia and death as a result of plumbing mishaps involving reversal of the gas sources to the apparatus [12]. Dislodging of the pins from the pin index connector of portable units and crossing the connections of oxygen and nitrous oxide lines in facilities with central gas plumbing are the most likely causes of these types of mishaps.

Health hazards associated with nitrous oxide and their prevention

Although nitrous oxide is not acutely toxic, several reports have alerted healthcare professionals that there are significant risks associated with chronic exposure to nitrous oxide. Operating room personnel (eg, anesthesiologists, operating room nurses) and dentists seem to be at the greatest risk for chronic exposure because of the frequency that this anesthetic gas is used in their working environments. Because nitrous oxide is the fifth most common inhalant used for recreational purposes in the United States, adolescents are also at risk for the manifestations of toxicity secondary to chronic exposure [13].

The health hazards that have been indicated with acute and chronic nitrous oxide in the dental office have been extensively explored [14]. The health hazards most frequently associated with nitrous oxide are the production of adverse neurologic symptoms, impaired reproductive capability, and teratogenicity. The neurologic symptoms resemble those caused by a vitamin B12 deficiency. These symptoms include paresthesias, diminished proprioception and vibration sensation, cutaneous sensation, motor weakness, clonus or hyperreflexia, areflexia, autonomic dysfunction, gait disturbance, intellectual or behavioral impairment, and impaired visual acuity [15]. The mechanism through which chronic nitrous oxide exposure produces these symptoms is the irreversible oxidation of the cobalt ion of cyanocobalamin, thus preventing it from acting as a coenzyme in the production of methionine [14,16]. Clearly, many of these neurologic symptoms are not conducive to the practice of dentistry, so all members of the dental staff need to be aware of these risks and take appropriate measures to prevent inadvertent and intentional (recreational) chronic exposure.

The relationship between nitrous oxide exposure in the workplace and reproductive health is among the most frequently studied topics in reproductive epidemiology. Despite this attention, no clear consensus exists about the risk for outcomes like spontaneous abortion in humans [17]. It is clear that nitrous oxide exposure in laboratory animals causes malformations and decreases live litter size. The results of epidemiologic research suggest that exposure to unscavenged nitrous oxide for as little as 5 hours per week is associated with reduced fertility in women [18]. Similarly, unscavenged nitrous oxide also increases the risk for spontaneous abortion [17]. These are difficult studies to perform and analyze because of the possibility of selection bias in identifying the study population and recall bias among the participants. Additionally, improvements in the scavenging of nitrous oxide in dental offices make it difficult to compare the results of older studies with those conducted more recently. Despite these difficulties and possible limitations, it is prudent to have an effective scavenging method to protect the reproductive health of women in the office who are of reproductive age. Additionally, pregnant patients should not be administered nitrous oxide, and any pregnant office staff should not work directly with patients who are receiving nitrous oxide.

Active scavenging of nitrous oxide in the dental environment is the most effective way for minimizing one's chronic exposure to nitrous oxide. Current guidelines from the National Institute for Occupational Safety and Health (NIOSH) recommend that the time-weighted exposure to nitrous oxide not exceed 25 ppm for any healthcare worker. Because closed systems with endotracheal tubes are used when administering anesthetic gases to patients in the operating room environment, scavenging nitrous oxide and other gases is fairly easy, leading to minimal pollution of the workplace with traces of these gases. The dental operatory, however, offers a unique set of challenges for keeping the exposure at less than 25 ppm. For starters, the "open" system for administering the gas offers plenty of opportunities for gases to escape into the operatory. A good fit of the mask over the patient's nose is critical. The total gas flow also should not be excessive. Excessive gas flow through the system (as indicated by a fully inflated/distended reservoir bag) facilitates leaking of gas between the mask and the patient's face. Patients who talk a lot during nitrous oxide administration also contribute to pollution of the operatory. The scavenging mechanism for many analgesia machines occurs exclusively at the nosepiece, removing most of the nitrous oxide during patient exhalation. Talking and mouth breathing result in a fair amount of gas being exhaled through the mouth into the open air. The analgesia machine connections and its tubing also should be regularly inspected for leaks.

Enteral sedation with a single agent

Similar to N_2O/O_2 sedation, oral sedatives also have a place in the practice of dentistry. Several characteristics of the enteral route of administration make this route of administration for sedatives well suited for dentistry. Perhaps the most favorable characteristic of this administration route is the ease of administering the agents to most adult populations. Oral drug administration is not technically difficult and does not require special instrumentation to deliver the sedatives. Equally important is the high level of patient acceptance to receiving sedatives by mouth, compared with more invasive techniques required for parenteral sedative administration.

Despite the many favorable characteristics of enteral sedation, there are a few disadvantages that are inherent with this method. The prolonged latency to the onset of sedative effects introduces some inconvenience that can be overcome with adequate consideration given to the timing of drug administration. The most problematic aspect of the disadvantages, however, is the inability to titrate the drug administration to a desired endpoint of sedation. Accordingly, careful consideration needs to be given to determining the appropriate dose for each patient situation. There is also a great deal of inter- and intrapatient variability in the response to oral sedatives, adding to the unpredictability of the sedative effect. Variability in drug absorption across the gastrointestinal mucosa and the hepatic first-pass effect are among the factors that lead to the unpredictable nature of this mode of sedation. In the most serious of situations, a relative overdose of the sedative may be given, resulting in too much CNS depression, the loss of consciousness, and the ability of the patient to maintain their protective reflexes (eg, patent airway). At the other end of the variability spectrum is the relative underdosing of the patient. An apparent lack of efficacy occurs in these situations, leading to patient and dentist dissatisfaction. Patient recovery after enteral sedation presents another disadvantage. Unlike N_2O/O_2 sedation, the patient must have a responsible adult escort to take them home at the end of the procedure because of lingering blood concentrations of the drug that impair judgment.

Most states permit dentists to prescribe and administer single enteral agents (either alone or in combination with N_2O/O_2) without additional training or credentialing beyond their undergraduate dental school curriculum. If a dentist wishes to administer multiple enteral sedatives concomitantly, however, additional training and certification is necessary. This discussion focuses on the delivery of single sedative agents, either by oral ingestion or absorption across intraoral mucosa (transmucosal absorption). The following discusses the attributes and disadvantages of producing sedation in adults with the benzodiazepines, an imidazopyridine, antihistamines, and barbiturates. A discussion of the use of chloral hydrate for producing sedation can be found elsewhere in this issue.

Benzodiazepines

Perhaps the most used and safest group of sedative drugs found in dentistry are the benzodiazepines. To fully appreciate the many pharmacologic properties of the benzodiazepine drug class, a brief review of the gamma-aminobutyric acid (GABA) system of neurotransmission is necessary. GABA is one of the primary inhibitory neurotransmitters within the CNS. GABA is the ligand for a heterogenous group of membrane-bound receptors (GABA$_A$) found in several CNS regions. Activation of GABA-dependent pathways within the CNS results in many effects that may be beneficial to capitalize on in the dental setting. These beneficial effects of GABA-mediated neurotransmission include anxiolysis, muscle relaxation, and generalized CNS depression. Of particular importance is the GABA$_A$ receptor activation of cerebral cortex regions that formulate emotional responses, such as the limbic system. GABA$_A$ receptors are associated with opening chloride ion channels on postsynaptic neurons. The net result is an increase in the conductance of chloride ions to the intracellular space of neurons (hyperpolarization), and the accompanying increase in stimulus strength needed to activate the affected postsynaptic neurons.

There are many different benzodiazepines, each having its own subtle pharmacologic difference. In general, the benzodiazepine drug class has a wide margin of safety, making them ideal for many dental applications. This wide margin of safety for benzodiazepines is because of their indirect mechanism that increases GABA-mediated effects. Rather than binding directly to the GABA$_A$ receptor-binding site, benzodiazepines bind to the omega receptor (formerly known as the "benzodiazepine receptor") of the GABA$_A$ receptor complex [19]. Benzodiazepine binding to the omega receptor increases the binding affinity of GABA for its binding site on the GABA$_A$ receptor complex, resulting in an increased frequency in opening of its associated chloride channel [20]. This increase in intracellular chloride ions produces a state of neuronal hyperpolarization and the apparent inhibition of the postsynaptic neuron with the usual amount of synaptic activity.

The benzodiazepines have a wide variety of uses. They have selective antianxiety properties, some somnolence, strong anticonvulsant properties, and centrally mediated muscle relaxation. Some of the benzodiazepines also produce mild to profound anterograde amnesia. The effects the dentist wishes the patient to experience greatly influence which benzodiazepine to dispense. Table 1 compares the benzodiazepines commonly used dentistry.

A significant part of the decision-making process when selecting a benzodiazepine for conscious sedation should include the drug's pharmacokinetic properties (ie, getting the drug to and from the receptor) and its pharmacodynamic properties (ie, the drug effect occurring at the receptor). Once in the bloodstream, most of the benzodiazepines are heavily bound to plasma proteins such as albumin, resulting in less than 5% of the ingested dose being free to bind to the receptor and exert an effect. This means that in patients

Table 1
Enteral sedatives used for conscious sedation in dentistry that bind to the omega (benzo-diazepine) receptor

Omega receptor agonist	Suggested adult enteral dose	Estimated working time	Miscellaneous
Diazepam (Valium®)	5–15 mg	1–2 h	Prototypic benzodiazepine Needs to be taken 1 h before appointment Active metabolites that can produce sedation for 2–3 days Excellent muscle relaxant Not recommended for elderly patients or those with impaired liver function
Triazolam (Halcion®)	0.25–0.5 mg	1 h	Rapid onset Needs to be taken 30–45 min before appointment Excellent anxiolytic Frequently produces amnesia Works well with N_2O/O_2
Midazolam (Versed®)	0.5 mg/kg	1 h	Rapid onset Excellent anxiolytic Frequently produces amnesia Available as an oral suspension (2 mg/ml) Works well with N_2O/O_2 Expensive
Alprazolam (Xanax®)	0.5–1 mg	1–2 h	Needs to be taken 1 h before appointment Excellent anxiolytic
Lorazepam (Ativan®)	1–2 mg	2–3 h	Needs to be taken 1–2 h before appointment Excellent anxiolytic
Zolpidem (Ambien®)	10 mg	1 h	Imidazopyridine drug class, NOT a benzodiazepine Rapid onset Needs to be taken 20–30 min before appointment Excellent anxiolytic Works well with N_2O/O_2
Receptor antagonist Flumazenil (Romazicon®)	0.2–1.0 mg	1 h	Best if given IV Acceptable absorption when given sublingual or IM[a] Dose should be increased if given Sublingual or IM[a] Because of the possibility of rebound sedation, the patient must be monitored for 60–75 min after antagonist administration

[a] *From* Heniff MS, Moore GP, Trout A, et al. Comparison of routes of flumazenil administration to reverse midazolam-induced respiratory depression in a canine model. Acad Emerg Med 1997;4:1115–8.

with reduced plasma protein (elderly patients, abusers of ethanol, patients suffering from malnutrition resulting in emaciation, and patients with severe liver disease), the benzodiazepine dose needed to achieve the desired effect may be considerably less than normal. As discussed later, the various benzodiazepines have distinct pharmacokinetic "personalities" that dictate their onset and duration of action profiles. The dentist should consider these "personality profiles" when selecting a benzodiazepine for a particular patient and procedure.

Another consideration when using benzodiazepines for conscious sedation is that many of them undergo oxidative metabolism by way of the hepatic cytochrome P450 enzymes. As a result, other medications the patient may be taking might significantly alter the amount of benzodiazepine that is available by either delaying the metabolism of the benzodiazepine or accelerating it. Thus, the dentist prescribing benzodiazepines should always refer to cytochrome P450 drug interaction tables when making decisions about administering benzodiazepines.

The adverse effect profile of benzodiazepines is minimal. Excessive CNS depression and respiratory depression occur in overdose situations. Excessive CNS depression is usually manifest as severe alterations in consciousness, ranging from weak or inappropriate responses to verbal commands or stimulation to the loss of consciousness. Depression of respiration (eg, patency of the airway, rate or depth of breathing) that requires intervention is an indication that an overdose has occurred. Careful dosing of the benzodiazepines decreases the likelihood of these adverse effects, but additive or supra-additive CNS depression is a reality with other drugs that produce CNS depression (ethanol, opioids, antidepressants). In situations in which a benzodiazepine is likely to contribute to severe respiratory depression and the inadequate oxygenation of the patient, the benzodiazepine receptor antagonist flumazenil may need to be administered in conjunction with positive pressure ventilation. Flumazenil needs to be readily available when using benzodiazepines to produce sedation (for review, see articles by Jackson and Johnson, and Haas in this issue). An interesting and not wholly unusual adverse reaction is simply paradoxic in nature. Instead of becoming more sedate and relaxed, affected patients become more agitated or fearful than they were before dosing with the benzodiazepine.

Benzodiazepines exhibit weak dependence liability, but addiction can occur with their prolonged use (addictions to benzodiazepines are among the most difficult to break). This class of sedative should be used with caution in patients with hepatic or renal disease because of obvious metabolism and excretion concerns, respectively. Similarly, caution is necessary when considering benzodiazepine sedation for patients with narrow-angle glaucoma because of their mild anticholinergic properties. All of these conditions should alert the dentist to the need for a consultation with the patient's physician. Given the high teratogenesis potential, benzodiazepines are not to be used with women who are or might be pregnant.

Diazepam (Valium®)

Perhaps the most familiar sedative agent in dentistry, diazepam has a long and successful record in helping relieve mild to moderate dental procedure-evoked anxiety. The "personality" of diazepam includes strong anti-anxiety effects but minimal somnolence and virtually no amnesia at orally prescribed doses. Diazepam is lipid soluble, which is important in the sedative's onset. Diazepam has long-acting metabolites (oxazepam and desmethyldiazepam), however, that have sedative properties. Consequently, the clinical duration of diazepam sedation tends to be moderate to long in length. Diazepam readily redistributes into lipid structures, and a clinical "rebound" effect can occur when this sequestered drug is re-released into the bloodstream after a meal. It is not uncommon for patients who have been sedated earlier to get drowsy after eating, so they should be warned of this possibility. Diazepam is supplied in 5- and 10-mg tablets. The typical adult dose is 5–10 mg daily (PO) 1 hour before the procedure. If patient sedation with this dose range is not successful (eg, patient experiences minimal signs of sedation), the dose can be cautiously increased to a total of 15–20 mg for subsequent sedations, paying close attention for the onset of unwanted side effects (eg, unresponsive to verbal commands). Diazepam is classified as Pregnancy Risk Category D. It is a substrate of the cytochrome P450 isozymes 2C19 and 3A4, so medications that activate or retard the activity of those isozymes affect the metabolism of diazepam.

Diazepam is an ideal medication for patients who are a bit anxious about the procedure and want "the edge taken off." It does not cause significant somnolence or amnesia, and is a poor choice when those are the desired effects. Another indication for diazepam is the patient who has been successfully sedated with it in the past and has great personal confidence in its ability to provide sedation for future treatments. Patients, especially the elderly and physically debilitated, should be warned that residual sedative effects are likely for the few days after the procedure. Accordingly, patients should exercise caution in making important decisions and may wish to refrain from driving and operating machinery during this period.

Triazolam (Halcion®)

Triazolam is one of the more potent benzodiazepines. It has a short half-life because it is rapidly redistributed and rapidly metabolized. Similar to the other benzodiazepines, triazolam is a full agonist at the omega receptor and potentiates the CNS depression produced by other sedatives. Triazolam's personality is one of rapid onset, short duration of action, and profound anterograde amnesia. Originally developed as a medication for treating insomnia, it has the ability to induce a somnolent state. Unfortunately, the suggested dose of triazolam for treating insomnia was too high when the drug was first introduced to the market, and the importance of medical supervision was not emphasized adequately [21]. Consequently, the early occurrence of unwanted side effects prompted many to question triazolam's safety. Careful review of the problems resulted in many changes in the way triazolam was prescribed, and the drug's safety is no longer in question.

The combination of probable amnesia and somnolence has brought triazolam into the forefront as a preferred sedative among dentists who use oral sedation in their practices [22,23]. Triazolam is supplied in 125 μg (0.125 mg) and 250 μg (0.25 mg) tablets. The typical adult dose is 250–375 μg PO or sublingual 30–45 minutes before the procedure. Clinical research suggests that the sublingual route for triazolam administration may be slightly more efficacious secondary to slightly higher plasma concentrations compared with the oral route [24]. Triazolam carries a Pregnancy Risk Category X, and must not be used if there is any possibility the patient might be pregnant. It is metabolized by the cytochrome P450 enzyme system.

Triazolam is well suited for the average dental appointment that lasts no more than 1 hour. The patient can come to the office early, take the sedative in the waiting room, and be comfortably sedate for their appointment within 30–45 minutes. Most appealing for this benzodiazepine is its profound amnesia. Patients have little or no recall the following day of details associated with their appointment. If coadministered with N_2O/O_2 inhalational sedation, the sedative effects can be as profound as a combined benzodiazepine/opioid intravenous sedation.

Some dentists have recently started to administer additional sublingual doses of triazolam when the clinical effects begin to wane and they want to perform additional dentistry during the appointment. There are little or no data to support the safety of this practice, and there is growing concern that many of these patients may become profoundly sedate, perhaps even losing consciousness, with more than one sedative administration within such a short window of time. Also, although many state laws allow "single oral agent" sedation, those laws were written with the intent that the "single agent" would be given as a "single dose." Although the practice of oral re-dosing may seem reasonable to those with a naive background in pharmacology, we urge dentists *not* to adopt this practice until scientific and legal issues regarding the method can be sorted out. Given the numerous scientific questions that remain with this practice, dentists choosing to adopt the technique of oral re-dosing with triazolam or any other oral sedative should obtain the additional training necessary to administer deeper levels of sedation and obtain a permit through their region's quality assurance division (eg, state licensing bureau). Additionally, we strongly recommend that physiologic monitoring be used and recorded at least every 15 minutes (preferably every 5 minutes during the procedure). This should most importantly include monitoring of airway patency and respiratory function (by way of a precordial/pretracheal stethoscope), tissue oxygenation (by way of pulse oximetry), blood pressure, and heart rate. This degree of monitoring is necessary when using sedation techniques with a greater risk for rendering the patient unconscious. Although probably not intentional, the practice of re-dosing falls into this category of risk.

Midazolam (Versed®)

Midazolam has been a popular benzodiazepine for parenteral sedation in dentistry since the mid 1980s. Midazolam has recently been gathering favor as an oral/transmucosal sedative also. Midazolam is known to have a marked first-pass effect in the liver, making the transmucosal route slightly preferable for achieving sedation. This can be either from nasal inhalation, rectal administration, or PO (with emphasis on maximizing the time spent retaining the solution in the mouth before swallowing). The typical dose is 0.25–0.5 mg/kg PO, maximum 20 mg 20–30 minutes before a procedure. Midazolam is supplied as an elixir (2 mg/mL) exclusively for oral administration, or as a 5-mg/mL solution (formulated for injection) that can be combined with a vehicle such as nonparticulate fruit juice or sugary powder (eg, Kool-Aid®) to make a reasonably palatable mixture. The drug is highly distasteful without some sort of alteration.

Because midazolam is expensive compared with other orally administered sedatives, often it is not cost effective to use in the adult population. Most of the oral/transmucosal administration of midazolam for dental sedation takes place in the pediatric dental environment. Although effective in the adult patient, midazolam by way of the enteral route is best for short procedures. The medication is classified as Pregnancy Risk Category D, and is a substrate for the CYP 3A4 isozyme. It has a personality similar to triazolam in that it can induce profound amnesia, moderate somnolence, and is short acting.

Lorazepam (Ativan®)

Lorazepam is one of the more hydrophilic benzodiazepines that are available for PO administration. The hydrophilic property of lorazepam makes it more difficult for this benzodiazepine to cross the blood–brain barrier. As a result, lorazepam has a longer time to the onset of sedation and requires a long time for recovery. Like diazepam, lorazepam has minimal somnolent and amnesic effects, giving a clinical profile of a long-acting anxiolytic agent. Unlike diazepam, it has no active metabolites, and is therefore devoid of rebound effects during the time surrounding the recovery. Lorazepam is supplied in 0.5-, 1-, and 2-mg tablets. The typical adult dose is 1–2 mg PO, 1–2 hours before the procedure. Lorazepam is also a Pregnancy Risk Category D drug. Lorazepam is not metabolized by the cytochrome P450 enzyme system.

Lorazepam is best suited for sedating the anxious patient who is undergoing long dental procedures (2–3 hours). Lorazepam is also a good sleep aid, taken at bedtime the night before the appointment, to help the anxious patient get a good night's sleep and be well rested before their appointment.

Alprazolam (Xanax®)

Alprazolam has the nice characteristic of having a half-life longer than triazolam but shorter than lorazepam. Alprazolam is almost a pure anxiolytic drug; it produces little or no amnesia or somnolence. It is supplied as 0.25-, 0.5-, 1-, and 2-mg tablets. The typical adult dose is 0.5–1 mg 1 hour before the procedure. It is classified as Pregnancy Risk Category D, and is a substrate of the CYP 3A4 isozyme. Recommendations for the use of alprazolam include when anxiolysis without somnolence is the major goal, and the dental appointment will be 1–2 hours in length.

Imidazopyridines

A novel addition to the sedative market is zolpidem (Ambien®). Zolpidem, a member of the imidazopyridine drug class, is distinct and unrelated to the benzodiazepines. Zolpidem binds to and stimulates a benzodiazepine omega receptor of the $GABA_A$ receptor complex, however. Similar to the benzodiazepines, zolpidem binding to the omega receptor increases the binding affinity of GABA for its binding site on the $GABA_A$ receptor complex, resulting in neuronal hyperpolarization and the apparent inhibition of the postsynaptic neuron with the usual amount of synaptic activity. Its clinical sedation actions therefore mimic those of the benzodiazepine family of sedatives (see Table 1). Classified as a hypnotic, one of zolpidem's most remarkable clinical attributes is its rapid onset and short duration of action. Clinically evident sedation is typically produced in approximately 20 minutes. Zolpidem's personality is such that it provides anxiety relief with strong hypnotic action. Some practitioners question, however, whether the anxiolytic actions of this medication are as profound as those of the benzodiazepines. In comparison with triazolam, zolpidem is less amnesic, provides less muscle relaxation, yet produces the same somnolence.

One of the greatest advantages and indications for zolpidem is in a busy dental practice, when a patient suddenly decides they would benefit from some anxiolysis. The rapid onset of sedative effects makes this an ideal consideration for an oral "rescue" medication in appropriate situations. Therefore, zolpidem is recommended for situations in which a rapid onset is advantageous and when amnesia is not necessary. Zolpidem is supplied as 5- and 10-mg capsules. Zolpidem is typically administered in a 10-mg dose at bedtime the night before the procedure to insure a good night's sleep, or the same dose 20 minutes before the procedure. It carries a Pregnancy Risk Category B.

Antihistamines

As commonly recognized, a side effect of antihistamines is sedation. Many dentists have come to rely on antihistamine-induced sedation, especially for treating pediatric patients. Although diphenhydramine (Benadryl®) is a good oral sedative for infants and toddlers, dentists more typically administer either promethazine (Phenergan®) or hydroxyzine (Vistaril®, Atarax®) for children and preteens. Orally administered antihistamines have limited efficacy for producing sedation. One method for improving the efficacy of orally administered antihistamines is to coadminister them with other sedatives. One popular antihistamine-containing "recipe" consists of meperidine, hydroxyzine, and scopolamine (also known as "DVS," an abbreviation for "Demerol®, "Vistaril®," and scopolamine). As discussed earlier, however, sedative combinations such as this one are classified as multi-agent sedation techniques and require more advanced training in conscious sedation and a special permit in most states and regions.

Promethazine is supplied as an elixir (5 mg/mL) or as suppositories (25 and 50 mg). The typical dose is 25–50 mg 1 hour before the procedure, resulting in a duration of sedative action approximately 4–5 hours in length. Hydroxyzine comes as a 2-mg/mL elixir and is typically administered at 2–4 mg/kg, (maximum dose of 75 mg). Hydroxyzine often works best in divided doses: 50 mg at bedtime the night before a procedure, 50 mg the morning of the appointment, and 50 mg 1 hour before the appointment. The duration of action for hydroxyzine is approximately 6 hours. Diphenhydramine is formulated as 25- and 50-mg tablets. Administering 25–50 mg 1 hour before the procedure results in adequate sedation.

As single oral agents, the antihistamines work well to produce a light and mild sedation with mostly somnolence. Although they are typically used to produce sedation with pediatric patients, their sedative effects are similar when used for adults. The most predictable and clinically useful sedative effects occur when antihistamines are combined with other sedative agents, requiring additional training and a special permit in most states and regions.

Barbiturates

The use of barbiturates (eg, pentobarbital, secobarbital) for their sedative properties has largely fallen out of favor in dentistry, and for good reason. Although the general mechanism by which barbiturates produce sedation at $GABA_A$ receptors is similar to that of the benzodiazepines, there are some important differences. Rather than binding directly to the $GABA_A$ receptor, barbiturates bind to another site on the $GABA_A$ receptor complex (not the omega receptor binding site used by benzodiazepines). Although barbiturate binding at this site also increases the binding affinity of GABA for its binding site on the $GABA_A$ receptor complex, the end result at the chloride channel is slightly different [19,25,26]. Rather than increasing the frequency at which the chloride channel opens like the benzodiazepines, barbiturates increase the duration of the channel opening, resulting in neuronal hyperpolarization. Unfortunately, barbiturates also have a direct effect on the chloride channel of the $GABA_A$ receptor complex. At higher doses, barbiturates can open the chloride channel directly, not requiring GABA. This direct mechanism makes it more likely that profound depression of the patient's CNS can occur, and if not recognized early and managed properly, severe disability, even death, can occur. Thus this class of sedatives is inherently more dangerous and does not offer any significant advantages. Accordingly, we do not recommend the use of enteral barbiturates in the dental setting unless there is physiologic monitoring of the patient's respiratory and cardiovascular systems and the dentist has sufficient advanced training in managing deeper levels of sedation and the complications that might be expected with profound CNS depression.

Administration technique and recovery

The induction of anesthesia with orally administered sedatives is not technically difficult because it only involves the swallowing of a pill or elixir by the patient. The timing of sedative administration in relation to when the dental treatment is to begin can be the greatest challenge. Ultimately, one would like the plasma concentrations of the sedative to be within the therapeutic range during the dental treatment. One would especially like the plasma concentrations of the sedative to be at their greatest during those parts of the treatment in which sedation helps the patient cope and the dentist perform the treatment. Decisions about when the sedative is to be taken by the patient should be based on the time required to reach peak plasma concentrations and when during the treatment this would be most beneficial. As was probably clear in the earlier sections on the individual oral sedative, the latency to reach peak plasma concentrations can be highly variable. Oral sedatives with latencies between 30–60 minutes have the greatest practicality for dentistry.

The latency for reaching plasma concentrations in the therapeutic range requires the dentist to make one important decision, specifically, should the sedative be taken at the office or at home (or en route to the office). Although there is great convenience in having the patient medicate on their own outside of the office, it is our recommendation that the patient take the sedative in the controlled environment of the dental office for reasons that involve risk management, for example, assessing the patient's baseline status and the effects (desired and undesired) of the sedative. Measuring and recording baseline vital signs is highly recommended immediately before administering any pharmacologic agent, especially sedatives. After verifying that the baseline vital signs are within normal limits and that all of the details surrounding the sedation have been taken care of (signing of consent documents, knowing that an adult escort will be present when the patient is to be dismissed), it is time to administer the sedative. By having the patient take the sedative in the office, one is also more sure about their level of compliance and understanding of the dosing instructions, such as when to take the medication and how much to take. The name of the sedative, the dose administered, and the time of administration need to be documented in the patient's chart. The patient should not be left unattended after taking the sedative. A family member, escort, or member of the office staff should be with the patient at all times.

Dental treatment delivery should begin once the patient reaches a comfortable level of sedation. The signs of sedation vary depending on the personality of the chosen sedative. Sometimes it takes a little longer than expected for the patient to reach this comfortable level of sedation, so patience may be warranted. If indicated, the efficacy of the oral sedative can be enhanced by the careful addition of nitrous oxide and oxygen in the manner described earlier. By varying the titration of N_2O/O_2, the depth of the sedation can be changed quickly on an as-needed basis. A tempting alternative method for increasing the efficacy of an oral sedative is to administer another dose of the same sedative. Considering the latency to reach therapeutic plasma concentrations, oral re-dosing is not practical. Additionally, there are likely to be situations in which this practice induces a greater level of CNS depression than is indicated or safe, which can be especially problematic if this occurs after the procedure's completion. Remember, the patient is to remain conscious, respond appropriately to verbal commands and stimuli, and maintain their protective reflexes. Failure to maintain any or all of these characteristics would suggest that an excessive amount of CNS depression is present and the patient's safety is in jeopardy unless the dentist has sufficient advanced training in managing deeper levels of sedation. Accordingly, we do not endorse the practice of re-dosing with any oral sedative as a method for increasing the efficacy or depth of the sedation.

Methods for monitoring physiologic status of the patient sedated with PO agents need to be in place during the procedure. The most important physiologic parameters that need monitoring include the level of CNS depression and the adequacy of respiratory function and ventilation of the lungs. Monitoring the status of the cardiovascular system is also important (blood pressure and heart rate), with the realization that it is not one of the organ systems that shows immediate changes as complications develop. Fortunately, the level of monitoring required for the patient who is receiving oral sedatives is not sophisticated, technically difficult to perform or interpret, or invasive for the patient.

Evaluating the patient's level of consciousness is generally sufficient for determining the amount of sedation-induced CNS depression present. As long as the patient retains the ability to respond appropriately to physical stimulation or verbal command, one is working within the range of conscious sedation. It is acceptable during conscious sedation for the latency of the patient's responses to be slower than normal, and their speech to be slurred in some situations.

The next most important physiologic parameter to monitor during sedation is the adequacy of respiratory function and ventilation of the lungs. The most serious of sedation-related complications is usually a consequence of the patient losing the ability to maintain their own airway without assistance.

As long as the patient maintains consciousness, the likelihood of this occurrence is small. If the patient lapses into a state of unconsciousness, however, the tongue and other soft tissues in the oropharynx loose their muscular tone and are able to partially or completely block the patency of the airway. If not corrected by positioning the head in a manner to relieve the blockage, a state of hypoxia develops quickly. There also is a concomitant build-up of carbon dioxide from cellular metabolism when the patency of the airway is blocked, resulting in an acidotic condition. With a prolonged combination of these two insults to homeostasis, the functioning of other systems becomes compromised. Most notably, neither neurons of the CNS nor cells of the myocardium tolerate these physiologic conditions well. Severe brain damage and death are likely consequences if the airway problems are not corrected.

Assessment of lung ventilation during oral sedation is simple and requires no special instrumentation. In the simplest of situations, talking with the patient, watching their chest rise and fall with each breath, feeling the warmth of expired air against your hand when it is passively in front of their mouth or nose, or watching the reflective surface of the dental mouth mirror alternate between foggy and clear when placed under the patients nose are all methods to evaluate ventilation of the lungs. The use of a pretracheal stethoscope connected to the operator's ear is another method for determining the patency of the airway and the rate and depth of the patient's breathing.

Although these methods are useful for determining whether the airway is open and capable of ventilating the lungs, they tell nothing about how well the tissue is being oxygenated. Pulse oximetry measures the percentage of oxygenated hemoglobin by evaluating the ratio of absorbed versus reflected light wavelengths at a peripheral site (fingertip, toe, bridge of the nose, or earlobe). Hemoglobin saturation of normal adults breathing room air is typically 97–100%. Although the hemoglobin saturation is likely to drop slightly in the sedated patient, it should NEVER decrease to less than 90%, because this equates to arterial oxygen tensions that would be approximately 60 mm Hg. Although the pulse oximeter is a valuable instrument for assessing oxygenation, direct techniques like assessing the movement of the chest and listening to the movement of air with a pretracheal stethoscope should be considered the "gold standard."

Dismissing the patient at the end of the procedure should only occur when the patient has recovered sufficiently from the effects of the sedative. Although a return to baseline levels of alertness are not likely because of the pharmacokinetics of oral sedation (eg, redistribution, hepatic metabolism), a certain level of recovery is necessary before dismissing the patient. This should minimally include the ability to hold a coherent conversation demonstrating that the patient is oriented to their surroundings, the ability to ambulate with minimal assistance, and vital signs that are close to those obtained at baseline. Once these criteria have been met, it is acceptable to dismiss the patient to a responsible adult escort. Documentation that supports your assessment of the patient's return to baseline and the adequate resolution of sedative effects should be recorded, together with any interventions that needed to be performed during the procedure or the recovery. Documentation in the patient's chart also needs to include the name of the adult escorting the patient from the office and the time they are dismissed.

Summary

There are clearly many safe and effective sedatives available to the dental practitioner for reducing patient fear and improving their level of comfort. Careful consideration needs to be given to the objectives of the sedation when deciding which pharmacologic agents to use because they all possess slightly different clinical characteristics and various degrees of risk. Patient selection also is critical when making decisions about sedation because the patient's expectations and general health status factor into keeping the procedure safe.

N_2O/O_2 sedation is an excellent choice for managing the mildly fearful dental patient or when minimal sedation is desirable. Among the sedatives administered enterally, the benzodiazepines are the most commonly used, and for good reason. These drugs are safe, effective, and offer a host of different personalities from which the dentist can choose. If used wisely and thoughtfully, the dentist can tailor the effects and duration of onset and recovery to the needs of the patient and the expected parameters of the appointment. When N_2O/O_2 sedation is combined with a single enteral sedative, a more profound level of CNS depression is achieved that can be modestly altered by changing the concentration of inhaled nitrous oxide.

With these many pharmacologic alternatives, many different dental patient populations can be sedated in a safe, effective manner, thus allowing the delivery of most dental treatments in a setting of reduced psychologic and physiologic stress. These pharmacologic sedatives have truly opened up a wonderful world of possibilities for the comfortable delivery of dental care, and should be integrated into every office's repertoire for delivery of care.

References

[1] Cahill FJ, Ellenberger EA, Mueller JL, et al. Antagonism of nitrous oxide antinociception in mice by intrathecally administered antisera to endogenous opioid peptides. J Biomed Sci 2000;7:299–303.

[2] Quock RM, Emmanouil DE, Vaughn LK, et al. Benzodiazepine receptor mediation of behavioral effects of nitrous oxide in mice. Psychopharmacology (Berl) 1992;107:310–4.

[3] Jevtovic-Todorovic V, Todorovic SM, Mennerick S, et al. Nitrous oxide (laughing gas) is an NMDA antagonist, neuroprotectant, and neurotoxin. Nat Med 1998;4:460–3.

[4] Neuman GG, Sidebotham G, Negoianu E, et al. Laparoscopy explosion hazards with nitrous oxide. Anesthesiology 1993;78:875–9.

[5] Eger II EI, Saidman LJ, Brandstater B. Equipotent alveolar concentrations of methoxy-flurane, halothane, diethyl ether, fluroxene, cyclopropane, xenon, and nitrous oxide in the dog. Anesthesiology 1965;26:756–63.

[6] Hohner P, Reiz S. Nitrous oxide and the cardiovascular system. Acta Anaesthesiol Scand 1994;38:763–6.

[7] Haas DA, Yagiela JA. Agents used in general anesthesia, deep sedation, and conscious sedation. In: Yagiela JA, Neidle EA, Dowd FJ, editors. Pharmacology and therapeutics for dentistry. 4th edition. St. Louis (MO): Mosby; 1998.

[8] Fink BR. Diffusion anoxia. Anesthesiol 1955;16:511–9.

[9] Einarsson S, Stenqvist O, Bengtsson A, et al. Nitrous oxide elimination and diffusion hypoxia during normo- and hypoventilation. Br J Anaesth 1993;71:189–93.

[10] Papageorge MB, Noonan LW, Rosenberg M. Diffusion hypoxia: another view. Anesth Pain Control Dent 1993;2:143–9.

[11] Quarnstrom FC, Milgrom P, Bishop MJ, et al. Clinical study of diffusion hypoxia after nitrous oxide analgesia. Anesth Prog 1991;38:21–3.

[12] Duncan GH, Moore PA. Nitrous oxide and the dental patient: a review of adverse reactions. J Am Dent Assoc 1984;108:213–9.

[13] McGarvey EL, Clavet GJ, Mason W, et al. Adolescent inhalant abuse: environments of use. Am J Drug Alcohol Abuse 1999;25:731–41.

[14] Yagiela JA. Health hazards and nitrous oxide: A time for reappraisal. Anesth Prog 1991;38:1–1.

[15] Iwata K, O'Keefe GB, Karanas A. Neurologic problems associated with chronic nitrous oxide abuse in a non-healthcare worker. Am J Med Sci 2001;322:173–4.

[16] Pema PJ, Horak HA, Wyatt RH. Myelopathy caused by nitrous oxide toxicity. Am J Neuroradiol 1998;19:894–6.

[17] Rowland AS, Baird DD, Shore DL, et al. Nitrous oxide and spontaneous abortion in female dental assistants. Am J Epidemiol 1995;141:531–8.

[18] Rowland AS, Baird DD, Weinberg CR, et al. Reduced fertility among women employed as dental assistants exposed to high levels of nitrous oxide. N Engl J Med 1992;327:993–7.

[19] Felpel LP. Antianxiety drugs and centrally acting muscle relaxants. In: Yagiela JA, Neidle EA, Dowd FJ, editors. Pharmacology and therapeutics for dentistry. 4th edition. St. Louis (MO): Mosby; 1998.

[20] Study RE, Barker JL. Cellular mechanisms of benzodiazepine action. JAMA 1982;247: 2147–51.

[21] Berthold CW, Schneider A, Dionne RA. Using triazolam to reduce dental anxiety. J Am Dent Assoc 1993;124:58–64.

[22] Bixler EO, Kales A, Manfredi RL, et al. Triazolam and memory loss. Lancet 1991; 338:1391–2.

[23] Weingartner HJ, Hommer D, Lister RG, et al. Selective effects of triazolam on memory. Psychopharmacology (Berl) 1992;106:341–5.

[24] Berthold CW, Dionne RA, Corey SE. Comparison of sublingually and orally administered triazolam for premedication before oral surgery. Oral Surg Oral Med Oral Pathol Oral Radiol Endod 1997;84:119–24.

[25] MacDonald RL, Olsen RW. GABA$_A$ receptor channels. Ann Rev Neurosci 1994;17: 569–602.

[26] Sieghart W. GABA$_A$ receptors: ligand-gated Cl⁻ ion channels modulated by multiple drug-binding sites. Trends Pharmacol Sci 1992;13:446–50.

THE DENTAL
CLINICS OF
NORTH
AMERICA

Dent Clin N Am 46 (2002) 803–814

Sedation for pediatric dental patients

Michael D. Webb, DDS[a,b,c],
Paul A. Moore, DMD, PhD, MPH[d,*]

[a]*Department of Pediatric Dentistry, Baylor College of Dentistry, USA*
[b]*Clinical Department of Dentistry, Children's Medical Center of Dallas, USA*
[c]*Texas Scottish Rite Hospital for Children, USA*
[d]*Department of Dental Public Health, University of Pittsburgh School of Dental Medicine,
552 Salk Hall, 3501 Terrace Street, Pittsburgh, PA 15261, USA*

There are few areas of dental therapeutics as controversial as the pharmacologic management of fearful and uncooperative pediatric dental patients. A pediatric dentist is faced with one of the most difficult tasks in our profession: maximizing comfort and cooperation while minimizing risks and costs of dental care for the unmanageable child. Pharmacosedation provides the means for children to avoid psychologically traumatic experiences that might inhibit regular oral health care when they become adults. By controlling disruptive behaviors, the pediatric dentist is able to provide quality dental care in an environment that is pleasant for the child, the parent, and the practitioner.

It is generally agreed that most fearful and uncooperative children can and should be managed with behavioral (nonpharmacologic) management procedures [1]. These include behavior modification techniques such as tell-show-do, positive reinforcement, controlled expectations, modeling, and suggestion. Unfortunately, there is a small percentage of the pediatric population that cannot be successfully managed solely through behavioral management techniques. When behavioral management strategies fail, some form of pharmacologic sedation or anesthesia may be a valuable and necessary alternative.

The sedative agents and techniques used by dentists who treat children vary with the practitioner's experience and training. Dentists with limited knowledge and experience in providing sedation to children should adhere to single drug regimens that have a wide margin of safety. Conversely,

---

* Corresponding author.
E-mail address: pam7@pitt.edu (P.A. Moore).

pediatric dentists and practitioners who have advanced training in anesthesiology and management of sedation complications in the pediatric population may elect to use multiple drug regimens that are likely to produce deeper levels of sedation.

Levels of sedation and anesthesia have been classified by the American Dental Association into three categories: conscious sedation, deep sedation, and general anesthesia [2]. None of these anesthetic strategies is ideal for treating all pediatric patients (see box below). Sedation regimens that provide conscious sedation for young, uncooperative patients are not effective for every child. Deep sedation techniques are also less than 100% successful and require added anesthesia training or certification for their safe and proper use. General anesthesia is an effective and reliable means of treating unmanageable pediatric patients but is expensive, inconvenient, and not without added risk [3].

Drugs commonly used to produce conscious sedation are nitrous oxide, opioids, benzodiazepines, chloral hydrate, barbiturates, and antihistamines (Table 1). Oral administration is the most common route of administering sedative agents to children. It is recommended that preoperative medications not be administered outside the treatment facility: chloral hydrate, opioids,

---

Definitions of sedation/anesthesia[a]

Conscious sedation

A minimally depressed level of consciousness that retains the patient's ability to independently and continuously maintain an airway and respond appropriately to physical stimulation and verbal command.

Deep sedation

An induced state of depressed consciousness accompanied by partial loss of protected reflexes, including the inability to continually maintain an airway independently and/or to respond purposefully to verbal command.

General anesthesia

An induced state of unconsciousness accompanied by partial or complete loss of protected reflexes, including the inability to independently maintain an airway and respond purposefully to physical stimulation or verbal command.

---

[a] American Dental Association. The use of conscious sedation, deep sedation, and general anesthesia in dentistry. Chicago: American Dental Association; 1996.

Table 1
Sedation regimens for pediatric dental patients

Agent	Formulation	Dosage	Route	Onset time	Comments
Chloral hydrate					
Chloral hydrate syrup	500 mg per 5 ml	50–60 mg/kg	PO	30–45 min	Chloral hydrate is irritating to mucosa Nausea and vomiting may occur Multiple drug interactions
Opioids					
Meperidine (Demerol®)	50 mg per 5 ml	2.0 mg/kg	PO	45–60 min	Poor bioavailability orally Respiratory depression may occur Increases local anesthetic toxicity
Fentanyl Oralet®	200 mcg 300 mcg 400 mcg	5–15 mcg/kg 5–15 mcg/kg 5–15 mcg/kg	Transmucosal Transmucosal Transmucosal	20–30 min 20–30 min 20–30 min	Child's minimum weight must be 15 kg Severe hypoventilation possible Limited to hospital setting only
Benzodiazepines					
Midazolam (Versed®)	5.0 mg per ml 1.0 mg per ml	0.5–0.75 mg/kg 0.2–0.3 mg/kg	PO Intranasal	15–20 min 10–15 min	Usual maximum dose is 15 mg Short half-life (106 min)
Diazepam (Valium®)	2-, 5-, 10-mg tablets 5 mg/5ml	0.15–0.25 mg/kg	PO PO	30–60 min	Effective for 6–12-year-old anxious children Usual maximum dose is 15 mg
Inhalational sedation					
Nitrous oxide/oxygen	Pure gases	25–60%	Inhalational	2–4 minutes	Effective for mild to moderate anxiety Waste gases must be controlled Rapid elimination and recovery

and other sedatives should be administered in the controlled environment of the dental facility. Many pediatric dentists have decreased their use of parenteral sedation in response to concerns of safety, state certification requirements, and malpractice costs. The goal of sedating the pediatric dental patient is to safely control the child's behavior so that quality dental care can be provided while helping the child cope with the stress of dental treatment. These goals may not always be met with conscious sedation techniques. Deeper forms of sedation or general anesthesia may be needed to provide necessary dental care to uncooperative children.

Sedation is not a substitute for effective local anesthesia. Dosage guidelines for local anesthesia based on weight should be strictly followed. Multiple drug techniques that include opioids seem to pose even greater problems when local anesthesia dosages are exceeded because of the significant incidence of serious side effects and the difficulty of managing the life-threatening respiratory emergencies that may develop [4,5]. A more detailed discussion of adverse reactions to local anesthetics is presented elsewhere in this issue of the *Dental Clinics of North America*.

Nitrous oxide inhalation sedation

Nitrous oxide is used in pediatric dentistry to induce relaxation and to modify the noxious stimuli of dental treatment. It may be used as the sole sedative agent or as an adjunct to other agents. Its unique pharmacokinetics and proven safety record support its continued use in pediatric dentistry [6].

The absorption of N_2O through the pulmonary alveoli is rapid, with blood levels and clinical effects being seen within minutes of its administration [7]. The distribution of N_2O is limited when compared with other anesthetic gases and therefore large tissue reservoirs of the gas that would delay recovery are not established. Metabolism of N_2O is essentially nonexistent and excretion rapidly occurs primarily through the lungs at a rate similar to its absorption. The clinical consequences of N_2O's unique pharmacokinetics include rapid induction and recovery, ability to titrate and adjust to desired sedative endpoint, and reversibility.

The induction process for a child who is familiar with nitrous oxide/ oxygen inhalation sedation can be nearly complete in 3–5 minutes. Children who have not experienced the effects of nitrous oxide need more explanation of the experience and require a slower, more controlled induction. Subjective symptoms such as tingling of the extremities or a feeling of warmth usually occur within the first few minutes.

Within 5–10 minutes after discontinuing nitrous oxide, the patient has eliminated most of the gas from the body. Because of a higher cardiac output, recovery may be more rapid in children than adults. After a 10–15 minute observation period, full recovery is apparent and the child may usually leave the office and return home.

Because of rapid elimination during the initial 3–5 minutes, large volumes of nitrous oxide are exhaled. As nitrous oxide leaves the plasma and enters the alveoli, it dilutes the ambient air (21% oxygen) that is being inhaled. The result is a theoretic drop in the oxygen concentration to hypoxic levels, frequently referred to as "diffusion hypoxia." In clinical practice, diffusion hypoxia is not a significant problem when administering N_2O sedation. A child who has received nitrous oxide:oxygen sedation has been breathing high concentrations of oxygen (at least 40–50%) and the excess oxygen prevents the dilution of oxygen in air [8]. Diffusion hypoxia is likely to be a problem only after general anesthesia in which the nitrous oxide:oxygen ratio is often higher (75%:25%) and other respiratory depressant drugs have been administered [6]. Nevertheless, a common practice in dentistry is to administer 100% oxygen at the conclusion of nitrous oxide sedation. This procedure has been recommended primarily because it is believed to prevent nausea [9].

The rapid elimination of nitrous oxide permits the pediatric dentist to reverse the effect of the sedation. This reversibility is one of the major reasons for nitrous oxide's record of safety. If a child becomes unexpectedly oversedated, the nitrous oxide concentration can be decreased and the child immediately returns to a more comfortable level of sedation.

One of the absolute advantages of nitrous oxide's rapid absorption and elimination is that the sedative effects can be adjusted to the amount of stimulation that occurs during the procedure. By adjusting the concentration, the sedation can be titrated to the child's moment-to-moment needs.

Pediatric dentists commonly use nitrous oxide/oxygen inhalational sedation. A survey of members of The American Academy of Pediatric Dentistry indicated that 85% of the respondents used nitrous oxide/oxygen analgesia with most using it more frequently than five times per week [10]. In a study that looked at the effect of nitrous oxide-oxygen on physiologic and behavioral parameters in children, there were significant reductions in adverse behavior with no effect on oxygen saturation when a nitrous oxide-oxygen mixture was compared with 100% oxygen [11]. Nitrous oxide has been combined with other agents to provide additive sedative effects. It has been found to augment the effects of diazepam and to result in "deep" rather than "conscious" sedation when combined with chloral hydrate [12–14]. Nitrous oxide-oxygen analgesia seems to be a safe and useful tool in the sedation of pediatric dental patients.

Opioid sedation

Opioid analgesics decrease a patient's psychologic reaction to painful stimuli, produce sedation, and reduce disruptive motor activity. Side effects of opioids include nausea and vomiting that is induced by direct stimulation of the chemoreceptor trigger zone [15]. Respiratory depression, a consequence of decreased sensitivity to CO_2, may also be seen [16]. An estimate of the comparative frequency of these two side effects reveals that mild respiratory depression is more commonly observed than nausea and vomiting [17].

When used for pediatric sedation, the dosage ranges for opioids are invariably higher than required for analgesia. For example, the recommended dosage guidelines in pediatric dentistry are up to 2.0 mg/kg for meperidine (Demerol®). When used concomitantly with other central nervous system (CNS) depressant drugs, these guidelines should be adjusted downward [4,18].

Sedation using opioids has maintained a degree of popularity among pediatric dentists. The most common opioid used for oral sedation in pediatric dentistry is meperidine. It is rapidly absorbed from the gastrointestinal tract and has an onset of 30–60 minutes. First-pass metabolism breaks down nearly 75% of the administered dose. The maximum clinical effect is seen after approximately 1 hour with a duration of action of less than 2 hours. Supplemental drugs frequently used for their added sedative effects and antiemetic effects are promethazine and hydroxyzine [4].

A less commonly used oral opioid sedation technique is oral transmucosal fentanyl citrate (OTFC). This formulation is available as a lozenge on a plastic stick (Fentanyl Oralet®). The child sucks on the lozenge and slowly releases the sedative drug, fentanyl, into saliva, that is then absorbed across the mucous membranes of the oral cavity. The advantages of the OTFC are patient acceptance, rapid onset, and a high bioavailability compared with oral administration that must undergo significant first-pass metabolism [19,20]. Three different formulations are available (200, 300, and 400 micrograms), depending on the child's weight. Dosing recommendations are for 5–15 mcg/kg; doses higher than 15 mcg/kg are contraindicated because they are associated with an excessive frequency of hypoventilation [21]. The use of a pulse oximeter is necessary during administration. Once the desired level of preoperative sedation is achieved, the lozenge should be removed. The formulation is marketed only to hospitals and monitored anesthesia care settings. Respiratory depression, hypotension, itching of the eyes and nose, nausea, and vomiting have been reported [20,22].

Benzodiazepine sedation

Although benzodiazepines have been used extensively in the management of adults who are anxious and fearful of dental procedures, their clinical use in pediatric dentistry has only recently been initiated. The benzodiazepines lack significant respiratory depressant effects at therapeutic doses. There is a specific benzodiazepine antagonist available (flumazenil) that can reverse the central nervous system (CNS) depressant effects seen with overdose [23,24].

Diazepam has been used to provide sedation of pediatric dental patients. Although the drug's elimination may be delayed in the neonate, the pharmacokinetics of diazepam seems to be similar for young children and adults. It has an apparent long duration of action caused by an active metabolite, des-methyldiazepam, that is slowly eliminated and retains some sedative activity.

In pediatric dentistry, diazepam seems to be an effective sedative, particularly if the lack of cooperation is from fear and apprehension [25]. Its large therapeutic index and linear dose-response relationship are valuable assets for a pediatric sedative that is administered orally [26,27]. The recommended dose for oral diazepam is 0.15–0.25 mg/kg given 1 hour before the appointment.

Newer benzodiazepine derivatives such as midazolam and triazolam are now being studied to determine appropriate dosages and to address safety concerns in younger children [28–30]. Midazolam offers the advantage of having a shorter onset and duration of action. It is commonly used as a pre-anesthetic sedative and is becoming popular in pediatric dentistry. There is a flavored oral preparation available that has eliminated the need to mix the intravenous formulation in a vehicle to make it palatable. The dosage regimen of midazolam for pediatric dentistry is 0.5–0.75 mg/kg, administered approximately 30 minutes before the procedure. Duration of action is approximately 30 minutes. A shorter onset period may be an advantage in some clinical situations. Triazolam has not gained widespread acceptance in pediatric dentistry in part because few studies have demonstrated its safety or efficacy in children undergoing dental procedures. The lack of a commercially available liquid formulation of triazolam also limits it usefulness as a pediatric premedicant.

In addition to oral administration of various benzodiazepines, intranasal administration of midazolam, a water soluble, short-acting benzodiazepine, has been evaluated clinically because of its rapid onset (10–15 minutes) and rapid elimination [31]. Although the drug is reliably absorbed, the formulation is somewhat irritating and may cause stinging and discomfort when initially administered. Dosages of 0.2–0.3 mg/kg have been reported to provide adequate sedation with rapid onsets and minimal delay in recovery [22].

Chloral hydrate sedation

Liebig first introduced chloral hydrate into practice in 1832 and it is the oldest and best-studied sedative-hypnotic used in pediatric dentistry. The sedative-hypnotic activity of chloral derivatives is probably caused by the active metabolite trichloroethanol. Following absorption, chloral hydrate is rapidly metabolized to trichloroethanol (TCE) and to a lesser extent to trichloroacetic acid (TCA). Plasma half-life of TCE is estimated to be 8 hours. Peak plasma concentrations of TCE are reached in 20–60 minutes. Plasma concentrations of chloral hydrate are nearly undetectable after oral dosing. Rectal absorption of chloral hydrate formulations containing polyethylene glycol vehicles is nearly as rapid as oral absorption, although somewhat less complete [32,33].

Although definitive studies in children are sparse, it is generally assumed that therapeutic doses of chloral hydrate have minimal effects on respiratory and cardiovascular function [34]. Changes in respiratory function (pCO_2, respiratory rate, tidal volume) are comparable to natural sleep. Asthmatic patients may be somewhat more sensitive to chloral hydrate's minimal respiratory depressive properties [35]. The CO_2 chemoreceptor response seems to be unchanged in infants administered 50 mg/kg chloral hydrate [36].

The primary pharmacologic effect of chloral hydrate is CNS depression. Signs and symptoms following ingestion of increasing doses of chloral hydrate progress from relaxation, lethargy, drowsiness, and hypnosis to loss of consciousness and coma. Given alone, chloral hydrate provides measurable sedation at doses more than 40 mg/kg with therapeutic doses ranging from 50–60 mg/kg. When administered in combination with other CNS depressants, a lower dose of chloral hydrate also may be effectively prescribed [37].

Adverse effects of chloral hydrate administration are rare. When used as a hypnotic, untoward reactions occur in approximately 2% of cases. Overt CNS depression, characterized by disorientation, and prolonged drowsiness account for half of these reactions. The reports of reactions in dental premedication are generally similar although dose-related reactions such as prolonged CNS depression and vomiting occur more frequently in younger ambulating populations. With extremely high doses of chloral hydrate (ie, 75 mg/kg) a significant incidence of vomiting has been reported [38]. The maximum recommended dose in children, irrespective of body weight, is 1000–1500 mg [39].

Chloral hydrate may induce cardiac arrythmias, and in overdose situations cardiac arrest has been reported [34]. Cutaneous reactions to chloral hydrate, although described frequently in textbooks, seldom occur. Skin eruptions are usually erythematous, eczematous, and scarlatiniform [40]. Fixed eruptions, skin lesions occurring at the same site on repeated administration, have also been reported [41].

Chloral hydrate has been implicated in a variety of drug interactions. As one might expect, chloral hydrate produces additive CNS depression when administered with other sedatives. This additive drug interaction permits one to decrease the dose of both depressants, thereby limiting the side effects of the drugs. The reduced dosages when chloral hydrate is combined with the antiemetic promethazine have been shown to appreciably decrease the incidence of nausea and vomiting [38,42]. Nitrous oxide/oxygen in combination with 60 mg/kg chloral hydrate may increase the level of CNS depression to such an extent that the child's protective reflexes may be compromised [14].

Three inadvertent overdose reactions have been described by Hayden [43]. These mishaps were caused by either incorrect calculation of dose or lack of communication among the dentist, staff, parent, and patient. A low dose (250 mg) has reportedly induced laryngospasm and cardiac arrest when chloral hydrate elixir, a known irritant to mucous membranes, was rapidly introduced into the oropharynx with a syringe.

Because vomiting is frequent with doses greater than 60 mg/kg, consumption of a large overdose is often prevented. In children, hypotension and cardiac arrhythmias commonly occur with overdose. These symptoms are distinctly different from local anesthetic or narcotic overdose in which convulsions and respiratory depression are usually reported. The high incidence of nausea and vomiting, concerns for its possible mutagenicity, and the risk for cardiovascular collapse have decreased the use of chloral hydrate in recent years.

Barbiturate sedation

The barbiturate sedative-hypnotics were the primary therapeutic agents for treating anxiety and induction of sleep before the introduction of benzodiazepines. As premedicants in pediatric dentistry, the most frequently prescribed agents are secobarbital and pentobarbital [44]. The barbiturates produce dose-dependent effects ranging from relaxation and sedation to hypnosis and general anesthesia. They have minimal effects on respiratory function at therapeutic doses although respiratory drive may be inhibited at higher doses.

The use of barbiturates in pediatric dentistry has been limited for two reasons: their reputed ability to induce paradoxic excitement and their limited therapeutic dosage range. Inadequate doses are ineffectual and may actually cause some uncooperative children to become more unmanageable. Even at higher doses in the therapeutic range, a few children, particularly when stimulated, demonstrate paradoxic excitation [45]. This reversal of sedative effects, seen with less than 5% of pediatric patients, may be caused by barbiturates' anti-analgesic properties or may be attributable to respiratory depression and subsequent agitation.

Precautions

Overall, the safety and efficacy of pediatric pharmacosedation is a function of a practitioner's ability and preparedness, drug and dosage selection, and awareness of a child's unique physical and psychologic makeup (see list below).

- Unique characteristics of pediatric sedation
- Child's weight and volume of distribution
- Unique physical anatomy
- Responsiveness to oral sedatives
- Limitations for route of drug administration
- Psychologic makeup and coping skills

When compared with adults, pediatric patients have unique characteristics that seem to increase the risks associated with sedation [3]. The most obvious anatomic difference between the adult and pediatric patient is body size. An increased awareness of dosage adjustment in pediatric patients has developed in the last few years within dentistry. Available data as reported by Aubuchon's survey [46], and by Moore and Goodson's case report analysis [5] reinforce the belief that serious adverse reactions in pediatric sedation are commonly caused by inadequate weight-based dosage reduction.

The pediatric airway anatomy is an important factor in airway complications when sedating children. Infants and young children have narrow nares, a large tongue, a high glottis, and slanting vocal cords. In an infant, the narrowest point of the upper airway may be at the level of the cricoid ring rather than the vocal cords. Airway obstruction is therefore more likely to occur below the vocal cords in pediatric patients [47]. Additionally, because of the smaller caliber of the airway passages, acute bronchial inflammation can present a significantly more severe obstruction in younger patients. Because children have significantly higher metabolic rates, hypoxia develops rapidly when airway obstructions occur.

Children's responsiveness to sedatives may differ from that of adults because of differences in pharmacokinetics or pharmacodynamics. Fortunately, differences in drug absorption, distribution, and excretion occur primarily in the perinatal period and are usually not relevant to office practice, where treatment is usually limited to children over 2 years of age.

It has been reported that young children may be unexpectedly sensitive to the CNS depressants used for sedation in pediatric dentistry. Transient airway obstruction was seen in 4 of 15 preschool children who were administered 60 mg/kg of chloral hydrate in combination with nitrous oxide. These four children were found to be among the youngest in this treatment group [14]. This finding supports empiric findings by Grimes, who recommends reducing weight-based dosages for patients under 2 years of age [48]. Wilson reported a similar response and believed that children with large tonsils and adenoids were most at risk [49].

Children, particularly uncooperative preschool children, come to a dental office under circumstances different from those of adults. Although children are anxious and fearful, unlike adults, they have not arrived at a dental office of their own desire. A 2- or 3-year-old does not consider acquiring good dental health a significant motivator to tolerate treatment and, in fact, sees no obvious benefits in cooperating with therapy. Additionally, children lack experience with uncomfortable situations and have inadequate coping skills with which to tolerate treatment. These differences in a child's psychologic development limit the success of any sedation therapy in many instances.

As a consequence of these differences, dose-response curves for sedatives used in pediatric dentistry are flat, placebo effects seem nearly comparable to effective doses, and high failure rates are frequently reported [14,50]. Strategies for correcting these pharmacologic inadequacies, such as remedicating unsuccessfully sedated patients and using a variety of drug combinations, may increase the likelihood of adverse responses. Using large doses of synergistic agents decreases the therapeutic index of sedation procedures and significantly affects the overall safety.

References

[1] Moore P, Houpt M. Sedative drug therapy in pediatric dentistry. In: Dionne RA, Phero JC, editors. Management of pain and anxiety in dental practice. New York: Elsevier; 1991. p. 239–66.
[2] American Dental Association policy statement. The use of conscious sedation, deep sedation and general anesthesia in dentistry. Chicago: American Dental Association; 1996.
[3] Moore PA. Pediatric sedation and anesthesia: monitoring and management considerations. In: Dionne RA, Laskin DM, editors. Anesthesia and sedation in the dental office. New York: Elsevier; 1986. p. 107–15.
[4] Goodson JM, Moore P. Life-threatening reactions following pedodontic sedation: an assessment of narcotic, local anesthetic and antiemetic drug interaction. J Am Dent Assoc 1983;107:239–45.
[5] Moore PA, Goodson JM. Risk appraisal of narcotic sedation for children. Anesth Prog 1985;32:129–39.
[6] Duncan GH, Moore PA. Nitrous oxide and the dental patient: potential hazards and complications. J Am Dent Assoc 1984;108:213–9.
[7] Moore PA. Psychomotor impairment due to N2O exposure. Anesth Prog 1983;30:72–5.
[8] Cassidy D, Nazif MM, Zullo T, et al. Transcutaneous oxygen monitoring of patients undergoing nitrous oxide-oxygen sedation. Ped Dent 1986;8:29–31.
[9] Langa H. Techniques of administration; possible reaction of the patient; indications and contraindications. In: Langa H, editor. Relative analgesia in dental practice: inhalational analgesia and sedation. Philadelphia: WB Saunders; 1976. p. 167–232.
[10] Wilson S. A survey of the American Academy of Pediatric Dentistry membership: nitrous oxide and sedation. Ped Dent 1996;18(4):287–93.
[11] Primosch RE, Buzzi IM, Jerrell G. Effect of nitrous oxide-oxygen inhalation with scavenging on behavioral and physiological parameters during routine pediatric dental treatment. Ped Dent 1999;21(7):417–20.
[12] Houpt MI, Kupietzky A, Koenigsberg SR. Effects of nitrous oxide on diazepam sedation of young children. Ped Dent 1996;18(3):236–41.
[13] Litman RS, Kottra JA, Verga KA, Berkowiz RJ, Ward DS. Chloral hydrate sedation: the additive and respiratory depressant effects of nitrous oxide. Anesth Analg 1998;86(4): 724–8.
[14] Moore PA, Mickey EA, Hargreaves JA, et al. Sedation in pediatric dentistry: a practical assessment procedure. J Am Dent Assoc 1984;109:564–9.
[15] Jaffe JH, Martin WR. Opioid analgesics and antagonists. In: Gilman AG, Rall TW, Nies AS, Taylor P, editors. Goodman and Gilman's the pharmacologic basis of therapeutics. 8th edition. New York: Pergamon Press; 1990. p. 493.
[16] Lambertsen CJ, Wendel H, Longenhagen JB. The separate and combined respiratory effects of chlorpromazine and meperidine in normal men controlled at 46 mm Hg alveolar pCO$_2$. J Pharmacol Exp Ther 1961;131:381–93.
[17] Eckenhoff JE, Helrich M. Study of narcotics and sedatives for use in preanesthetic medication. J Am Med A 1958;167:415–22.
[18] Moore PA. Clinical pharmacology of opioid analgesics. Dent Clin N Am 1984;28: 389–400.
[19] Streisand JB, Stanley TH, Hague B, et al. Oral transmucosal fentanyl citrate premedication in children. Anesth Analg 1989;69:28.
[20] Moore PA, Cuddy MA, Magera JA, et al. Oral transmucosal fentanyl pretreatment for outpatient general anesthesia. Anesth Prog 2000;47(2):29–34.
[21] Fentanyl Oralet Package Insert. Abbott Laboratories, Hospital Products Division Medical Department. North Chicago (IL) 60064.
[22] Wilton NCT, Leigh J, Rosen DR, et al. Preanesthetic sedation of preschool children using intranasal sedation. Anesthesiol 1988;169:972.

[23] Flumazenil in Intravenous Conscious Sedation with Diazepam Multicenter Study Group II, Moore PA. Reversal of central benzodiazepine effects by flumazenil after intravenous conscious sedation with diazepam and opioids. Clin Ther 1993;14:910–23.

[24] Finder RL, Moore PA. Benzodiazepines for intravenous conscious sedation: agonists and antagonists. Comp Cont Ed Dent 1993;14:972–82.

[25] Boyd JD, Manford ML. Premedication in children. Brit J Anesth 1973;45:501–6.

[26] Auil B, Cornejo G, Gallardo F. Flunitrazepam and diazepam compared as sedatives in children. J Dent Child 1983;50:442–4.

[27] Kopel HM. The pharmacodynamics of pedodontic sedative premedication. Cal Dent A J 1984;12:23–30.

[28] McMillan CO, Spahr-Schopferl A, Sikich H. Premedication of children with oral midazolam. Can J Anesth 1992;39:545.

[29] Stopperich DS, Moore PA, Finder RL, et al. Oral triazolam pretreatment for intravenous sedation. Anesth Prog 1993;40:117–21.

[30] Quarnstrom FC, Milgrom P, Moore PA. Clinical experience with oral triazolam in preschool children. Anesth Pain Control Dent 1992;1:157–9.

[31] Wolbergh EJ, Willis RJ, Eckhert J. Plasma concentrations of midazolam in children following intranasal midazolam. Anesthesiol 1991;74:233.

[32] Breimer DD. Clinical pharmacokinetics of hypnotics. Clinic Pharmacokin 1977;2:93–109.

[33] Marshall EK, Owens AH. Absorption, excretion and metabolic fate of chloral hydrate and trichloroethanol. Bull John Hopkins Hosp 1954;95:1–18.

[34] Nordenberg A, Delisle G, Izukawa T. Cardiac arrhythmias in a child due to chloral hydrate ingestion. Pediatrics 1971;47:134–5.

[35] Aldrete JA, Itkin IH. Effects of chloral hydrate on the respiration of nonasthmatic and asthmatic patients. J Allergy Clin Immunol 1969;43:343–8.

[36] Lees MH, Olsen GD, McGilliard KL, et al. Chloral hydrate and the carbon dioxide chemoreceptor response: a study of puppies and infants. Pediatrics 1982;72:447–50.

[37] Moore PA. Therapeutic assessment of chloral hydrate premedication for pediatric dentistry. Anesth Prog 1984;31:191–6.

[38] Houpt MI, Weiss NJ, Koenigsberg SR, et al. Comparison of chloral hydrate with and without promethazine in the sedation of young children. Ped Dent 1985;7:41–6.

[39] Smith RC. Chloral hydrate sedation for handicapped children: double-blind study. Anesth Prog 1977;24:159–62.

[40] Almeyda J, Levantine A. Drug reactions XVII: cutaneous reaction to barbiturates, chloral hydrate and its derivatives. Br J Dermatol 1972;86:313–6.

[41] Miller LH, Brownstein MH, Hyman AB. Fixed eruption due to chloral hydrate. Arch Dermatol 1966;94:60–1.

[42] Robbins MB. Chloral hydrate and promethazine as premedicants for the apprehensive child. J Dent Child 1967;34:327–31.

[43] Hayden J. Chloral hydrate as a sedative in dentistry. Colo Dent A J 1982;61:3–4.

[44] Barenie JT, Ripa L. Sedative-hypnotics. In: Management of dental behavior in children. Littleton (MA): PSG Publishing Co; 1979.

[45] Nazif M. Thioridazine and secobarbital as premedicating agents. J Dent Child 1971;38:704.

[46] Aubuchon RW. Sedation liabilities in pedodontics. Ped Dent 1982;4:171–80.

[47] Motoyama EK. Respiratory physiology in infants and children. In: Motoyama EK, Davis PJ, editors. Smith's anesthesia for infants and children. St. Louis (MO): CV Mosby Company; 1996. p. 33.

[48] Grimes JG. Oral premedication in children. Anesth Analg 1962;41:201–2.

[49] Wilson S, Creedon RL, George M, et al. A history of sedation guidelines: where we are headed in the future. Ped Dent 1996;18:194–9.

[50] Leelataweedwud P, Vann WF. Adverse events and outcomes of conscious sedation for pediatric patients: study of an oral sedation regimen. J Am Dent Assoc 2001;132:1531–9.

THE DENTAL
CLINICS OF
NORTH
AMERICA

Dent Clin N Am 46 (2002) 815–830

Emergency drugs

Daniel A. Haas, DDS, PhD, FRCD(C)*

*Department of Clinical Sciences, Discipline of Anesthesia, Faculty of Dentistry,
University of Toronto, 124 Edward Street, Toronto, Ontario, M5G 1G6, Canada
Department of Pharmacology, Faculty of Medicine, University of Toronto,
Toronto, Ontario, M5S 1A8, Canada
Department of Dentistry, Sunnybrook and Women's College Health Sciences Centre,
Toronto, Ontario, M4N 3M5, Canada*

Dentists must be prepared to manage medical emergencies that may arise in practice. This need is supported by surveys that have shown that dental office emergencies are not uncommon, with syncope being the most frequent event cited [1]. When syncope is excluded, it is estimated that an average of one other medical emergency arises approximately every 4 years in practice [2]. Therefore, dentists should be ready to manage these events. Preparation focuses primarily on prevention but should also include the presence of specific equipment and emergency drugs.

There are numerous proposals for lists of drugs that a dentist should have readily available for the management of medical emergencies [3–11]. These suggested lists share similarities but they are not identical. These recommendations can differ from what is actually found in dental practice [12]. Ultimately it is the individual dentist's own decision as to which drugs are appropriate for his or her particular practice. This article reviews the drugs that should be considered for this purpose.

Basic principles

The dentist's role in the handling of any medical emergency begins with prevention by following basic principles, such as conducting a thorough medical history with appropriate alterations to dental treatment as necessary [13]. It is usually considered essential that the dentist be trained and

---

* Department of Clinical Sciences, Discipline of Anesthesia, University of Toronto, 124 Edward Street, Toronto, Ontario, M5G 1G6, Canada.
  E-mail address: daniel.haas@utoronto.ca (D.A. Haas).

competent in basic life support (BLS), or cardiopulmonary resuscitation (CPR) [7]. This provides the dentist with the skills to manage most medical emergencies, starting with the assessment, and if necessary, the treatment of airway, breathing, and circulation (the ABCs of CPR). In most cases, only after these basics are addressed should the dentist consider the use of emergency drugs. Nevertheless, acknowledging the importance of prevention and competency in BLS, a core group of drugs must be readily accessible.

There are many potential emergencies and protocols to follow. Ideally, a dentist should be aware of all of them; yet, the reality is that when the emergency first develops, the precise diagnosis may not be clear. Without a diagnosis, how can one formulate a treatment plan? This problem can be circumvented by following the key principle that the most important aspect of nearly all medical emergencies in the dental office is to prevent or correct insufficient oxygenation of the brain and heart. On a simple level, if a patient has lost consciousness, it is a result of lack of oxygenated blood in the brain. If a patient is having an episode of acute angina pectoris, it is a result of relative lack of oxygenated blood to specific sites in cardiac muscle. The management of all medical emergencies occurring in a dental office should include ensuring that oxygenated blood is being delivered to the brain and heart. Beginning with an ABC approach is always prudent, particularly if the diagnosis is not clear. Furthermore, an ABC approach should always be considered before the administration of a drug.

Drugs that should be promptly available to the dentist can be divided into two categories. The first category represents those drugs that may be considered essential. These drugs are summarized in Table 1. The second category contains drugs that are also helpful and should be considered as part of the emergency kit. These supplementary drugs are summarized in Table 2. The precise composition of the drug kit can vary as the presence of the drugs in this latter group may depend on the nature of the dental practice. Those with training in Advanced Cardiac Life Support would also have additional drugs, including vasopressin, amiodarone, lidocaine, norepinephrine, verapamil, adenosine, procainamide, magnesium, and others [14]. This latter group is not discussed in this article.

Dentists who are trained to administer general anesthesia or intravenous sedation would be expected to have additional drugs commensurate with the modality practiced. These dentists would be expected to have a patent intravenous line in place and therefore drug administration could use this route, which may be considered ideal. It may be assumed that dentists without advanced training in anesthesia or sedation may not be proficient in venipuncture. In this case the intramuscular route of administration, which can include the intralingual injection, would be appropriate. The intralingual intramuscular injection should provide a more rapid onset of action compared with the more traditional sites, although not as rapid as intravenous. This article assumes the intramuscular route is the one most likely to be used.

Table 1
Essential emergency drugs

Drug	Indication	Initial adult dose
Oxygen	Almost any medical emergency	100%: inhalation
Epinephrine	Anaphylaxis	0.1 mg IV or 0.3–0.5 mg IM
	Asthma unresponsive to albuterol	0.1 mg IV or 0.3–0.5 mg IM
	Cardiac arrest	1 mg IV
Nitroglycerin	Pain of angina	0.3–0.4 mg sublingual
Antihistamine	Allergic reactions	
(diphenhydramine or		25–50 mg IV, IM
chlorpheniramine)		10–20 mg IV, IM
Albuterol	Asthmatic bronchospasm	2 sprays (180 µg–200 µg) inhalation
Aspirin	Myocardial infarction	160 mg–325 mg

Pediatric doses (approximate, not to exceed the adult doses listed above)
  Epinephrine = 0.01 mg/kg
  Diphenhydramine = 1 mg/kg
  Albuterol = 1 spray (90–100 µg)

Essential drugs

Oxygen

Oxygen is indicated for every emergency except hyperventilation. Understanding the basic pharmacology of oxygen resides in knowledge of the oxyhemoglobin dissociation curve. Room air contains 20.9% oxygen, and this

Table 2
Supplementary emergency drugs

Drug	Indication	Initial adult dose
Glucagon	Hypoglycemia in unconscious patient	1 mg IM
Atropine	Clinically significant bradycardia	0.5 mg IV or IM
Ephedrine	Clinically significant hypotension	5 mg IV, or 10–25 mg IM
Hydrocortisone	Adrenal insufficiency Recurrent anaphylaxis	100 mg IV or IM
Morphine or nitrous oxide	Angina-like pain unresponsive to nitroglycerin	Titrate 2 mg IV, 5 mg IM ~35%, inhalation
Naloxone	Reversal of opioid overdose	0.1 mg IV or 0.4 mg IM
Lorazepam or midazolam	Status epilepticus	4 mg IM or IV 5 mg IM or IV
Flumazenil	Benzodiazepine overdose	0.1 mg IV

The final composition of the supplementary emergency drugs depends on the individual dentist's needs and the nature of the practice. The drugs listed above should be considered. Dental offices that provide conscious sedation, deep sedation or general anaesthesia require additional drugs.

normally results in oxyhemoglobin saturation approximating 98%. At this level the curve is stable. When mouth to mask or mouth to mouth ventilation is carried out as part of basic CPR, the exhaled carbon dioxide results in a reduction in the amount of oxygen delivered, to a level approximating 16%. Therefore, the patient is immediately at a disadvantage even when being ventilated adequately. As oxyhemoglobin saturation starts to decrease to less than 90%, the sigmoid shape of this curve results in a progressively more rapid decrease. Cardiac compressions carried out as part of CPR are meant to simulate cardiac output. Even when these compressions are being done ideally, they achieve only approximately 25–30% of the normal cardiac output [14]. This puts the patient at a further disadvantage. If cardiac arrest has been present for a period of time, acidosis may begin that will shift the oxyhemoglobin dissociation curve to the right. This results in a lower oxyhemoglobin saturation for a given partial pressure of oxygen being delivered to the lung alveoli. This further decreases the amount of oxygen available to be delivered to the tissues.

The accumulation of these facts points to the need to improve oxygen delivery by whatever means are available. This should be done with a clear full-face mask for the spontaneously breathing patient and a bag-valve-mask device for the apneic patient. Therefore whenever possible, with the exception of the patient who is hyperventilating, oxygen should be administered. For the management of a medical emergency it should not be withheld for the patient with chronic obstructive lung disease, even though they may be dependent on low oxygen levels to breathe if they are chronic carbon dioxide retainers. Short-term administration of oxygen to get them through the emergency should not depress their drive to breathe.

Oxygen should be available in a portable source, ideally in an "E"-size cylinder that holds more than 600 liters. This should allow for more than enough oxygen to be available for the patient until resolution of the event or transfer to a hospital. If the typical adult has a minute volume of 6 liters per minute, then this flow rate should be given as a minimum. If the patient is conscious, or unconscious yet spontaneously breathing, oxygen should be delivered by a full-face mask; a flow rate of 6–10 liters per minute is appropriate for most adults [15]. If the patient is unconscious and apneic, it should be delivered by a bag-valve-mask device with which a flow rate of 10–15 liters per minute is appropriate [15]. A positive pressure device may be used in adults, provided that the flow rate does not exceed 35 liters per minute.

Epinephrine

Epinephrine is the drug of choice for the emergency treatment of anaphylaxis and asthma that does not respond to its drug of first choice, albuterol. Epinephrine also is indicated for the management of cardiac arrest, but in the dental office setting, it may not be as likely to be given, because intravenous access may not be available. Its administration intramuscularly is not as likely to be effective in this latter emergency, in which adequate oxygenation and early defibrillation is most important for the cardiac arrest dysrhythmias with the best prognoses, namely ventricular fibrillation or pulseless ventricular tachycardia [16].

Epinephrine, an endogenous catecholamine, is an agonist at all adrenoceptors. When considering its use in emergencies, the effects on the cardiovascular and respiratory systems are most important.

The actions on the heart are mediated primarily by the stimulation of β-1 receptors. This results in an increase in heart rate, force of contraction and automaticity. The combination of increased rate and stroke volume leads to an increase in cardiac output. In turn, this should lead to improved perfusion. This increase in cardiac output may be required to reverse the hypotension that can accompany anaphylaxis. Increased myocardial automaticity can predispose to dysrhythmias in a beating heart, but may be advantageous during cardiac arrest. Myocardial oxygen requirement increases as a result of the greater work of the heart. This can be an adverse effect, particularly in the compromised heart in which an increased demand for oxygen in the presence of diminished supply may predispose to ischemia, with subsequent angina or infarction.

The effects on the vasculature are primarily caused by either α-1 stimulation that induces constriction mainly in skin and mucous membranes, or β-2 effects that include vasodilatation of the blood vessels predominantly in skeletal muscle. The increased peripheral vasoconstriction is beneficial during management of a cardiac arrest [14].

The effects on the respiratory system are also of importance. The stimulation of β-2 receptors causes bronchorelaxation. This is beneficial in the emergency treatment of a bronchoconstriction as found during an acute asthmatic attack when bronchorelaxation cannot be induced by a β-2 agonist alone. This action is also required in the management of anaphylaxis.

As a drug, epinephrine has a rapid onset and short duration of action, usually 5–10 minutes when given intravenously. For emergency purposes, epinephrine is available in two formulations. It is prepared as 1:1,000, which equals 1 mg per mL, for intramuscular, including intralingual, injections. More than one ampule or prefilled syringe should be present, as multiple administrations may be necessary. It also is available as 1:10,000, which equals 1 mg per 10 mL, for intravenous injection. Autoinjector systems are also available for intramuscular use (such as the EpiPen) that provide one dose of 0.3 mg as 0.3 ml of 1:1,000, or the pediatric formulation that is one dose of 0.15 mg as 0.3 ml of 1:2,000.

Initial doses for the management of anaphylaxis are 0.3–0.5 mg intramuscularly or 0.1 mg intravenously [7,16–18]. These doses should be repeated as necessary until resolution of the event. Similar doses should be considered in asthmatic bronchospasm that is unresponsive to a beta-2 agonist, such as albuterol. Dose in cardiac arrest is 1 mg intravenously.

Intramuscular administration during cardiac arrest has not been studied, but would seem to be unlikely to render significant effect.

Epinephrine is clearly a highly beneficial drug in these emergencies. Concurrently, however, it can be a drug with a high risk if given to a patient with ischemic heart disease. Nevertheless, it is the primary drug needed to reverse the life-threatening signs and symptoms of anaphylaxis or persistent asthmatic bronchospasm.

Nitroglycerin

This drug is indicated for acute angina or myocardial infarction. It is characterized by a rapid onset of action. Its primary mechanism of action is through vasodilation, which results in a decrease in venous return to the heart and therefore a reduction in the work of cardiac muscle. In turn, this reduces myocardial oxygen consumption. Given that angina pectoris arises from an imbalance in the supply and demand of oxygen in the heart, this action is beneficial.

Nitroglycerin presents little in the way of adverse reactions. Because it decreases blood pressure, it should not be administered if systolic blood pressure is less than 90 mm Hg. It may lead to headache if given to a patient with chest pain of noncardiac origin.

For emergency purposes it is available as 0.3-, 0.4-, or 0.6-mg sublingual tablets or a 0.4-mg sublingual spray. One important point to be aware of is that the tablets have a short shelf life of approximately 3 months once the bottle has been opened and the tablets have been exposed to air or light. The spray has the advantage of having a shelf life that corresponds to that listed on the bottle. Therefore, if a patient uses his or her own nitroglycerin, there is a possibility of the drug being inactive. This supports the need for the dentist to always have a fresh supply available. With signs of angina pectoris, 0.3 or 0.4 mg should be administered sublingually. Relief of pain should occur within minutes. If necessary, this dose can be repeated twice more in 5-minute intervals provided that systolic blood pressure remains above 90 mm Hg.

Injectable antihistamine

An antihistamine is indicated for the management of allergic reactions. Whereas mild non-life-threatening allergic reactions may be managed by oral administration, life-threatening reactions necessitate parenteral administration. Antihistamines may be classified as those that block either H-1 or H-2 histamine receptors. Whereas a case can be made for the use of both classes of drugs [19], the H-1 antagonist is commonly considered the first line antihistamine [6,18]. The H-1 antagonist therefore would be the more essential of the two. These drugs block the action of histamine at the H-1 receptor; they do not inhibit the release of histamine.

Two injectable agents may be considered, either diphenhydramine (Benadryl) or chlorpheniramine. Parenteral diphenhydramine is available as either a 10 or a 50 mg per mL solution. Parenteral chlorpheniramine is available as a 10 mg per mL solution. They may be administered as part of the management of anaphylaxis or as the sole management of less severe allergic reactions, particularly those with primarily dermatologic signs and symptoms such as urticaria. Recommended doses for adults are 25–50 mg of diphenhydramine or 10–20 mg of chlorpheniramine.

Albuterol

A selective β-2 agonist such as albuterol (Ventolin) is the first choice for management of bronchospasm. When administered by an inhaler, it provides selective bronchodilation with minimal systemic cardiovascular effects. It has a peak effect in 30–60 minutes, with a duration effect of 4–6 hours. Other inhalational selective β-2 agonists could also be considered for emergency management of an acute asthmatic attack. Examples include metaproterenol (Alupent) or terbutaline (Brethaire, Bricanyl).

Albuterol is available as a metered dose inhaler that provides 90 or 100 micrograms of drug per administration. Adult dose is 180 to 200 micrograms, which is two sprays, to be repeated as necessary. Pediatric dose is 90 to 100 micrograms, or one spray, repeated as necessary.

Aspirin

Aspirin is one of the more newly recognized life-saving drugs, as it has been shown to reduce overall mortality from acute myocardial infarction [20,21]. This drug is well known in dentistry. Aspirin blocks the cyclooxygenase enzymes, leading to a reduction in prostaglandins, prostacyclins, and thromboxanes. Thromboxanes potently constrict arteries and promote platelet aggregation. Aspirin's role as a drug in medical emergencies is derived from this inhibition of thromboxane, as it inhibits platelet aggregation.

The purpose of its administration during an acute myocardial infarction is to prevent the progression from cardiac ischemia to injury to infarction. There is a brief period of time early on during a myocardial infarction during which aspirin can show this benefit. For emergency use there are few contraindications. These would include known hypersensitivity to aspirin, severe asthma, or history of significant gastric bleeding.

Aspirin is available as 81-, 162.5-, 325-, 500-, or 650-mg tablets. The lowest effective dose is not known with certainty, but a minimum of 162 mg should be given immediately to any patient with pain suggestive of acute myocardial infarction.

Oral carbohydrate

An oral carbohydrate source, such as fruit juice or nondiet soft drink, should be readily available. Whereas this is not a drug, and perhaps should not be included in this list, it should be considered essential. If this sugar source is kept in a refrigerator it may not be appreciated that it is a key part of the emergency equipment. Therefore, consideration should be given to making this part of the emergency kit. Its use is indicated in the management of hypoglycemia in conscious patients.

Supplementary drugs

In addition to the six drugs discussed above, several other drugs should be considered as part of an emergency kit, as shown in Table 2.

Glucagon

The presence of this drug allows intramuscular management of hypoglycemia in an unconscious patient. The ideal management of severe hypoglycemia in a diabetic emergency is the intravenous administration of 50% dextrose. Glucagon is indicated if an intravenous line is not in place and venipuncture is not expected to be accomplished, as may often be the case in a dental office. It has actions that oppose insulin and its administration raises plasma glucose. Its anti-hypoglycemic effect occurs within 15 minutes if given intramuscularly. Its duration of action is approximately 90 minutes. Adverse effects are not expected.

The dose for an adult is 1 mg. If the patient weighs less than 20 kg, the recommended dose is 0.5 mg. Glucagon is available as a 1-mg formulation that requires reconstitution with its diluent immediately before use.

Atropine

This antimuscarinic, anticholinergic drug is indicated for the management of hypotension that is accompanied by bradycardia. By blocking cardiac muscarinic receptors, atropine will increase heart rate. Hypotension is normally accompanied by a reflex increase in heart rate. If hypotension is accompanied by a slow heart rate, correction of this bradycardia may resolve the low blood pressure. Conversely, one should be concerned about too great an increase in heart rate in patients with ischemic heart disease. Similarly, there should be concern with any patient in whom anticholinergic effects may be problematic, such as those patients with acute narrow angle glaucoma, prostatic hypertrophy, or urinary retention. It has a rapid onset and short duration of action.

The dose recommended is 0.5 mg initially, followed by increments as necessary until reaching a maximum of 3 mg. Paradoxically, doses of less than 0.4 mg have been associated with induction of bradycardia, likely caused by atropine's central nervous system's actions. Atropine is available in numerous strengths, ranging from 50 micrograms per mL to 1 mg per mL. A concentration approximating 0.5 mg per mL would be suitable for emergency purposes.

Ephedrine

This drug is a vasopressor that may be used to manage significant hypotension. Ephedrine is a sympathomimetic that directly and indirectly leads to stimulation of all adrenoceptors. It has similar cardiovascular actions as epinephrine, except that ephedrine is less potent and has a prolonged duration of action, lasting from 60–90 minutes. That α and β receptors are stimulated is an advantage over other commonly recommended vasopressors such as phenylephrine or methoxamine, which are selective α-1 agonists. These latter agents are effective provided adequate intravenous fluids are being coadministered, a situation that may not occur in the dental office. The β-1 stimulation causes an increase in heart rate and stroke volume, thereby increasing cardiac output, which in turn should help maintain perfusion. The result is an improvement in blood pressure and perfusion, thereby improving tissue oxygenation, one of the primary goals in the handling of any medical emergency. Similar precautions as noted with epinephrine administration should be considered when given to a patient with ischemic heart disease.

For the treatment of severe hypotension, it is ideally administered in 5-mg increments intravenously. Intramuscularly it should be given in a dose of 10–25 mg. It is formulated as either a 25- or 50-mg per mL solution.

Corticosteroid

Administration of a corticosteroid such as hydrocortisone may be indicated for the prevention of recurrent anaphylaxis. Hydrocortisone may also play a role in the management of an adrenal crisis. Corticosteroids provide membrane-stabilizing effects, reduce leukotriene formation, and reduce histamine release from mast cells. These actions are therefore beneficial in allergic reactions. The notable drawback to their use in emergencies is their slow onset of action, that approaches 1 hour even when administered intravenously. This is the reason these drugs are not considered essential, as they are of minimal benefit in the acute phase of the emergency. There is low likelihood of an adverse response with one dose.

The prototype for this group is hydrocortisone (Solu-Cortef) that may be administered in a dose of 100 mg as part of the management of these emergencies.

Morphine

Morphine is indicated for the management of severe pain that occurs with a myocardial infarction. ACLS recommendations list morphine as the analgesic of choice for this purpose [14]. It has the beneficial effects of being an excellent analgesic and having good mood-altering properties to help manage the stress that accompanies this event. This reduction in pain and stress should minimize endogenous epinephrine release. Morphine increases venous capacitance and therefore decreases systemic vascular resistance that reduces preload, a beneficial effect during a myocardial infarction, as it reduces the work of the heart. In turn, less oxygen is needed. It can be used if systolic blood pressure is more than 90 mm Hg and the patient is not hypovolemic.

The dose involves titration in 1–3-mg increments intravenously until pain relief is accomplished. This should be guided by a decrease in blood pressure and respiratory depression. Extreme caution should be used in the elderly. If an intravenous line is not in place, consideration can be given to administering morphine in a dose of approximately 5 mg intramuscularly. Again, lower doses need to be considered for the older patient. As a narcotic, it requires separate storage and recording, consistent with legal regulations.

Naloxone

If morphine is included in the emergency kit or opioids are used as part of a sedation regimen, then naloxone (Narcan) should also be present for the emergency management of inadvertent overdose. Naloxone is an antagonist at all opioid receptors, and therefore blocks all of the actions of morphine or any other opioid. Following intravenous administration, it has an onset of action of 1–2 minutes and a peak effect in 5–15 minutes. Its duration of action depends on the extent of the overdose it is reversing, and may range from 5–45 minutes. Naloxone must be used cautiously, as there is the potential for significant adverse effects. Particular concern should be given to patients with cardiac irritability, as this may be worsened and result in alterations in blood pressure, ventricular tachycardia, or ventricular fibrillation. Its short duration of action necessitates appropriate monitoring beyond its termination of effect.

Doses ideally should be titrated slowly in 0.1-mg increments to effect. It is formulated as either a 0.02-, 0.4-, or 1.0-mg per mL solution.

Nitrous oxide

Nitrous oxide is a reasonable second choice if morphine is not available to manage pain from a myocardial infarction. Its good analgesic and anxiolytic effects are advantageous to the patient having an acute myocardial infarction. As with morphine, this reduction in pain and stress should minimize endogenous epinephrine release. Nitrous oxide's effects on the cardiovascular system are negligible, although it is a mild myocardial depressant and mild sympathomimetic. It lacks morphine's beneficial effects on the cardiovascular system.

For management of pain associated with a myocardial infarction, it should be administered with oxygen, in a concentration approximating 35%, or titrated to effect.

Injectable benzodiazepine

The management of seizures that are prolonged or recurrent, also known as status epilepticus, may require administration of a benzodiazepine. All benzodiazepines share the effects of anxiolysis, sedation, anterograde amnesia, skeletal muscle relaxation, and an anticonvulsant action. It is this latter action that makes benzodiazepines valuable drugs during emergencies. Diazepam is often listed as the drug of choice for status epilepticus. This, however, should be administered intravenously, as the onset of action following intramuscular administration is unpredictable. In most dental practices, it would not be realistic to assume that the dentist could achieve venipuncture in a patient having an active seizure. This leads to the need for a water-soluble agent such as midazolam or lorazepam. Lorazepam has been reported as the drug of choice for status epilepticus [22] and can be administered intramuscularly. Midazolam, however, is another alternative that is water-soluble and could be considered. Sedation would be an expected side effect and patients should be appropriately monitored.

Adult doses to consider for lorazepam are 4 mg intramuscularly, or midazolam 5 mg intramuscularly. If an intravenous line is in place, these drugs should be slowly titrated to effect.

Flumazenil

Flumazenil (Romazicon) should be part of the emergency kit when oral or parenteral sedation is used [23]. This specific antagonist to the benzodiazepine receptor reverses benzodiazepine-induced unconsciousness, sedation, and amnesia. The duration of action is dose-dependent and dependent on the dose and specific agonist being reversed. As with naloxone, the potential for resedation requires that whenever this agent is used to reverse overdose, the patient should be monitored in recovery beyond the duration of action of flumazenil. There should be caution if the patient has a seizure disorder treated by benzodiazepines.

Dosage is 0.1 to 0.2 mg intravenously, incrementally. The total dose usually does not exceed 1.0 mg. Its effectiveness when given intramuscularly has not been established.

Drug use for specific emergencies

It is beyond the scope of this article to provide a detailed rationale and description of each treatment protocol or algorithm to be followed. The following is a synopsis of specific emergencies that incorporate the drugs discussed above. The etiologies and recognition are not discussed, but may be found in other excellent sources [6,7]. The management of all emergencies shares the need to assess and treat the ABCs as necessary and administration of oxygen (except for hyperventilation). One must also consider if and when to call for help and activate the local emergency medical system.

Syncope

No drugs other than oxygen are required to manage this most common emergency seen in dentistry [1]. As it is a transient period of unconsciousness, it is truly an emergency as the airway may be obstructed. The management includes positioning the patient to maximize blood flow to the brain by laying the patient supine with the legs slightly elevated. Attention to the ABCs must be carried out to ensure an open airway. Oxygen should be administered. The initial steps of the management of all unresponsive patients should begin with this protocol. When recovered, offering the patient a source of oral glucose should be considered.

Anaphylaxis

The drugs to be considered for this emergency are summarized in Table 3. Anaphylaxis is a severe allergic reaction [18,24]. It can be life-threatening if it manifests as any combination of bronchospasm, laryngeal edema, or hypotension. Each one of these three signs can be life-threatening on their own. When found in combination, and in particular, when these signs develop rapidly, the level of concern must be heightened. Timing is an important factor. With anaphylaxis to the penicillin family, 96% of all deaths occurred within the first hour.

Once anaphylaxis is apparent, one should follow basic principles and administer epinephrine. This should be an initial dose of 0.1 mg intravenously or 0.3–0.5 mg intramuscularly, repeated as necessary. Once stable, either diphenhydramine in a dose of 25–50 mg or chlorpheniramine in a dose of 10–20 mg may be given intramuscularly. If available, hydrocortisone in a dose of 100 mg may be given. Oxygen should be administered throughout.

For less severe allergic reactions, particularly when there are no signs of airway compromise, diphenhydramine or chlorpheniramine may be administered alone.

Bronchospasm (acute asthma)

Albuterol, epinephrine, and oxygen may be required for this emergency. The drug of first choice is the β-2 agonist, such as albuterol, although

Table 3
Drugs grouped by emergency

Emergency	Essential drugs	Supplementary drugs
Allergy/anaphylaxis	Epinephrine	Hydrocortisone
	Diphenhydramine or chlorpheniramine	
Asthma	Albuterol	
	Epinephrine	
Angina/myocardial infarction	Nitroglycerin	Morphine
	Aspirin	Nitrous oxide
Hypotension		Atropine
		Ephedrine
Diabetic hypoglycemia	Oral carbohydrate	Glucagon
Status epilepticus		Lorazepam or midazolam

The above table assumes that oxygen is being administered and that intravenous access is not necessarily available.

metaproterenol and terbutaline also can be considered. An adult should receive two sprays; a young child should receive one spray. This should be repeated as necessary. If there is no response then epinephrine should be administered in the same dosage as described for anaphylaxis.

Cardiac arrest

This is managed consistent with the principles of BLS, or ACLS if appropriately trained individuals are present. If there is skill at using a bag-valve-mask device, then 100% oxygen should be administered. If available, an automated external defibrillator can be used. It has been stated that even without electrocardiogram (ECG) monitoring, 1 mg epinephrine can be administered, as it is indicated for all pulseless rhythms [3]. The fundamental aspect in its management is rapid defibrillation and ventilation.

Angina/myocardial infarction

Nitroglycerin, oxygen, and aspirin may be required for these emergencies. If available, morphine or nitrous oxide is indicated if myocardial infarction is diagnosed. Management of angina pectoris depends on whether or not there is a positive history of ischemic heart disease. The algorithm is summarized in Table 4. Those patients who are known angina patients should be administered sublingual nitroglycerin and may take their own. Oxygen should be administered. Relief should result within minutes following nitroglycerin administration. If no relief ensues, a second dose should be given. A fresh supply of nitroglycerin should be used for the second dose to rule out ineffectiveness caused by deterioration of the drug, which may occur if the patient had opened the bottle more than 3 months ago and exposed the drug to air or light. Therefore, the dentist should use the fresh supply from the emergency kit. The steps outlined in Table 4 should be followed. If there is no relief after three administrations, a diagnosis of myocardial infarction should be assumed and the patient transferred and managed accordingly.

Table 4
Management of angina pectoris/myocardial infarction

Ischemic heart disease history: positive	Ischemic heart disease history: negative
ABCs and O_2	ABCs and O_2
	Call 911 (assume myocardial infarction)
Nitroglycerin	Nitroglycerin
If no relief after 3–5 minutes:	If no relief after 3–5 minutes:
Repeat	Repeat
If no relief after 3–5 minutes:	If no relief after 3–5 minutes:
Repeat	Repeat
If no relief after 3–5 minutes:	If no relief after 3–5 minutes:
Call 911 (assume myocardial infarction)	Call 911 (assume myocardial infarction)
Aspirin 162 or 325 mg	Aspirin 162 or 325 mg
Morphine 2 mg IV or 5 mg IM or $N_2O:O_2$	Morphine 2 mg IV or 5 mg IM or $N_2O:O_2$

If there is no history of ischemic heart disease, the protocol is the same, except that the emergency medical system should be called immediately, as the patient needs to be transferred and assessed in hospital.

Hypotension

If the patient is symptomatic and the blood pressure has dropped significantly from baseline, hypotension may be assumed. The management begins with the syncope protocol as described above. One should then reassess blood pressure and perfusion. The ideal management at this point is the administration of intravenous fluids, but that is not realistic in most dental offices where venipuncture may not be likely. If a drug is to be used, atropine at 0.5 mg can be considered if heart rate is less than 60 beats per minute. Otherwise, ephedrine may be considered in doses ranging from 5–25 mg. As described above, these agents should be used cautiously.

Diabetic emergencies

The management of emergencies associated with diabetes is summarized in Table 5. Hypoglycemia and hyperglycemia are serious and can be fatal if left untreated. With that in mind, hypoglycemia is often considered the more serious because of the rapidity of onset of signs. If the patient is conscious, the treatment is easy. The hypoglycemic patient should be given an oral source of carbohydrate, such as a fruit juice or nondiet soft drink. The hyperglycemic patient should be given insulin if the dose is known, as provided by an accompanying caregiver for example. If not, the patient should be transferred to hospital. The unconscious hypoglycemic patient is best managed with basic ABCs, followed by oxygen and 50% dextrose if an intravenous line is in place. If not, glucagon can be administered intramuscularly in a dose of 1 mg.

Seizures

Management should begin with the protection of the patient. If status epilepticus develops, as determined by seizures that are prolonged or

Table 5
Management of diabetic emergencies

Hypoglycemia	Hyperglycemia
If conscious	If conscious
Oral carbohydrates	Hospitalize
If unconscious	If unconscious
ABCs	ABCs
Oxygen	Oxygen
Call 911	Call 911
50% dextrose IV or	
1 mg glucagon IM	

repeated, then an injectable benzodiazepine can be administered. Either lorazepam at 4 mg or midazolam at 5 mg may be given intramuscularly if a patent intravenous line is not present. If given, one should continue to monitor for deep sedation and the potential loss of protective reflexes.

Summary

There is universal agreement that dentists require emergency drugs to be readily available. Opinions differ as to the specific drugs that should comprise an emergency kit. This article has provided one opinion. Oxygen, epinephrine, nitroglycerin, injectable diphenhydramine or chlorpheniramine, albuterol, and aspirin should be readily available in a dental office. Other drugs such as glucagon, atropine, ephedrine, hydrocortisone, morphine or nitrous oxide, naloxone, midazolam or lorazepam, and flumazenil should also be considered.

There are differences in the level of training of dentists in the management of medical emergencies [25]. Therefore the final decision should be made by the individual dentist who is in the best position to determine the appropriateness of these agents for the particular practice. Despite the best efforts at prevention, emergencies may still arise. Plans to manage these events are needed and there is the possibility that the drugs discussed above may be required. Their presence may save a life.

References

[1] Fast TB, Martin MD, Ellis TM. Emergency preparedness: a survey of dental practitioners. J Am Dent Assoc 1986;112:499–501.

[2] Atherton GJ, McCaul JA, Williams SA. Medical emergencies in general dental practice in Great Britain. Part 1: their prevalence over a 10-year period. Br Dent J 1999;186:72–9.

[3] Becker DE. Assessment and management of cardiovascular urgencies and emergencies: cognitive and technical considerations. Anesth Prog 1988;35:212–7.

[4] Dym H. Stocking the oral surgery office emergency cart. Oral Maxillofacial Surg Clin N Am 2001;103–18.

[5] Haas DA. Drugs in dentistry. In: Compendium of pharmaceuticals and specialties. 37th edition. Toronto: Webcom Ltd; 2002. p. L26–9.

[6] Malamed SF. Emergency medicine: beyond the basics. J Am Dent Assoc 1997;128:843–54.

[7] Malamed SF. Medical emergencies in the dental office. 5th edition. St. Louis: Mosby; 2000. p. 58–91.

[8] McCarthy FM. Emergencies in dental practice. 3rd edition. Philadelphia: Saunders; 1979.

[9] Morrow GT. Designing a drug kit. Dent Clin N Am 1982;26:21–33.

[10] Poswillo DE. Standing Dental Advisory Committee. General anaesthesia, sedation and resuscitation in dentistry: report of an expert working party. London: HMSO; 1990.

[11] Rosenberg MB. Drugs for medical emergencies. In: Yagiela JA, Neidle EA, Dowd FJ, editors. Pharmacology and therapeutics for dentistry. 4th edition. St. Louis: Mosby; 1998. p. 689–95.

[12] Atherton GJ, McCaul JA, Williams SA. Medical emergencies in general dental practice in Great Britain. Part 2: drugs and equipment possessed by GDPs and used in the management of emergencies. Br Dent J 1999;186:125–30.

[13] Little JW, Falace DA, Miller CS, Rhodus NL. Dental management of the medically compromised patient. 6th edition. St. Louis: Mosby; 2002.

[14] American Heart Association. In: Cummins RO, editor. Advanced cardiac life support provider manual. Dallas: American Heart Association; 2001.

[15] Becker DE. Management of respiratory complications in clinical dental practice. Anesth Prog 1990;37:169–75.

[16] Eisenberg MS, Mengert TJ. Cardiac resuscitation. New Engl J Med 2001;344:1304–13.

[17] Davis WH. Emergency drugs and allergy. In: McCarthy FM, editor. Emergencies in dental practice. 3rd edition. Philadelphia: Saunders; 1979. p. 232–53.

[18] Ewan PW. ABC of allergies. Anaphlylaxis. Brit Med J 1998;316:1442–5.

[19] Zeitler DL. Drugs for treating allergic reactions. Oral Maxillofacial Surg Clin N Am 2001; 13:43–7.

[20] Gunnar TM, Bourdillon PO, Dixon DW, et al. ACC/AHA guidelines for the early management of patients with acute myocardial infarction. Circulation 1990;82:664–707.

[21] ISIS (Second International Study of Infarct Survival) Collaborative Group. Randomized trial of intravenous streptokinase, oral aspirin, both, or neither among 17,187 cases of suspected acute myocardial infarction: ISIS-2. Lancet 1988;2:349–60.

[22] Alldredge BK, Gelb AM, Isaacs M, et al. A comparison of lorazepam, diazepam, and placebo for the treatment of out-of-hospital status epilepticus. N Engl J Med 2001;345: 631–7.

[23] Haas DA. Oral and inhalation conscious sedation. Dent Clin N Am 1999;43:341–59.

[24] Neuget AI, Ghatak AT, Miller RL. Anaphylaxis in the United States. An investigation into its epidemiology. Arch Intern Med 2001;161:15–21.

[25] Atherton GJ, McCaul JA, Williams SA. Medical emergencies in general dental practice in Great Britain. Part 3: perceptions of training and competence of GDPs in their management. Br Dent J 1999;186:234–7.

THE DENTAL
CLINICS OF
NORTH
AMERICA

Dent Clin N Am 46 (2002) 831–846

Practitioner's guide to fluoride

Erik Scheifele, DMD[a],*,
Deborah Studen-Pavlovich, DMD[b],
Nina Markovic, PhD[c]

[a]*Division of Pediatric Dentistry, Temple University School of Dentistry,
3223 North Broad Street, Philadelphia, PA, USA*
[b]*Department of Pediatric Dentistry, School of Dental Medicine, University of Pittsburgh,
3501 Terrace Street, Pittsburgh, PA 15261, USA*
[c]*Department of Dental Public Health, School of Dental Medicine,
Department of Epidemiology, Graduate School of Public Health, University of Pittsburgh,
3501 Terrace Street, Pittsburgh, PA 15261, USA*

Fluoride has been the cornerstone for dental caries prevention saving the United States an estimated \$40 billion in oral health care delivery over the past 40 years [1]. Dental caries is a multi-factorial infection of the teeth characterized by demineralization of the dental hard tissues caused by repeated acid attacks with the potential for remineralization. Demineralization can progress, causing loss of tooth structure. Once cavitation occurs, there is no healing mechanism that can replace lost tooth structure [2,3].

Fluoride exerts its caries-protective properties in several ways. The primary anticaries effect is topical (posteruptive) [4,5]. Fluoride concentrated in plaque and saliva can inhibit the demineralization of enamel [6,7]. Fluoride taken up, along with calcium and phosphate by demineralized enamel (remineralization), forms an enamel crystalline structure that is more resistant to bacterial acid dissolution [6,8–12].

The systemic incorporation of fluoride into the developing enamel is thought to provide caries inhibition; however, evidence suggests that systemic fluoride (preeruptive) plays a more minor role in caries inhibition than previously thought [11]. The systemic ingestion of fluoride may also have a topical effect on enamel by passing through the digestive tract to the serum and then to the saliva [13].

Fluoride has been shown to inhibit the process by which cariogenic bacteria metabolize carbohydrates to produce acid and affect the bacterial

---

* Corresponding author.
E-mail address: escheifele@dental.temple.edu (E. Scheifele).

production of adhesive polysaccharides [14]. The current view, however, is that fluoride's antibacterial effects occur at higher levels than those that prevail in the oral cavity [15].

Prescription fluorides

Dietary fluoride supplements

Fluoridated drinking water is the most effective and efficient strategy to reduce dental caries [16]. Supplements were designed to mimic the effects of fluoridated water. Since around 1950, fluoride supplements have been used in areas where there is little or no fluoride in the drinking water [17]. There is mixed opinion regarding the use of fluoride supplementation for caries prevention. Although there is evidence supporting the incorporation of fluoride into developing enamel [18–20], the systemic or preeruptive effect may play a modest role in caries prevention. Research suggests that fluoride's primary effect is topical or posteruptive [5].

Supplements can be as effective as fluoridated water in preventing caries [11,21,22]. There is concern, however, regarding the risk of enamel fluorosis. The prevalence of fluorosis has increased [23–25], and numerous studies have reported the association between supplementation and fluorosis [12,26–41]. Determination of the appropriate dosage schedule is based on the concentration of fluoride in the community drinking water and the age of the child. The current fluoride schedule has been jointly recommended by the American Dental Association (ADA), the American Academy of Pediatric Dentistry (AAPD), and the American Academy of Pediatrics (AAP) since 1994 [42–45] (Table 1). It is important to know the concentration of fluoride in the child's primary drinking water and from other sources (eg, day care, baby sitter, school, or bottled water) prior to supplementation. The fluoride concentration of community water can be determined by contacting the local water supplier or the local or state department of health. If the child's drinking water is from another source (eg, private well or bottled water), testing may be available through the local or state department of health, private laboratories, or dental schools. Fluoride acquisition indirectly by consuming foods and beverages processed in fluoridated areas is known as the "halo or diffusion" effect [46]. Practitioners should be aware

Table 1
Dietary fluoride supplementation schedule

Age	Less than 0.3 ppm F	0.3–0.6 ppm F	More than 0.6 ppm F
Birth–6 mos	0	0	0
6 mos–3 yrs	0.25 mg	0	0
3 yrs–6 yrs	0.50 mg	0.25 mg	0
6 yrs–up to at least 16 yrs	1.0 mg	0.50 mg	0

(*From* American Academy of Pediatric Dentistry. Reference manual 1999–2000. Pediatr Dent 1999; 21(Special issue):40; with permission.)

that the distillation and reverse-osmosis home-water filtration systems may remove 90% or more of the fluoride; whereas, the less expensive carbon or charcoal filter systems remove little, if any, fluoride [47–49].

A dentist or physician must prescribe dietary fluoride supplements. Fluoride supplements are available in liquid, tablet, and lozenge form both with and without vitamins (Table 2). The fluoride-vitamin combination may improve parental compliance, thereby providing a greater benefit [50]. Fluoride tablets and lozenges should remain in contact with the teeth for as long as possible before swallowing (chew and swish or dissolve) to maximize both the topical and systemic effect. The primary teeth of children 1–6 years old would benefit from the posteruptive effect of fluoride, and the

Table 2
Common fluoride compounds

Compound		Fluoride content	pH
Supplements:			
0.275 mg NaF	Drops	0.125 mg F	Neutral
0.55 mg NaF	Drops, tablets, lozenges	0.25 mg F	Neutral
1.1 mg NaF	Drops, tablets, lozenges	0.5 mg F	Neutral
2.2 mg NaF	Tablets, lozenges	1.0 mg F	Neutral
Fluoride supplements may be combined with vitamins:			
0.022% APF	Rinse	200 ppm	Acid
Professionally applied:			
0.31% APF		3100 ppm	Acid
&	Sequential rinse	&	
0.1% SnF_2		1000 ppm	
2.0% NaF	Gel, foam	9040 ppm	Neutral
1.23% APF	Gel, foam	12,300 ppm	Acid
8.00% SnF_2	Rinse	19,400 ppm	Acid
0.4–2% NaF or APF	Prophy paste	4000–20,000 ppm	Neutral or acid
5.0% NaF	Varnish	22,600 ppm	Neutral
Self applied rinses:			
0.05% NaF	Daily	230 ppm	Neutral
0.1% SnF_2	Daily	240 ppm	Acid
0.2% NaF	Weekly (Rx)	905 ppm	Neutral
0.1% APF	Weekly (Rx)	1000 ppm	Acid
Self applied gels:			
0.4% SnF_2		970 ppm	Acid
1.1% NaF	(Rx)	5000 ppm	Neutral
1.1% APF	(Rx)	5000 ppm	Acid
Dentifrices:			
0.13–0.15%	NaF	1000–1500 ppm	Neutral
0.12–0.15%	Na_2FPO_3 (MFP)	1000–1500 ppm	Neutral

Supplements are intended for children <16 years old. Professional topical fluoride applications or prophylaxis use about 5 g or 5 mL of compound. Mouthrinsing uses about 5–10 mL of solution. Toothbrushing uses about 1 g of material per brushing. Fluoride contents are approximate values. This list is not intended to be comprehensive.

developing permanent teeth may derive some preeruptive benefit; however, fluoride supplements could also increase the risk for enamel fluorosis [51,52]. Fluoride supplements taken after the teeth erupt in children 6–16 years old reduce caries experience [53–55].

There is little support for prenatal fluoride supplementation because the use of fluoride supplements by pregnant women does not benefit their off-spring [56], even though studies suggest fluoride can cross the placenta from mother to fetus [57,58].

Self-applied fluorides

Patients perceived to be at high risk for developing caries or who have experienced severe caries may receive additional topical fluoride. Risk factors may include orthodontic or prosthetic appliances, xerostomic patients (eg, head and neck radiation, medications, medical conditions such as Sjogren's syndrome), physically or mentally disabled patients unable to clean their teeth, poor diet, and hygiene. Fluoride mouthrinses and gels are concentrated fluoride preparations designed for home use.

Fluoride mouth rinses are designed for daily or weekly use in patients ≥ 6 years old. The age recommendation is due to an increased risk of ingestion and fluorosis. Fluoride rinses are available as stannous fluoride, acidulated phosphate fluoride, and sodium fluoride, which is the most common preparation. Several nonprescription or over-the-counter (OTC) preparations of 0.05% NaF are available for daily use. The 0.2% NaF preparation is a prescription mouthrinse intended for weekly use.

Studies from the 1970s and early 1980s indicated that fluoride mouthrinse reduced the caries experience among school children [59–66]. The National Preventive Dentistry Demonstration Program (NPDDP) compared the cost and effectiveness of combinations of caries-preventive procedures during 1976–1981 and documented only a limited reduction in dental caries attributed to fluoride mouthrinse, especially when children were also exposed to fluoridated water [67].

Fluoride gel is intended for daily use and is available as stannous fluoride and sodium fluoride (neutral and acidulated) preparations. Application is by custom tray or by brushing preferably at bedtime to allow prolonged exposure of fluoride to teeth. The research to support the efficacy of fluoride rinses and gels is promising but not definitive [68].

Restorative materials

Replacement of existing restorations accounts for almost 75% of all restorative procedures [69]. The reason most commonly cited for restoration replacement is secondary caries, which accounts for about 40% of such replacements [70]. In light of these observations and the known anti-caries activity of fluoride, fluoride has been incorporated into many restorative materials. The concept is for the fluoride-containing restorative material to release fluoride into the surrounding tooth, preventing demineralization [71] and enhancing remineralization of the enamel and dentin. Since the mid-1980s, a wide variety of fluoride-releasing dental restorative materials have been available to dentists and dental consumers [72]. The box below contains a list of several fluoride-containing materials. In vitro studies indicate that fluoride release from certain restorative materials can reduce the severity of recurrent caries [73–79]. Caries inhibition and remineralization potential have been shown in vitro by many fluoride-containing restorative materials when release levels have been equal to or exceeded 1 µg/mL [72]. All fluoride-containing materials release fluoride in an initial burst and then reduce exponentially to a much lower steady-state level of release [72]. Various types of aesthetic restorative dental materials showed a potential for fluoride recharge [80] after exposure to external sources of fluoride (ie, topical fluoride applications). The recharging effect of the restorative material is thought to occur when external fluoride is incorporated into the restorative material and then re-released.

Because of the small number of controlled clinical studies, it is difficult to say with certainty whether fluoride-releasing dental materials increase the remineralization of carious enamel and dentin, and whether these materials increase the resistance of enamel and dentin to caries [68]. Long-term, controlled clinical trials are needed to determine if fluoride incorporated into dental materials inhibits or reduces dental caries.

Professionally applied fluorides

For over 50 years, professionally applied topical fluorides have been used in dental offices. The premise for their efficacy was based primarily on the assumption that the fluoride would be incorporated into the crystalline

---

Fluoride containing dental materials

- Adhesives/bonding agents
- Bases and liners
- Bleaching/whitening materials (home and in-office products)
- Cavity varnishes
- Cements
  Temporary (ie, ZOE, ZnPO4)
  Permanent (ie, GI/hybrids, polycarboxylate, ZOE, ZnPO4)
- Compomers
- Composite resin materials
- Core build-up materials
- Sealants

structure of the enamel, and with the incorporation of the fluoride, the enamel would become more resistant to acid destruction [81]. Traditionally, the topical fluoride would be applied following the prophylaxis to ensure a cleaner surface for its uptake. Recent evidence has suggested, however, that high concentrations of fluoride are not incorporated into the crystalline structure of enamel [81]. Rather, fluoride combines with calcium from the enamel to form a salt that adheres to the enamel surface. When the pH in the mouth becomes acidic, fluoride is released [82]. Presently, a professional cleaning is unwarranted to prepare the teeth to receive fluoride.

Fluoride gels and foams

Professionally applied fluoride gels and foams deliver a high concentration of fluoride (9040–12,300 parts per million [ppm]) at a low frequency (annual or semiannual application). In early clinical studies, professionally applied topical fluoride gels had shown to reduce dental caries effectively [83]. Recently, the caries reduction has decreased to 26%, with its primary effect on permanent teeth of children living in nonfluoridated areas [62,84,85]. Additionally, the optimal interval between professionally applied fluorides has not been established through clinical trials. Studies regarding these topical fluorides in the prevention of dental caries have been mixed at best [86]. According to the latest evidence, semiannual frequency can be recommended for children who will benefit from the therapy [86].

Fluoride foams (1.23% APF and 2% NaF) were introduced to dental professionals in 1993. Several advantages exist for using the foam. They include:

(1) requiring a smaller quantity of fluoride to fill the tray
(2) decreased risk of fluoride ingestion
(3) less clogging of suction lines in the dental operatory [84].

Additionally, the foamy consistency may have a greater appeal for the pediatric population. The enamel uptake of the foam is similar to the gel preparation [87].

Whether to apply the topical fluoride for 4 minutes or 1 minute has not been proven in human clinical trials [67]. During the first minute of application is when the greatest percentage of fluoride uptake occurs [85]. Certainly, a 1-minute topical fluoride application would be desirous for the younger population, but the evidence has not been demonstrated to make this recommendation.

Fluoride prophylaxis pastes

Many prophylaxis pastes containing fluoride ranging from 4000–20,000 ppm are used professionally. None of these pastes has been recommended, however, by the Food and Drug Administration (FDA) or the ADA as caries preventive products. Except for several Scandinavian studies involving a professional prophylaxis with a fluoridated paste (2200 ppm) every 2–4 weeks, no data document efficacy from annual or semiannual use of the pastes [88–90]. Even though chronic fluoride ingestion rarely occurs, the wide range of fluoride content in these products is without any basis [91]. Manufacturers of these types of fluoride products should be required to justify their recommendations.

Fluoride varnishes

Fluoride varnishes were developed as alternative topical products to the conventional fluoride gels and foams. They first appeared in Europe in 1964 as a 2.26% fluoride product and have had wide acceptance in Europe and Canada to prevent dental caries [92]. For almost 30 years in Europe, fluoride varnishes have been the modality of choice for professionally applied topical fluorides [93]. The premise for their effectiveness is the adherence of a high concentration of fluoride onto the enamel for up to 24 hours. Fluoride is deposited as calcium fluoride, and its ions are slowly released into the oral cavity. Advantages of the varnishes include an acceptable taste, rapid setting time, ease of application, and use of smaller amounts of fluoride when compared with professionally applied topical gels and foams [94].

Two types of varnishes, sodium fluoride or a difluorosilane, are available in the United States today. Their approval from the FDA is for use as a cavity varnish or as a dentinal hypersensitivity agent [95]. Because caries prevention is considered to be a drug claim, manufacturers of fluoride varnishes would need to submit evidence from clinical trials to receive FDA approval as anticaries agents [96]. In the United States the therapeutic use of fluoride varnishes for caries prevention is referred to as "off-label" because the product is being used for purposes other than originally approved [97]. This does not imply that professionally applied fluoride varnishes for caries prevention are illegal or unethical practices. Studies by Weinstein et al and Domoto et al have demonstrated promising caries prevention results [98,99]. In Washington and North Carolina, treatment with fluoride varnishes is a Medicaid-covered service [100]. In the near future, fluoride varnishes should become a vital part of the caries prevention plan.

Fluoride varnishes are applied onto the fissures, proximal surfaces of primary molars, and sometimes incisors with a small disposal brush and a saliva ejector. The frequency of application is based on the patient's caries risk assessment. The most frequently prescribed regimen is a semiannual application [101]. In order for fluoride varnishes to be effective, reapplication is required. Professional prophylaxis of the teeth is not essential prior to varnish application, even though most manufacturers recommend one. This ease of application makes it quite attractive for use with precooperative pediatric dental patients. The teeth should be dried with compressed air or with cotton gauze. Then, the varnish is applied and sets on contact with oral fluids.

Fluoride varnishes are another modality to deliver and retain fluoride onto the enamel surface of teeth. Varnishes may provide an alternative for caries control in patients with special needs, those receiving head and neck radiation, those undergoing orthodontic treatment, and those on chronic oral medications [100]. As more clinical trials are completed in the United States, fluoride varnishes should become an important component of caries prevention.

OTC fluorides

Fluoride has been incorporated into OTC, commercial dentifrices for over 40 years and accounts for approximately 98% of all dentifrices sold in the United States [102]. The use of OTC fluoride dentifrices along with community water fluoridation correlates with a significant decline in caries prevalence and extent among children and young adults [103–106]. Children in the United States have experienced a 36% decline in mean decayed, missing, and filled surfaces (DMFS) between 1980 and 1986 [107]. This reduction in caries is largely attributed to declines in smooth surface caries when compared with occlusal surfaces [108]. Individuals at greatest risk for caries include those without access to an optimally fluoridated water supply and those of lower socioeconomic status [109]. As a public health measure, fluoride in community water supplies and fluoride dentifrices have been repeatedly demonstrated as the most cost-effective measures for preventing dental caries [110].

Effectiveness of OTC preparations compared with placebos has demonstrated the effectiveness of fluoride dentifrices in caries reduction. In a review of published 2–3 year clinical studies comparing placebo and 0.243% sodium fluoride (NaF) dentifrices, Biesbrock found a mean dental caries reduction of 32% [111]. Fluoride dentifrices in the United States usually contain sodium fluoride (NaF) or sodium monofluorophosphate (MFP). In their review of studies comparing NaF and MFP formulations, Stookey et al concluded that NaF was significantly more effective than MFP in preventing caries by 5–10% in trials of 2–3 years duration [110]. Finally, a significant dose response of decreasing incident caries with increasing fluoride concentrations in dentifrices has been found for both NaF [111,112] and MFP [113,114]. A twofold or more concentration of currently marketed fluorides were compared in these trials, and the reduction of incident caries was in the range of 12–20% over the 3 years of the study, with a significant reduction in occlusal caries [103,111,113,114].

High fluoride products may be beneficial to individuals at high risk for caries, including those living in nonfluoridated areas. High fluoride dentifrices are counter-indicated, however, for use in the general population where fluoridated drinking water is available and among young children, where the risk of dental fluorosis may be high. In a review of fluoride dentifrice use in early childhood with subsequent development of dental fluorosis, summarized results of these studies conducted since the 1990s have identified an association between dental fluorosis and the use of fluoride dentifrice [115]. Findings from studies of lower-dose fluoride dentifrices' anticaries activity also were reviewed by these researchers. They concluded that there are important gaps in the knowledge about the effectiveness of lower-concentration fluoride dentifrices and their use.

Daily use of OTC fluoride mouthrinses used in conjunction with fluoride dentifrices has demonstrated additional benefit in caries reduction [116,117]. Currently, 0.05% NaF rinses are available and have shown a 65% reduction in caries when used twice daily [116] and appear particularly efficacious in root caries reduction [117]. Caries incidence is reduced generally by about 10–20% when rinses are utilized in unsupervised oral hygiene as an adjunct to fluoride dentifrices [117].

Ideally, loosely bound fluoride reservoirs that can maintain the concentration of fluoride in the oral cavity following product use would have a significant impact on caries inhibition [118–120]. Currently, controlled-release fluoride rinses and dentifrices are being evaluated for their effectiveness for sustained bioavailability in salivary fluoride to improve the de- and remineralization processes. Current findings indicate that a lower-concentrated fluoride dentifrice with controlled release of fluoride that can be incorporated into dental plaque when acidified to a critical pH may be appropriate for caries prevention [119]. This dentifrice could be developed in the near future as an effective OTC product [119].

Toxicity

Fluoride's caries preventive effects are well known; however, the potential toxic effects of fluoride must be considered. The optimal daily fluoride intake is considered to be 0.05–0.07 mg F/kg of body weight [46]. Ingestion of large amounts of fluoride may cause acute toxic reactions involving the gastrointestinal, neurological, cardiovascular, and blood chemistry systems and ultimately death [121–123]. Toxic reactions may occur with ingestion of about 5–8 mg F/kg [124,125]. A certainly lethal dose is considered to be 32–64 mg F/kg [124].

Dental fluorosis occurs as a result of excessive ingestion of fluoride during tooth development [126]. The severity of the fluorosis depends on the dose, duration, and timing of the fluoride ingestion [127]. Because enamel is not susceptible to fluorosis once its pre-eruptive maturation is complete, the risk of fluorosis is limited to children ≤ 8 years old [128]. Regardless of the severity, enamel fluorosis is considered a cosmetic rather than a functional effect [24,128–130].

Skeletal fluorosis, a crippling bone disease, has been associated with high levels of fluoride. Bone health, according to accepted scientific knowledge, is not adversely affected by ingestion of optimally fluoridated water [131–135]. Ingestion of fluoride has also been suggested to cause cancer; however, the American Cancer Society has stated "Scientific studies show no connection between cancer rate in humans and adding fluoride to drinking water" [136]. Several reviews have also concluded that there is no relationship between fluoridation and cancer [137–140].

Caution must be exercised with all fluoride-containing products, especially professionally applied fluoride treatments that may pose the greatest risk of acute toxicity. Practitioners prescribing or administering fluoride need to be aware of the potential acute and chronic toxic reactions associated with the various treatment modalities.

Acknowledgments

The authors would like to thank Ms. Sharon Hohman, secretary to the Department of Pediatric Dentistry, for her contribution in the completion of this manuscript. Her attention to details, accuracy, and word-processing agility are greatly appreciated.

References

[1] National Institute of Dental and Craniofacial Research. Research on fluorides to improve oral health. Available at: http.grants.nih.gov/grants/guide/pa-files/PA-01-121.html. Accessed September 1, 2002.

[2] Anusavice KJ. Efficacy of nonsurgical management of the initial carious lesion. J Dent Ed 1997;61:895–905.

[3] Makinen KK, Hujoel PP, Bennett CA, et al. A descriptive report of the effects of a 16-month xylitol chewing gum programme subsequent to a 40-month sucrose gum programme. Caries Res 1998;32:107–12.

[4] Burt BA, Eklund SA. Fluoride: human health and caries prevention. In: Burt BA, Eklund SA, editors. Dentistry, dental practice and the community. 5th edition. Philadelphia: WB Saunders; 1999. p. 279–96.

[5] Clarkson BH, Fejerskov O, Ekstrand J, Burt BA. Rational use of fluorides in caries control. In: Fejerskov O, Ekstrand J, Burt BA, editors. Fluorides in dentistry. 2nd edition. Copenhagen: Munksgaard; 1996. p. 347–57.

[6] Featherstone JDB. Prevention and reversal of dental caries: role of low level fluoride. Community Dent Oral Epidemiol 1999;27:31–40.

[7] Koulourides T. Summary of session II: fluoride and the caries process. J Dent Res 1990; 69(Special issue):558.

[8] Chow LC. Tooth-bound fluoride and dental caries. J Dent Res 69 1990;(Special issue): 595–600.

[9] Ericsson SY. Cariostasis mechanisms of fluorides: clinical observations. Caries Res 1977; 11(suppl 1):2–23.

[10] Kidd EAM, Thylstrup A, Fejerskov O, et al. Influence of fluoride in surface enamel and degree of dental fluorosis on caries development in vitro. Caries Res 1980;14:196–202.

[11] Thylstrup A. Clinical evidence of the role of pre-eruptive fluoride in caries prevention. J Dent Res 1990;69(Special issue):742–50.

[12] Thylstrup A, Fejerskov O, Bruun C, et al. Enamel changes and dental caries in 7-year-old children given fluoride tablets from shortly after birth. Caries Res 1979;13:265–76.

[13] Leverett DH, Adair SM, Proskin HM. Dental fluorosis among children in fluoridated and non-fluoridated communities. J Dent Res 1988;67(Special issue):230.

[14] Hamilton IR. Biochemical effects of fluoride on oral bacteria. J Dent Res 1990;69(Special issue):660–7.

[15] ten Cate JM. Current concepts on the theories of the mechanism of action of fluoride. Acta Odontol Scand 1999;57:325–9.

[16] Graves RC, Bohannan HM, Disney JA, et al. Recent dental caries and treatment patterns in US children. J Public Health Dent 1986;46:23–9.

[17] Burt BA. The case for eliminating the use of dietary fluoride supplements for young children. J Public Health Dent 1999;59(4):269–74.

[18] Groeneveld A, van Eck AAMJ, Backer Dirks O. Fluoride in caries prevention: is the effect pre- or post-eruptive? J Dent Res 1990;69(Special issue):751–5.

[19] Marthaler TM. Fluoride supplements for systemic effects in caries prevention. In: Johansen E, Taves DR, Olsen TO, editors. Continuing evaluation of the use of fluorides. Boulder (CO): Westview; 1979. p. 33–59.

[20] Murray JJ. Efficacy of preventive agents for dental caries. Systemic fluorides: water fluoridation. Caries Res 1993;27(Suppl 1):2–8.

[21] Driscoll W. The use of fluoride tablets for the prevention of dental caries. In: Forrester D, Schultz E, editors. International Workshop on Fluorides and Dental Caries Reductions. Baltimore: University of Maryland; 1974. p. 25–96.

[22] Hargreaves JA. Water fluoridation and fluoride supplementation: considerations for the future. Proceedings of a Joint IADR/ORCA International Symposium on Fluorides: mechanisms of action and recommendations. J Dent Res 1990;69(Special issue):765–70.

[23] Clark DC. Trends in prevalence of dental fluorosis in North America. Community Dent Oral Epidemiol 1994;22:148–52.

[24] Public Health Service Committee to Coordinate Environmental Health and Related Programs. Review of fluoride: benefits and risk. Washington (DC): US Department of Health and Human Services, Public Health Service; 1991.

[25] Szpunar SM, Burt BA. Trends in the prevalence of dental fluorosis in the United States: a review. J Public Health Dent 1987;47:71–9.

[26] Aasenden R, Peebles TC. Effects of fluoride supplementation from birth on human deciduous and permanent teeth. Arch Oral Biol 1974;19:321–6.

[27] Awad MA, Hargreaves JA, Thompson GW. Dental caries and fluorosis in 7–9- and 11–14-year-old children who received fluoride supplements from birth. J Can Dent Assoc 1994;60:318–22.

[28] D'Hoore W, Van Nieuwenhuysen J-P. Benefits and risks of fluoride supplementation: caries prevention versus dental fluorosis. Eur J Pediatr 1992;151:613–6.

[29] de Liefde B, Herbison GP. The prevalence of developmental defects of enamel and dental caries in New Zealand children receiving differing fluoride supplementation in 1982 and 1985. N Z Dent J 1989;85:2–8.

[30] Holm AK, Andersson R. Enamel mineralization disturbances in 12-year-old children with known early exposure to fluorides. Community Dent Oral Epidemiol 1982;10:335–9.

[31] Ismail AI, Brodeur J-M, Kavanagh M, et al. Prevalence of dental caries and dental fluorosis in students, 11–17 years of age, in fluoridated and non-fluoridated cities in Quebec. Caries Res 1990;24:290–7.

[32] Kalsbeek H, Verrips GH, Backer Dirks O. Use of fluoride tablets and effect on prevalence of dental caries and dental fluorosis. Community Dent Oral Epidemiol 1992;20:241–5.

[33] Lalumandier JA, Rozier RG. The prevalence and risk factors of fluorosis among patients in a pediatric dental practice. Pediatr Dent 1995;17:19–25.

[34] Larsen MJ, Kirkegaard E, Poulsen S, et al. Dental fluorosis among participants in a non-supervised fluoride tablet program. Community Dent Oral Epidemiol 1989;17:204–6.

[35] Pendrys DG, Katz RV. Risk for enamel fluorosis associated with fluoride supplementation, infant formula, and fluoride dentifrice use. Am J Epidemiol 1989;130:1199–208.

[36] Pendrys DG, Katz RV, Morse DE. Risk factors for enamel fluorosis in a fluoridated population. Am J Epidemiol 1994;140:461–71.

[37] Pendrys DG, Katz RV, Morse DE. Risk factors for enamel fluorosis in a non-fluoridated population. Am J Epidemiol 1996;143:808–15.

[38] Riordan PJ, Banks JA. Dental fluorosis and fluoride exposure in Western Australia. J Dent Res 1991;70:1022–8.

[39] Suckling GW, Pearce EIF. Developmental defects of enamel in a group of New Zealand children: their prevalence and some associated etiological factors. Community Dent Oral Epidemiol 1984;12:177–84.

[40] Wöltgens JHM, Etty EJ, Nieuwland WMD. Prevalence of mottled enamel in permanent dentition of children participating in a fluoride programme at the Amsterdam dental school. J Biol Buccale 1989;17:15–20.

[41] Woolfolk MW, Faja BW, Bagramian RA. Relation of sources of systemic fluoride to the prevalence of dental fluorosis. J Public Health Dent 1989;49:78–82.

[42] American Academy of Pediatric Dentistry. Reference manual 1995. Pediatr Dent 16 1994–5 (Special issue):1–96.

[43] American Academy of Pediatrics Committee on Nutrition. Fluoride supplementation for children: interim policy recommendations. Pediatrics 1995;95:777.

[44] American Dental Association. New fluoride schedule adopted. ADA News 1994.

[45] Meskin LH, editor. Caries diagnosis and risk assessment: a review of preventive strategies and management. J Am Dent Assoc 1995;126(Suppl):15–245.

[46] Warren JJ, Levy SM. Systemic fluoride sources, amounts, and effects of ingestion. Dent Clin North Am 1999;43:695–711.

[47] Levy SM, Kiritsy MC, Warren JJ. Sources of fluoride intake in children. J Public Health Dent 1995;55:39–52.

[48] Nowak A, Nowak MV. Fluoride concentration of bottled and processed waters. Iowa Dent J 1989;75:28.

[49] Tate WH, Chan JT. Fluoride concentrations in bottled and filtered waters. Gen Dent 1994;42:362–6.

[50] Hennon DK, Stookey GK, Muhler JC. The clinical anticariogenic effectiveness of supplementary fluoride-vitamin preparations. Results at the end of three years. J Dent Child 1966;33:3–11.

[51] Levy SM. Review of fluoride exposures and ingestion. Community Dent Oral Epidemiol 1994;22:173–80.

[52] Margolis FJ, Burt BA, Schork A, et al. Fluoride supplements for children: a survey of physicians' prescription practices. Am J Dis Child 1980;134:865–8.

[53] DePaola PF, Lax M. The caries-inhibiting effect of acidulated phosphate-fluoride chewable tablets: a two-year double-blind study. J Am Dent Assoc 1968;76:554–77.

[54] Driscoll WS, Heifetz SB, Korts DC. Effect of chewable fluoride tablets on dental caries in school children: results after six years of use. J Am Dent Assoc 1978;97:820–4.

[55] Stephen KW, Campbell D. Caries reduction and cost benefit after 3 years of sucking fluoride tablets daily at school: a double-blind trial. Br Dent J 1978;144:202–6.

[56] Leverrett DH, Adair SM, Vaughn BW, et al. Randomized clinical trial of the effect of prenatal fluoride supplements in preventing caries. Cares Res 1997;31:174–9.

[57] Ekstrand J, Whitford GM. Fluoride metabolism. In: Ekstrand J, Fejerskow O, Siluentone LM, editors. Fluoride in dentistry. Copenhagen: Munksgaard; 1988. p. 165–6.

[58] Shen YW, Taves DR. Fluoride concentrations in the human placenta and maternal and cord blood. Am J Obstet Gynecol 1974;119:205–9.

[59] DePaola PF, Soparkar P, Foley S, et al. Effect of high concentration ammonium and sodium fluoride rinses in dental caries in school children. Community Dent Oral Epidemiol 1977;5:7–14.

[60] Horowitz HS, Creighton WE, McClendon BJ. The effect on human dental caries of weekly oral rinsing with a sodium fluoride mouthwash: a final report. Arch Oral Biol 1971;16:609–16.

[61] Leverett DH, Sveen OB, Jensen ØE. Weekly rinsing with a fluoride mouthrinse in an unfluoridated community: results after seven years. J Public Health Dent 1985;45:95–100.

[62] Ripa LW. A critique of topical fluoride methods (dentifrices, mouthrinses, operator -, and self-applied gels) in an era of decreased caries and increased fluorosis prevalence. J Public Health Dent 1991;51:23–41.

[63] Ripa LW, Leske G. Effect on the primary dentition of mouthrinsing with a 0.2 percent neutral NaF solution: results from a demonstration program after four school years. Pediatr Dent 1981;3:311–5.

[64] Ripa LW, Leske GS, Sposato A, et al. Supervised weekly rinsing with a 0.2 percent neutral NaF solution: final results of a demonstration program after six school years. J Public Health Dent 1983;43:53–62.

[65] Ripa LW, Leske GS, Sposato A, et al. Supervised weekly rinsing with a 0.2% neutral NaF solution: results after 5 years. Community Dent Oral Epidemiol 1983;11:1–6.

[66] Rugg-Gunn AJ, Holloway PJ, Davies TGH. Caries prevention by daily fluoride mouthrinsing: report of a three-year clinical trial. Br Dent J 1973;135:353–60.

[67] Centers for Disease Control and Prevention. MMWR—Morbidity and Mortality Weekly Report: recommendations and reports 2001;50(RR-14): 1–42.

[68] Tinanoff N, Douglass JM. Clinical decision-making for caries management in primary teeth. J Dent Educ 2001;65:1133–42.

[69] Kidd EAM, Toffenetti F, Mjör IA. Secondary caries. Int Dent J 1992;42:127–38.

[70] MacInnis WA, Ismail A, Brogan H. Placement and replacement of restorations in a military population. J Can Dent Assoc 1991;57:227–31.

[71] Hörsted-Bindslev P. Fluoride release from alternative restorative materials. J Dent 1994;22(suppl 1):S17–20.

[72] Eichmiller FC, Marjenhoff WA. Fluoride-releasing dental restorative materials. Oper Dent 1998;23:218–28.

[73] Benelli EM, Serra MC, Rodrigues Jr, AL, et al. In situ anticariogenic potential of glass ionomer cement. Caries Res 1993;27:280–4.

[74] Dijkman GE, de Vries J, Arends J. Secondary caries in dentine around composites: a wavelength—independent microradiographical study. Caries Res 1994;28:87–93.

[75] Dionysopoulos P, Kotsanos N, Pagadogiannis Y, et al. Artificial secondary caries around two new F-containing restoratives. Oper Dent 1998;23:81–6.

[76] Gilmour AS, Edmunds DH, Newcombe RG. Prevalence and depth of artificial caries-like lesions adjacent to cavities prepared in roots and restored with glass ionomer or a dentin-bonded composite material. J Dent Res 1997;76:1854–61.

[77] Hatibovic-Kofman S, Koch G. Fluoride release from glass ionomer cement in vivo and in vitro. Swed Dent J 1991;15:253–8.

[78] Peveira PN, Inokoshi S, Tagami J. In vitro secondary caries inhibition around fluoride releasing materials. J Dent 1998;26:505–10.

[79] Serra MC, Cury JA. The in vitro effect of glass-ionomer cement restoration on enamel subjected to demineralization and remineralization model. Quintessence Int 1992;23: 143–7.

[80] Preston AJ, Higham SM, Agalamanyi EA, et al. Fluoride recharge of aesthetic dental materials. J Oral Rehab 1999;26:936–40.

[81] Dijkman TG, Arends J. The role of 'Ca-F$_2$-like' material in topical fluoridation of enamel in situ. Acta Odontol Scand 1988;46:391–7.

[82] Houpt M, Koenigsberg S, Shey Z. The effect of prior tooth cleaning on the efficacy of topical fluoride treatment: two year results. Clin Prev Dent 1983;5:8–10.

[83] Ripa LW. Professionally (operator) applied topical fluoride therapy: a critique. Int Dent J 1981;31:105–20.

[84] Ripa LW. An evaluation of the use of professional (operator-applied) topical fluorides. J Dent Res 1990;69(Special issue):786–96.

[85] Wei SHY, Yiu CKY. Evaluation of the use of topical fluoride gel. Caries Res 1993; 27(Suppl I):29–34.

[86] Johnston DW, Lewis DW. Three-year randomized trial of professionally applied topical fluoride gel comparing annual and biannual application with/without prior prophylaxis. Caries Res 1995;29:331–6.

[87] Wei SHY, Hattab FN. Enamel fluoride uptake from a new APF foam. Pediatr Dent 1988;10:111–4.

[88] Axelsson P, Lindhe J. The effect of a preventive programme on dental plaque, gingivitis and caries in schoolchildren. Results after one and two years. J Clin Periodontol 1974; 1:126–38.

[89] Axelsson P, Lindhe J, Waseby J. The effect of various plaque control measures on gingivitis and plaque in schoolchildren. Comm Dent Oral Epidemiol 1976;4:232–9.

[90] Poulson S, Agerbaek N, Melsen B, et al. The effects of professional tooth cleansing on gingivitis and dental caries in children after 1 year. Comm Dent Oral Epidemiol 1976; 4:195–9.

[91] Newbrun E. Current regulations and recommendations concerning water fluoridation, fluoride supplements, and topical fluoride agents. J Dent Res 1992;71:1255–65.

[92] Peterson LG. Fluoride mouthrinses and fluoride varnishes. Caries Res 1993;27(Suppl 1): 35–42.

[93] Bawden JW. Fluoride varnish: a useful new tool for public health dentistry. J Public Health Dent 1998;58:266–9.

[94] Seppä L. Efficacy and safety of fluoride varnishes. Compend Contin Educ Dent 1999; 20(Special issue):18–26.

[95] Beltran-Aguilar ED, Goldstein JW, Lockwood SA. Fluoride varnishes: a review of their clinical use, cariostatic mechanism, efficacy and safety. J Am Dent Assoc 2000;131: 589–96.

[96] Wakeen LM. Legal implications of using drugs and devices in the dental office. J Public Health Dent 1992;52:403–8.

[97] Food and Drug Administration. The FDA Modernization Act of 1997. Available at:http://www.fda.gov/opacom/backgrounders/modact.htm. Accessed September 1, 2002.

[98] Domoto P, Weinstein P, Leroux B, et al. White spot caries in Mexican-American toddlers and parental preference for various strategies. J Dent Child 1994;61:343–6.

[99] Weinstein P, Domoto P, Wohlers K, et al. Mexican American parents with children at risk for baby bottle tooth decay: pilot study at migrant farmworkers clinic. J Dent Child 1992;59:376–83.

[100] Vaikuntam J. Fluoride varnishes: should we be using them? Pediatr Dent 2000;22:513–6.

[101] Bravo M, Baca P, Llodra JC, et al. A 24-month study comparing sealants and fluoride varnish in caries reduction on different permanent first molar surfaces. J Public Health Dent 1997;57:184–6.

[102] Stamm JW. The value of dentifrices and mouthrinses in caries prevention. Int Dent J 1993;43:517–27.

[103] Brown LJ, Swangeo PA. Trends in caries experience in US employed adults from 1971–74 to 1985: cross sectional comparisons. Adv Dent Res 1993;7:52–60.

[104] Brunelle JA, Carlos JP. Changes in the prevalence of dental caries in US schoolchildren, 1961–1980. J Dent Res 1982;61:1346–51.

[105] Brunelle JA, Carlos JP. Recent trends in dental caries in US children and the effect of water fluoridation. J Dent Res 1990;69(Special issue):728–32.

[106] Newbrun E. Effectiveness of water fluoridation. J Pub Health Dent 1989;49:279–89.

[107] Brunelle JA. Dental caries survey in United States children 1986–1987. Oral health of US children national and regional findings. Bethesda (MD): US Department of Health and Human Services; NIH Publication 1989;89–2247:3–9. Publication No. 89–2247.

[108] Brown LJ, Selwitz RH. The impact of recent changes in the epidemiology of dental caries on guidelines for the use of dental sealants. J Public Health Dent 1995;55(Special issue):274–91.

[109] US Department of Health and Human Services. Oral health in America: a report of the Surgeon General. Rockville (MD): US Department of Health and Human Services, National Institute of Dental and Craniofacial Research. National Institutes of Health 2000;63–65:158–66. Publication No. 00–4713.

[110] Stookey GK, DePaola PF, Featherstone JDB, et al. A critical review of the relative anticaries efficacy of sodium fluoride and sodium monofluorophosphate dentifrices. Caries Res 1993;27:337–60.

[111] Biesbrock AR, Gerlach RW, Bollmer BW, et al. Relative anti-caries efficacy of 1100, 1700, 2200, and 2800 ppm fluoride ion in a sodium fluoride dentifrice over 1 year. Community Dent Oral Epidemiol 2001;29:382–9.

[112] Lu KH, Ruhlman CD, Chung KL, et al. A three year clinical comparison of sodium monofluorophosphate dentifrice with sodium fluoride dentifrices on dental caries in children. J Dent Child 1987;54:242–5.

[113] Marks RG, Conti RJ, Moorhead JEE, et al. Results for a three-year caries clinical trial comparing NaF and SMFP fluoride formulations. Int Dent J 1994;44:275–85.

[114] Stephen KW, Creanor SL, Russell JI, et al. A 3-year health dose response study of sodium monofluorophosphate dentifrices with and without zinc citrate; anti-caries results. Community Dent Oral Epidemiol 1988;16:321–5.

[115] Warren JJ, Levy SM. A review of fluoride dentifrice related to dental fluorosis. Pediatr Dent 1999;21:265–71.

[116] Fure S. Five year incidence of caries, salivary and microbial conditions in 60-, 70-, and 80-year old Swedish individuals. Caries Res 1998;32:166–74.

[117] Zimmer S. Caries preventive effects of fluoride products when used in conjunction with fluoride dentifrice. Caries Res 2001;35:18–21.

[118] ten Cate JM, Duijsters PP. Influence of fluoride in solution on tooth demineralization. I. Chemical data. Caries Res 1983;26:176–82.

[119] Vogel GL, Zhang A, Chow LC, et al. Effect of a water rinse on "labile" fluoride and other ions in plaque and saliva before and after conventional and experimental fluoride rinses. Caries Res 2001;35:116–24.

[120] White DJ, Nelson DG, Faller RV. Mode of action of fluoride: application of new techniques and test methods to the examination of the mechanism of action of topical fluoride. Adv Dent Res 1994;8:166–74.

[121] Beal JF, Rock WP. Fluoride gels. A laboratory and clinical investigation. Br Dent J 1976;140:307–10.

[122] Ekstrand J, Koch G. Systemic fluoride absorption following fluoride gel application. J Dent Res 1980;59:1067–70.

[123] Rubenstein LK, Avent MA. Frequency of undesirable side effects following professionally applied topical fluoride. J Dent Child 1987;54:245–7.

[124] Heifetz SB, Horowitz HS. The amounts of fluoride in current fluoride therapies: safety considerations for children. J Dent Child 1984;51:257–69.

[125] Shulman JD, Wells LM. Acute fluoride toxicity from ingesting home-use dental products in children, birth to 6 years of age. J Public Health Dent 1997;57:150–8.

[126] Bawden JW. Where is Waldo? The timing of fluorosis. J Public Health Dent 1996;56:5.

[127] DenBesten PK, Thariani H. Biological mechanisms of fluorosis and level and timing of systemic exposure to fluoride with respect to fluorosis. J Dent Res 1992;71:1238–43.

[128] Institute of Medicine. Fluoride. In: Dietary references intakes for calcium, phosphorous, magnesium, vitamin D, and fluoride. Washington (DC): National Academy Press; 1997. p. 288–313.

[129] Clark DC, Hann HJ, Williamson MF, Berkowitz J. Aesthetic concerns of children and parents in relation to different classifications of the Tooth Surface Index of Fluorosis. Community Dent Oral Epidemiol 1993;21:360–4.

[130] Kaminsky LS, Mahoney MC, Leach J, et al. Fluoride: benefits and risks of exposure. Crit Rev Oral Biol Med 1990;1:261–81.

[131] Cauley JA, Murphy PA, Riley TJ, et al. Effects of fluoridated drinking water on bone mass and fractures: the study of osteoporotic fractures. J Bone Min Res 1995;10:1076–86.

[132] Gordon SL, Corbin SB. Summary of workshop on drinking water fluoridation influence on hip fracture on bone health. Osteoporos Int 1992;2:109–17.

[133] Jacobsen SJ, O'Fallon WM, Melton LJ. Hip fracture incidence before and after fluoridation of the public water supply, Rochester, Minnesota. Am J Public Health 1993; 83:743–55.

[134] Karagas MR, Baron JA, Barrett JA, et al. Patterns of fracture among the United States elderly: geographic and fluoride effects. Ann Epidemiol 1996;6:209–16.

[135] Suarez-Almazor ME, Flowerdew G, Saunders LD, et al. The fluoridation of drinking water and hip fracture hospitalization rates in two Canadian communities. Am J Public Health 1993;83:689–93.

[136] American Cancer Society. A statement on fluoride and drinking water fluoridation by Clark W. Heath, Jr, MD, Vice President of Epidemiology and Surveillance Research of American Cancer Society. February 17, 1998.

[137] International Agency for Research on Cancer. IARC monographs on the evaluation of the carcinogenic risk of chemicals to humans, vol 27. Lyon: International Agency for Research on Cancer; 1982.

[138] Knox EG. Fluoridation of water and cancer: a review of the epidemiological evidence. Report of the Working Party. London: Her Majesty's Stationary Office; 1985.

[139] National Research Council. Health effects of ingested fluoride. Report of the Subcommittee on Health Effects of Ingested Fluoride. Washington (DC): National Academy Press; 1993.

[140] US Department of Health and Human Services. Review fluoride: benefits and risks. Report of the Ad Hoc Subcommittee on Fluoride. Washington (DC): US Department of Health and Human Services, Public Health Service; 1991.

Dent Clin N Am 46 (2002) 847–856

THE DENTAL
CLINICS OF
NORTH
AMERICA

Treatment of xerostomia: a systematic review of therapeutic trials

Michael T. Brennan, DDS, MHS*, Galib Shariff, DDS,
Peter B. Lockhart, DDS, Philip C. Fox, DDS

*Department of Oral Medicine, Carolinas Medical Center, Post Office Box 3280,
Charlotte, NC 28232, USA*

Xerostomia, the perception of dry mouth, may result from a range of etiologic factors. Although not always directly linked, xerostomia is commonly associated with salivary gland dysfunction [1]. It has been demonstrated that specific subjective complaints of oral dryness are related to a reduction in salivary flow [2], although in general xerostomia cannot be considered synonymous with salivary dysfunction. The lack of a strong association between the subjective perception of a dry mouth and decreased salivary flow is likely related to the finding that 50% of salivary function must be lost before subjective changes are recognized [3].

When xerostomia is related to salivary gland dysfunction, the cause will often fall into one of the following categories: medication side effects, autoimmune exocrinopathies (eg, Sjögren's syndrome), radiation-induced salivary gland dysfunction, dehydration, or salivary gland trauma. Other less common causes of salivary dysfunction include: salivary gland tumors, infectious processes (bacterial, viral), endocrine disease, dementia of the Alzheimer's type, cystic fibrosis, sarcoidosis, and amyloidosis [4]. Nonsalivary causes of xerostomia include cognitive or neurologic dysfunction, psychologic conditions, and idiopathic causes.

Over the years, a wide variety of agents and techniques have been used to manage patients with dry mouth complaints. In general, treatment is nonspecific, with the same therapeutic agents being applied in all cases. The range of systemic treatment options has been reviewed recently [5]. Although there are many published clinical trials and proposed therapies, the experimental quality varies considerably. The purpose of the present article is to systematically assess the level of evidence available in therapeutic

---

* Corresponding author.
E-mail address: mike.brennan@carolinashealthcare.org (M.T. Brennan).

clinical trials for the management of xerostomia. Specifically, we examine and rate the quality of randomized controlled trials in peer-reviewed journals, using established objective criteria. Our goal is to determine the strength of the clinical trial evidence for proposed xerostomia therapies.

Methods

Literature search

Articles were identified through the Pub Med search engine, http://www.ncbi.nlm.nih.gov/PubMed. The MESH terms "xerostomia" and "therapeutics" or "xerostomia" and "therapy" were used to identify published articles. Additionally, the following search limits were utilized: randomized controlled trial, human subjects, and the English language. We identified 52 articles classified as randomized controlled clinical trials for the treatment of xerostomia from 1966 to 2001 (Table 1). A wide variety of therapies assessed in randomized controlled trials were identified. Local therapies for xerostomia have ranged from saliva substitutes to electrostimulation, whereas systemic therapies have included agents from pilocarpine to acupuncture. Any therapy used for the treatment of dry mouth tested in a randomized clinical trial was included in the present article.

Quality assessment criteria

We utilized the criteria proposed by Hadorn to evaluate each clinical trial [6]. Assessment was completed for the following eight categories: selection of patients, allocation of patients to treatment groups, therapeutic regimen, study administration, patient withdrawals, patient blinding, blinding of outcome measures, and statistical analysis. Bias identified in each category was further classified into major and minor flaws. Examples of major flaws included: patients not randomly assigned, no placebo in the control group, and investigators not blinded to the patient treatment group. Minor flaws included items such as: nonideal randomization, imperfect blinding (eg, a patient could likely discern what was active treatment versus placebo), and withdrawals not handled appropriately in statistical analysis.

Two reviewers assessed each article. Discrepancies were resolved by a consensus meeting of reviewers. The sample size (number of subjects) was also recorded for each clinical trial.

Collectively, the major and minor flaws in the eight categories allow for clinical trials to be categorized into three levels: A, B, and C [6]. Level A, the highest quality evidence, requires a well-conducted clinical trial with no evidence of major flaws and less than three minor flaws. Level B includes more poorly controlled trials with one or more major or three or more minor flaws. Level C represents expert opinion derived from nonrandomized trials.

Table 1
Interventions assessed in clinical trials for xerostomia

Condition	Clinical trial intervention	References
Sjögren's syndrome	Pilocarpine	[10,20]
	Interferon alpha	[14,21,22]
	Longovital®	[23]
	Acupuncture	[24]
	Saliva substitutes	[25]
	Mucin-containing lozenges	[26]
	Mucin-containing gum vs. Carbamide-containing gum	[27]
	Electrostimulation	[18,28]
	Evening primrose oil	[29]
	N-Acetylcysteine	[30]
	Bromhexine	[17,31–33]
	Efamol	[16]
	Azathioprine	[34]
	Hydroxychloroquine	[35]
	Prednisone vs. Piroxicam	[36]
	Nandrolone decanoate	[37]
Radiotherapy damage	Pilocarpine	[8,9,38–43]
	Acupuncture	[44]
	Vegetable oil vs. Xerolube	[45]
	Linseed extract (Salinum®) vs. Methyl cellulose	[46]
	Saliva substitute	[38,47]
	Coumarin/troxerutine (Venalot®)	[48]
	Amifostine	[12,15]
	Oral balance gel and Biotene®	[49]
Radioiodine treatment	Amifostine	[50]
Xerostomia[a]	Anethole Trithione	[51]
	Lemon lozenge	[52]
	Saliva substitute	[19,52–54]
	Pilocarpine	[7,11,54]
	Oral lubricants	[55]
	Yohimbine vs. Anetholtrithione	[56]
	Acupuncture	[57]
	Chewing gum	[52,53,58]
	Anhydrous crystalline maltose	[13]

[a] Xerostomia trials represent inclusion of patients with dry mouth complaints from a wide variety of etiologies.

Results

For randomized controlled trials, the maximum number of major flaws using Hadorn criteria is 18, whereas the maximum number of minor flaws is 20. In the 52 articles reviewed, the mean $\pm$ SD number of major flaws was 2.2 ± 1.7 (range $= 0$–5), of minor flaws 4.3 ± 1.6 (range $= 1$–7). Of the 52 clinical trials assessed, only 4 could be classified as A-level evidence (ie, no major flaws and <3 minor flaws) [7–10]. Each of A level trials assessed pilocarpine treatment of xerostomia. The remaining 48 trials were classified as B level evidence. Because our search strategy selected only randomized controlled trials, no C level (expert opinion) studies were present.

A further analysis of individual major and minor flaws demonstrated common biases in the xerostomia literature (Table 2). The most frequent major flaws included the lack of a placebo control and inappropriate or absent measurement of baseline confounders or prognostic factors. A failure to ensure investigator blinding to treatment group was also a common major flaw. The most common minor flaw was a lack of details on treatment compliance (such as a pill count), which was found in 71% of clinical trials. Additional minor flaws found in the majority of the xerostomic literature included an inadequate explanation of admission and exclusion criteria as well as an incomplete explanation of the randomization method.

Wide variations in sample size were found (range; 10–373). Many studies were small; 16 (31%) had a sample size ≤25. Eight studies had a sample size >100 [8–15]. Three studies judged to be A level evidence had a sample size >100 [8–10], whereas the other A level study had a sample size of 39 [7].

Based on this review, pilocarpine is the only therapeutic agent that has a strong evidence base supporting its use for treatment of xerostomia. There are well-controlled clinical trials demonstrating efficacy of pilocarpine in at least two xerostomic conditions: Sjögren's syndrome (SS) and postradiation

Table 2
Common major and minor flaws in the xerostomia literature

	% (n) of trails
Major flaw	
Placebo not used for control group	35% (n = 18)
Prognostic factors or confounders not measured at baseline	35% (n = 18)
Investigator not blinded to patient treatment group	31% (n = 16)
Study population was not representative of majority of patients with condition under investigation[a]	25% (n = 13)
Analytical techniques described are incorrect	21% (n = 11)
Patients withdrew with reasons not listed	17% (n = 9)
Patients not randomly assigned	13% (n = 7)
Minor flaw	
Actual dose taken by patients was not recorded (e.g. pill count)	71% (n = 37)
Criteria for admission to and exclusion not adequately described	65% (n = 34)
Method of randomization inadequately described or not truly randomized	58% (n = 30)
Diagnostic criteria inadequately described	50% (n = 26)
Excessive withdrawal[b]	40% (n = 21)
Withdrawals not handled appropriate in statistical analysis	35% (n = 18)

[a] Sample size of <10/treatment group was placed in this category.

[b] >10% withdrawal for study duration ≤3 months and >15% withdrawal for study duration >3 months.

salivary dysfunction [7–10]. Other interventions appear promising (see below) but presently lack a strong evidence base in the published literature. Further well-designed and carefully conducted studies will be necessary to establish the efficacy of these interventions.

Discussion

A wide range of interventions for the management of xerostomia has been studied (see Table 1). Evidence in the form of randomized clinical trials to support the efficacy of most of these interventions is limited or of less than optimal quality. Only four randomized clinical trials in the xerostomia literature met an A level of evidence. All four of these studies, discussed below, assessed the efficacy of pilocarpine in the treatment of xerostomia.

In the SS literature, two studies met the highest level of evidence. In the first study, Vivino et al compared the efficacy of 2.5 mg pilocarpine, 5.0 mg pilocarpine, and placebo given 4× daily for 12 weeks in a multi-center trial of 373 patients. Results demonstrated that patients in the 5.0 mg pilocarpine group had greater global improvement of dry mouth and dry eyes symptoms compared with placebo. Additionally, salivary flow was significantly higher in the 5.0 mg pilocarpine group compared with the placebo group [10].

The second study was by Fox et al [7]. This clinical trial examined the safety and efficacy of 5.0 mg pilocarpine given for a range of xerostomia etiologies: 18 primary SS, 3 secondary SS, 12 cancer radiotherapy, and 6 idiopathic. Results demonstrated a significant increase in both parotid and submandibular flow rates in the pilocarpine compared with the placebo group. Subjective improvements in oral dryness, speaking, chewing, and swallowing were reported as well [7].

Two clinical trials of pilocarpine for treatment of radiotherapy-induced xerostomia also met the highest level of evidence. In the first study by Johnson et al, 207 patients with previous radiotherapy ≥4000 cGy were randomized to 5 mg pilocarpine, 10 mg pilocarpine, or placebo tid for 12 weeks [8]. Both pilocarpine groups had a significant improvement in symptoms of oral dryness, as well as improved mouth comfort. Although a significant increase in whole saliva was noted for the pilocarpine compared with the placebo group, this was not consistent for all individual study visits [8].

The other A level study in the radiation-induced xerostomia literature by LeVeque et al was a multicenter study of 162 patients that had received ≥4000 cGy for head and neck cancer [9]. In this dose-escalation trial, patients were randomized to receive active treatment with 2.5 mg pilocarpine tablets tid, titrated first to 5.0 mg and then to 10 mg or a placebo, over a 12-week period. A significant improvement in the overall global assessment of xerostomia was demonstrated in patients receiving the 5 mg and 10 mg pilocarpine doses. A significant increase in whole saliva production for pilocarpine compared with placebo was found at each study visit [9].

Although the remainder of clinical trials met the B level of evidence, five were close to the highest level of evidence, having no major flaws and only 3 or 4 minor flaws [14,16–19]. These trials looked at a variety of interventions for xerostomia. Four were SS studies, and the fifth enrolled hospice patients with a complaint of dry mouth. The first study examined the efficacy of very low-dose interferon-alpha, 150 or 450 IU once a day or three times a day, compared to placebo, given orally for 12 weeks in 109 patients with primary SS. Although no changes were demonstrated in the primary endpoints of symptomatic oral dryness and unstimulated whole saliva, a secondary analysis did show a significant benefit of 150 IU interferon-alpha tid over placebo, with increased stimulated whole salivary flow rates at 12 weeks [14].

The next study in the higher range of B level evidence examined the effect of an electrical simulation device on whole salivary flow rates in SS patients [18]. Results demonstrated a small yet significant increase in flow rates in patients utilizing the electrical stimulation device compared with a nonactive placebo device. It was noted, however, that significant differences could be attributed to the responses of only 3 of 14 subjects assigned to the active device [18].

Another study in the Sjögren's literature with higher B level evidence examined the efficacy of Efamol® (evening primrose oil) in a randomized, double-blind, cross-over study [16]. Results demonstrated no significant differences in xerostomia outcome measures with active drug compared with a placebo [16].

The final Sjögren's study with higher B level evidence and xerostomia outcome measures assessed bromhexine in a randomized placebo-controlled study [17]. Although an improvement in ocular measures was demonstrated, the bromhexine group had no improvement in mouth dryness [17].

The fifth study compared the effects of a mucin-based saliva substitute to a mucin-free placebo saliva substitute in patients with advanced malignant disease with dry mouth complaints [19]. No differences between the two saliva substitutes were found [19].

One of the most frequent major flaws in the xerostomia literature was a failure to use a placebo control. Although ethical concerns may preclude the use of a placebo control in some conditions (eg, cancer therapy), few arguments can be made to exclude a placebo in xerostomia clinical trials. As with the use of a placebo control, the other common major and minor flaws identified can be eliminated with appropriate clinical trial design and data collection.

The very frequently found minor flaw of excessive withdrawal of patients is likely related to the inherent logistic difficulties of clinical trials: the severity of side effects with some treatment regimens or the frustration of patients with no apparent treatment response. This often unavoidable loss of patients during a clinical trial is evidenced by the finding that all four A level studies in the xerostomia literature demonstrated this minor flaw.

One notable therapy not included in the present systematic review was cevimeline, a muscarinic agonist with a spectrum of activity similar to pilocarpine. Although this drug is United States Food and Drug Administration approved for the treatment of xerostomia in Sjögren's syndrome, and phase 3 clinical trials have been conducted, no studies had been published in a peer-reviewed journal at the time this article was written.

Summary

The results of the present systematic review of randomized controlled trials published in peer-reviewed journals demonstrate the presence of a wide variety of biases and the weakness of the existing literature of xerostomia treatment. The report of statistically significant efficacy on an outcome measure is only meaningful in the setting of a well-controlled, appropriately designed clinical trial. This points to the importance of evaluating the quality of the clinical trial closely when deciding if study results are applicable to a specific patient population.

Future studies in the management of xerostsomia will require an increased effort on the part of investigators to eliminate easily recognized flaws during the planning stages of a clinical trial. Minimizing bias in clinical studies will allow for easier interpretation and comparisons of different studies. Better clinical trial design is vital to provide maximal confidence in the efficacy of xerostomia interventions.

References

[1] Fox PC, van der Ven PF, Sonies BC, et al. Xerostomia: evaluation of a symptom with increasing significance. J Am Dent Assoc 1985;110:519–25.

[2] Fox PC, Busch KA, Baum BJ. Subjective reports of xerostomia and objective measures of salivary gland performance. J Am Dent Assoc 1987;115:581–4.

[3] Dawes C. Physiological factors affecting salivary flow rate, oral sugar clearance, and the sensation of dry mouth in man. Journal of Dental Research 1987;66(Special issue):648–53.

[4] Atkinson JC, Fox PC. Salivary gland dysfunction. Clin Geriatr Med 1992;8:499–511.

[5] Grisius MM. Salivary gland dysfunction: a review of systemic therapies. Oral Surg Oral Med Oral Pathol Oral Radiol Endod 2001;92:156–62.

[6] Hadorn DC, Baker D, Hodges JS, et al. Rating the quality of evidence for clinical practice guidelines. J Clin Epidemiol 1996;49:749–54.

[7] Fox PC, Atkinson JC, Macynski AA, et al. Pilocarpine treatment of salivary gland hypofunction and dry mouth (xerostomia). Arch Intern Med 1991;151:1149–52.

[8] Johnson JT, Ferretti GA, Nethery WJ, et al. Oral pilocarpine for post-irradiation xerostomia in patients with head and neck cancer. N Engl J Med 1993;329:390–5.

[9] LeVeque FG, Montgomery M, Potter D, et al. A multicenter, randomized, double-blind, placebo-controlled, dose-titration study of oral pilocarpine for treatment of radiation-induced xerostomia in head and neck cancer patients. J Clin Oncol 1993;11:1124–31.

[10] Vivino FB, Al-Hashimi I, Khan Z, et al. Pilocarpine tablets for the treatment of dry mouth and dry eye symptoms in patients with Sjögren syndrome: a randomized placebo-controlled fixed-dose multicenter trial. Arch Intern Med 1999;159:174–81.

[11] Björnström M, Axéll T, Birkhed D. Comparison between saliva stimulants and saliva substitutes in patients with symptoms related to dry mouth. A multi-centre study. Swed Dent J 1990;14:153–61.

[12] Brizel DM, Wasserman TH, Henke M, et al. Phase III randomized trial of amifostine as a radioprotector in head and neck cancer. J Clin Oncol 2000;18:3339–45.

[13] Fox PC, Cummins MJ, Cummins JM. Use of orally administered anhydrous crystalline maltose for relief of dry mouth. J Altern Complement Med 2001;7:33–43.

[14] Ship JA, Fox PC, Michalek JE, et al. Treatment of primary Sjögren's syndrome with low-dose natural human interferon-alpha administered by the oral mucosal route: a phase II clinical trial. J Interferon Cytokine Res 1999;19:943–51.

[15] Wasserman T, Mackowiak JI, Brizel DM, et al. Effect of amifostine on patient assessed clinical benefit in irradiated head and neck cancer. Int J Radiat Oncol Biol Phys 2000; 48:1035–9.

[16] Manthorpe R, Hagen-Petersen S, Prause JU. Primary Sjögren's syndrome treated with Efamol/Efavit. A double-blinded cross-over investigation. Rheumatol Int 1984;4:165–7.

[17] Prause JU, Frost-Larsen K, Hoj L, et al. Lacrimal and salivary secretion in Sjögren's syndrome: the effect of systemic treatment with bromhexine. Acta Ophthalmol. 1984; 62:489–97.

[18] Steller M, Chou L, Daniels TE. Electrical stimulation of salivary flow in patients with Sjögren's syndrome. J Dent Res 1988;67:1334–7.

[19] Sweeney MP, Bagg J, Baxter WP, et al. Clinical trial of a mucin-containing oral spray for treatment of xerostomia in hospice patients. Palliat Med 1997;11:225–32.

[20] Rhodus NL, Schuh MJ. Effects of pilocarpine on salivary flow in patients with Sjögren's syndrome. Oral Surg Oral Med Oral Pathol 1991;72:545–9.

[21] Ferraccioli GF, Salaffi F, DeVita S, et al. Interferon alpha-2 (IFN alpha 2) increases lacrimal and salivary function in Sjögren's syndrome patients. Preliminary results of an open pilot trial versus OH-chloroquine. Clin Exp Rheumatol 1996;14:367–71.

[22] Shiozawa S, Tanaka Y, Shiozawa K. Single-blinded controlled trial of low-dose oral IFN-alpha for the treatment of xerostomia in patients with Sjögren's syndrome. J Interferon Cytokine Res 1998;18:255–62.

[23] Pedersen A, Gerner N, Palmvang I, et al. LongoVital in the treatment of Sjögren's syndrome. Clin Exp Rheumatol 1999;17:533–8.

[24] List T, Lundeberg T, Lundstrom I, et al. The effect of acupuncture in the treatment of patients with primary Sjögren's syndrome. A controlled study. Acta Odontol Scand 1998;56:95–9.

[25] van der Reijden WA, van der Kwaak H, Vissink A, et al. Treatment of xerostomia with polymer-based saliva substitutes in patients with Sjögren's syndrome. Arthritis Rheum 1996;39:57–63.

[26] Gravenmade EJ, Vissink A. Mucin-containing lozenges in the treatment of intraoral problems associated with Sjögren's syndrome. A double-blinded crossover study in 42 patients. Oral Surg Oral Med Oral Pathol 1993;75:466–71.

[27] Aagaard A, Godiksen S, Teglers PT, et al. Comparison between new saliva stimulants in patients with dry mouth: a placebo-controlled double-blinded crossover study. J Oral Pathol Med 1992;21:376–80.

[28] Talal N, Quinn JH, Daniels TE. The clinical effects of electrostimulation on salivary function of Sjögren's syndrome patients. A placebo controlled study. Rheumatol Int 1992;12:43–5.

[29] Oxholm P, Manthorpe R, Prause JU, et al. Patients with primary Sjögren's syndrome treated for two months with evening primrose oil. Scand J Rheumatol 1986;15:103–8.

[30] Walters MT, Rubin CE, Keightley SJ, et al. A double-blind, cross-over, study of oral N-acetylcysteine in Sjögren's syndrome. Scand J Rheumatol Suppl 1986;61:253–8.

[31] Frost-Larsen K, Isager H, Manthorpe R. Sjögren's syndrome treated with bromhexine: a randomised clinical study. BMJ 1978;1:1579–81.

[32] Manthorpe R, Frost-Larsen K, Hoj L, et al. Bromhexine treatment of Sjögren's syndrome: effect on lacrimal and salivary secretion, and on proteins in tear fluid and saliva. Scand J Rheumatol 1981;10:177–80.

[33] Tapper-Jones LM, Aldred MJ, Cadogan SJ, et al. Sjögren's syndrome treated with brom-hexine: a reassessment. BMJ 1980;280:1356.

[34] Price EJ, Rigby SP, Clancy U, et al. A double blind placebo controlled trial of azathioprine in the treatment of primary Sjögren's syndrome. J Rheumatol 1998;25:896–9.

[35] Kruize AA, Hené RJ, Kallenberg CGM, et al. Hydroxychloroquine treatment for pri-mary Sjögren's syndrome: a two year double blind crossover trial. Ann Rheum Dis 1993;52: 360–4.

[36] Fox PC, Datiles M, Atkinson JC, et al. Prednisone and piroxicam for treatment of primary Sjögren's syndrome. Clin Exp Rheumatol 1993;11:149–56.

[37] Drosos AA, van Vliet-Dascalopoulou E, Andonopoulos AP, et al. Nandrolone decanoate (deca-durabolin) in primary Sjögren's syndrome: a double blind pilot study. Clin Exp Rheumatol 1988;6:53–7.

[38] Davies AN, Singer J. A comparison of artificial saliva and pilocarpine in radiation-induced xerostomia. J Laryngol Otol 1994;108:663–5.

[39] Hamlar DD, Schuller DE, Gahbauer RA, et al. Determination of the efficacy of topical oral pilocarpine for postirradiation xerostomia in patients with head and neck carcinoma. Laryngoscope 1996;106:972–6.

[40] Horiot JC, Lipinski F, Schraub S, et al. Post-radiation severe xerostomia relieved by pilocarpine: a prospective French cooperative study. Radiother Oncol 2000;55:233–9.

[41] Lajtman Z, Krajina Z, Krpan D, et al. Pilocarpine in the prevention of postirradiation xerostomia. Acta Med Croatica 1999;53:65–7.

[42] Sangthawan D, Watthanaarpornchai S, Phungrassami T. Randomized double blind, placebo-controlled study of pilocarpine administered during head and neck irradiation to reduce xerostomia. J Med Assoc Thai 2001;84:195–203.

[43] Schuller DE, Stevens P, Clausen KP, et al. Treatment of radiation side effects with oral pilocarpine. J Surg Oncol 1989;42:272–6.

[44] Blom M, Dawidson I, Fernberg JO, et al. Acupuncture treatment of patients with radiation-induced xerostomia. Eur J Cancer B Oral Oncol 1996;32B:182–90.

[45] Walizer EM, Ephraim PM. Double-blind cross-over controlled clinical trial of vegetable oil versus xerolube for xerostomia: an expanded study abstract. ORL Head Neck Nurs 1996;14:11–2.

[46] Andersson G, Johansson G, Attström R, et al. Comparison of the effect of the linseed extract Salinum® and a methyl cellulose preparation on the symptoms of dry mouth. Gerodontology 1995;12:12–7.

[47] Epstein JB, Stevenson-Moore P. A clinical comparative trial of saliva substitutes in radiation-induced salivary gland hypofunction. Spec Care Dentist 1992;12:21–3.

[48] Grotz KA, Wustenberg P, Kohnen R, et al. Prophylaxis of radiogenic sialadenitis and mucositis by coumarin/troxerutine in patients with head and neck cancer–a prospective, randomized, placebo-controlled, double-blind study. Br J Oral Maxillofac Surg 2001; 39:34–9.

[49] Epstein JB, Emerton S, Le ND, et al. A double-blind crossover trial of Oral Balance gel and Biotene® toothpaste versus placebo in patients with xerostomia following radiation therapy. Oral Oncol 1999;35:132–7.

[50] Bohuslavizki KH, Klutmann S, Brenner W, et al. Salivary gland protection by amifostine in high-dose radioiodine treatment: results of a double-blind placebo-controlled study. J Clin Oncol 1998;16:3542–9.

[51] Hamada T, Nakane T, Kimura T, et al. Treatment of xerostomia with the bile secretion-stimulating drug anethole trithione: a clinical trial. Am J Med Sci 1999;318:146–51.

[52] Stewart CM, Jones AC, Bates RE, et al. Comparison between saliva stimulants and a saliva substitute in patients with xerostomia and hyposalivation. Spec Care Dentist 1998; 18:142–8.

[53] Davies AN. A comparison of artificial saliva and chewing gum in the management of xerostomia in patients with advanced cancer. Palliat Med 2000;14:197–203.

[54] Davies AN, Daniels C, Pugh R, et al. A comparison of artificial saliva and pilocarpine in the management of xerostomia in patients with advanced cancer. Palliat Med 1998;12: 105–11.

[55] Furumoto EK, Barker GJ, Carter-Hanson C, et al. Subjective and clinical evaluation of oral lubricants in xerostomic patients. Spec Care Dentist 1998;18:113–8.

[56] Bagheri H, Schmitt L, Berlan M, et al. A comparative study of the effects of yohimbine and anetholtrithione on salivary secretion in depressed patients treated with psychotropic drugs. Eur J Clin Pharmacol 1997;52:339–42.

[57] Blom M, Dawidson I, Angmar-Mansson B. The effect of acupuncture on salivary flow rates in patients with xerostomia. Oral Surg Oral Med Oral Pathol 1992;73:293–8.

[58] Olsson H, Spak CJ, Axéll T. The effect of a chewing gum on salivary secretion, oral mucosal friction, and the feeling of dry mouth in xerostomic patients. Acta Odontol Scand 1991;49:273–9.

THE DENTAL
CLINICS OF
NORTH
AMERICA

Dent Clin N Am 46 (2002) 857–868

Oral manifestations of drug therapy

James Guggenheimer, DDS

*Departments of Oral Medicine, Pathology, and Otolaryngology, University of Pittsburgh
School of Dental Medicine, 3501 Terrace Street, G-137 Salk, Pittsburgh, PA 15261, USA*

During the course of providing patient care, the dental practitioner may encounter a variety of oral abnormalities. A number of these may have developed because of a complication of the patient's concurrent drug therapy for a medical condition. The probability that these drug reactions will occur is increased because of current, wide spread attitudes on the part of both patients and health care providers in the United States. These include a ubiquitous demand for and use of medications (prescription and/or over-the-counter) for the treatment of acute and chronic diseases, as well as a multitude of nonspecific and trivial ailments. In addition, the pharmaceutical manufacturers are engaged in mass marketing of their products that are being promoted for a plethora of diseases. A heightened awareness about health issues has also been stimulated by mass media coverage of health-related issues in the daily news reports. Internet web sites that are dedicated to health-oriented content are providing additional sources for information about diseases and treatment options.

This environment has heightened awareness about the practice of medicine and increased demands for treatment [1]. As a consequence, it has been estimated that at least 90% of office visits to a physician result in a prescription being given [2]. Another trend, the current and dramatic growth of our aging population with its better access to health care, will also intensify the need for medications for the management of acute and chronic diseases that are more prevalent in the elderly. A survey of a sample of Medicare subscribers found that more than 90% had visited a physician in 1997 [3]. Two recent indicators lend additional support to the prevalence of drug use in the United States. Data from pharmaceutical manufacturers revealed that more than 2.04 billion prescriptions were dispensed during the calendar year 2000 [4]. This was in addition to the $19 billion that were spent on over-the-counter medications that year [5].

E-mail address: guggen@pitt.edu (J. Guggenheimer).

In addition, economic constraints and other obstacles that may restrict access to health care providers, as well as a better-informed public, have increased the desire to engage in self-medication. As a consequence, there has been a proliferation of over-the-counter agents and herbal medicines that are available in growing numbers of retail distributors. These trends have been further stimulated by renewed interest in alternative or complementary medicine that promotes the use of a variety of "natural" therapeutic agents whose effects, potential side-effects, and interactions have not been tested or documented [6]. Finally, biological and technological advances that are advancing our understanding of disease mechanisms are also enabling the development of new drugs for specific disease intervention or prevention.

In the modern dental practice, therefore, the practitioner should anticipate and needs to determine if an oral symptom or abnormality is a manifestation of an adverse drug reaction.

Classification of drug reactions

An oral side effect of a drug is considered to be the consequence of an undesirable effect or one that is "noxious and unintended" [7,8].

A variety of oral conditions may develop as complications from the use of drugs. The older literature appropriately labeled one such oral manifestation "stomatitis medicamentosa." Among more recent reviews of medication side effects, one report cited 46 orofacial abnormalities that were attributed to more than 150 medications [9]. In another report, 259 oral side-effects were identified and attributed to 113 of the 200 medications that were most frequently prescribed in 1992 [10].

Because of the number and variability of clinical manifestations that drug side effects can induce in the oral cavity, efforts have been made to classify and delineate these abnormalities. When the topic of adverse drug reactions was previously reviewed in *The Dental Clinics of North America* in 1984, eight categories of clinical manifestations were described [11]. Another periodical that regularly reports on dental therapies has also categorized eight types of drug reactions that may be encountered [12].

For the purposes of this article, six categories or descriptions of oral complications have been selected. The criteria used included side effects that are more likely to be encountered by the general dental practitioner, and complications that may result from drugs that are more frequently prescribed, or which are used over the long term for the management of chronic diseases. The categories of drug reactions and the medications that may cause them are summarized in Table 1.

One of the most frequent complications of drug therapy, xerostomia or dry mouth, will be discussed elsewhere in this issue.

Table 1
Oral manifestations of drug therapies and their etiology

Gingival hypertrophy
    Phenytoin (Dilantin®)
    Calcium channel blockers
        Nifedipine (Procardia®, Adalat®), diltiazem (Cardizem®, Dilaclor®), verapamil (Calan®,
           Isoptin®, Verelan® and amlodipine (Norvas®)
    Cyclosporine (Neoral®, Sandimmune®)

Tooth discoloration
    Tetracyclines
        Minocycline (Minocin®)

Candidiasis
    Broad spectrum antibiotics (tetracyclines)
    Corticosteroids (prednisone)
    Cancer chemotherapeutic agents (alkylating agents, antimetabolites)
    Immunosuppressants
        Corticosteroids
        Antirejection drugs (Cyclosporine)
    Xerostomic medications

Burns
    Aspirin and OTC products containing phenol, eugenol, or hydrogen peroxide

Taste aberrations (metallic taste)
    Oral hypoglycemics (Metformin)
    Antimicrobial (Metronidazole, tetracycline)
    Antipsychotic (Lithium)
    Antirheumatic (Allopurinol, penicillamine, phenylbutazone, gold salts)
    Cardiovascular (Enalapril)
    Cancer chemotherapeutic agents (Methotrexate)
    Gold compounds (Auranofin)
    Immunosuppressants (Corticosteroids, antirejection drugs)
    Xerostomic medications

Lichenoid drug reactions
    Antibiotics
    Oral hypoglycemics
    Antihypertensives
    Nonsteroidal anti-inflammatory agents
    Gold compounds

OTC, over-the-counter.

Soft tissue abnormalities

Gingival hyperplasia

Enlargement or overgrowth of the gingiva is a recognized complication that has been associated with the administration of phenytoin (Dilantin®), some calcium channel blockers, and cyclosporine (Sandimmune®). Although the cause and effect relationship with phenytoin was identified more than 60 years ago, the mechanism by which these drugs induce the hyperplasia has not been determined.

Phenytoin

Recent estimates have found that epilepsy and other seizure disorders affect between 5–10% of the population [13]. The first drug to be used for these patients, phenytoin (Dilantin®), was still listed among the 200 most frequently prescribed drugs in the United States in 2000 [4]. Clinical studies have found that approximately one half of the patients who are on phenytoin therapy develop gingival hyperplasia [14,15]. The risk for and degree of phenytoin enlargement is increased by poor oral hygiene, accumulation of plaque, and subsequent gingival inflammation; therefore, maintenance of good home care can minimize the overgrowth. There is no evidence that the use of phenytoin in conjunction with the other drugs that cause gingival hyperplasia will have an additive effect on the overgrowth. Other pathophysiological processes, however, can result in enhancement of the hyperplasia (Fig. 1).

Calcium channel blockers

Calcium channel blockers have been used for more than 20 years for the treatment of a variety of cardiovascular diseases including angina, arrhythmias, and hypertension. These drugs may also be effective for the management of other conditions, such as atherosclerosis, Raynaud's phenomenon, migraine headaches, peripheral vascular disease, and stroke [16]. In addition, calcium channel blockers are being investigated for potential use to treat a number of other disorders [16]. Because cardiovascular disease is one of the most prevalent conditions in the United States (and remains the leading cause of death), it was estimated that in 1995 at least 6 million individuals were using a calcium channel blocker [17]. Among the 10 calcium channel blockers currently available, 3 have been found to induce gingival hyperplasia more frequently. They are nifedipine (Procardia®, Adalat®), diltiazem (Cardizem®, Dilaclor®), and verapamil (Calan®, Isoptin®, Verelan®) [18]. These three calcium channel blockers were

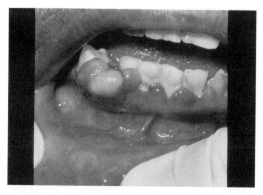

Fig. 1. Gingival hyperplasia with a concurrent pyogenic granuloma in a postpartum patient who was taking phenytoin (Dilantin®).

among the 200 most frequently prescribed medications in the United States in 2000 [4].

The effect of the calcium channel blockers on the gingiva is variable and unpredictable. A number of investigations have reported the incidence of hyperplasia to range from 20–83% [19,20]. The overgrowth is also influenced by the patient's compliance with oral hygiene (Fig. 2). If the patient can discontinue the therapy or be given an alternative medication, the hyperplasia will regress [18].

Cyclosporine

Cyclosporine (Sandimmune®, Neoral®) is an immunosuppressant drug that inhibits immune mechanisms that cause the rejection of transplanted organs. The drug was first used in 1978 for patients who had received kidney transplants [21]. Clinical studies have found that gingival hyperplasia develops in approximately 5–16% of patients who are taking cyclosporine [22], but in one report it occurred in 70% of the recipients [23]. The likelihood that the dental practitioner will encounter cyclosporine-induced gingival hyperplasia is increasing. In 2000, nearly 73,000 organ and bone marrow transplantations were performed in the United States [24], and patients who have received transplants are surviving for longer periods.

The clinical characteristics of cyclosporine-induced gingival hyperplasia are similar to those caused by phenytoin or the calcium channel blockers, and the overgrowth is also influenced by poor oral hygiene and the accumulation of dental plaque (Fig. 3). Discontinuance of therapy or a reduction of the cyclosporine dose may resolve the hyperplasia [25].

It has been reported that cyclosporine, when administered with a calcium channel blocker, can have an additive effect on the gingival hyperplasia [26]. This combined therapy is more likely to be used for patients who had cardiovascular disease and required a kidney, heart, or lung transplant. Corticosteroids may be used in conjunction with cyclosporine to enhance the

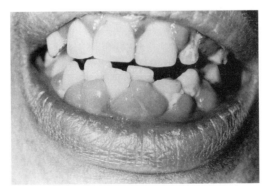

Fig. 2. Gingival hyperplasia in a patient who was taking the calcium channel blocker nifedipine.

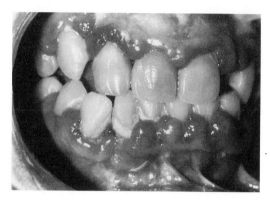

Fig. 3. A patient on cyclosporine therapy following kidney transplantation showing gingival hyperplasia, inflammation, and poor oral hygiene.

immunosupression and prevent organ rejection. This adjunctive therapy can increase the risk for oral candidiasis (see below).

Tooth discoloration

Tetracycline

In 1948, chlortetracycline, the first of the tetracyclines, was introduced. This group of antibiotics was only the fourth class of antimicrobial agents that were available at the time, which included the sulfonamides, penicillin, and streptomycin. The tetracyclines were the first "broad spectrum" antibiotics that were effective against both gram-positive and gram-negative bacteria as well as a number of other microorganisms [27]. Because of their wider range of antimicrobial activity, particularly for infections of the upper respiratory tract, and their availability for oral administration in the form of (liquid) suspensions, flavored syrups, or elixirs, they were frequently prescribed for pediatric patients.

Between 1961 and 1963, clinical evidence began to appear suggesting that tetracycline could cause tooth discoloration [28]. This association was subsequently substantiated by a number of clinical and laboratory studies demonstrating that tetracycline becomes irreversibly bound to calcified tooth structures if it is administered during the calcification stages of tooth development [28]. Following these disclosures, the pharmaceutical manufacturers of these antibiotics inserted warnings that the tetracyclines were contraindicated for use in children under 8 years of age.

Minocycline

A more recent concern, however, is tetracyclince-induced discoloration of the permanent dentition after its development has been completed. This phenomenon has been associated with another tetracycline product, mino-cycline (Minocin®) [29,30]. Minocycline is a semisynthetic tetracycline derivative that became available in 1972 [27]. Current indications for the use of minocycline include bronchitis, acne, genitourinary infections, and gas-trointestinal ulcers suspected to be caused by *Heliobacter pylori* [31]. Mino-cycline has also been assessed for use in conjunction with antirheumatic drugs for the treatment of rheumatoid arthritis [32]. Following minocycline therapy, pigmentation of the skin, nails, sclera, and gingiva has occurred, but these effects are reversible after treatment is discontinued [31].

The process by which this antibiotic penetrates permanent tooth structure has not been determined, but two theories have been proposed: (1) the anti-biotic is absorbed from the systemic circulation via the pulpal blood vessels into the dentin, and (2) it enters through defects in the enamel surface from the crevicular fluid [29]. Another possibility is that the drug enters the saliva from the systemic circulation and permeates exposed dentin tubules that have been exposed by attrition (Fig. 4).

The degree of minocycline discoloration can be very intense if the drug is incorporated into tooth structures during their development (Fig. 5). It has been suggested that this stain is a manifestation of drug degradation prod-ucts that consist of a minocycline-hemosiderin complex [31].

Altered immunity and candidiasis

The immune system protects the body from infection. A common oral manifestation of a loss of immunity is the development of an opportunistic infection by the fungus *Candida albicans*. Oral candidiasis has several clini-cal manifestations that are described as pseudomembranous (white patches), atrophic (erythematous, red, or inflamed), denture stomatitis, or median rhomboid glossitis [33].

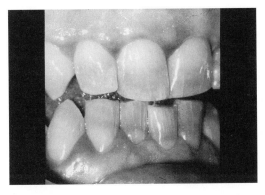

Fig. 4. Minocycline-induced discoloration of the permanent dentition in a 35-year-old patient who had been taking the medication for 3 years.

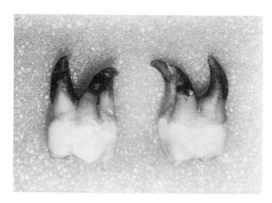

Fig. 5. Intense staining of the roots of two maxillary third molars. The patient began to take minocycline at age 17.

A number of drugs can suppress the body's immune responses and induce candidal overgrowth. These include the corticosteroids, cancer chemotherapeutic agents, and immunosuppressants (Table 1). The corticosteroids (glucocorticoids) are extensively used for their anti-inflammatory and immunosuppressant properties in the treatment of rheumatic, collagen, and similar autoimmune diseases, as well as asthma and other allergic disorders. Prednisone, a synthetic glucocorticoid was ranked 27th among the 50 most frequently prescribed drugs in 1999 [34].

Corticosteroids may be used in conjunction with anti-rejection drugs following organ and bone marrow transplantation (see cyclosporine, above). This combined immunosuppressive therapy may have an additive effect on the risk for developing oral candidiasis.

Systemic treatment with corticosteroids often entails long-term use that places patients at increased risk for developing oral candidiasis. This risk is increased by smoking, denture use, dry mouth, diabetes [35], and concurrent administration of other medications that can enhance the overgrowth of candidal organisms (see Table 1).

Corticosteroids are also administered by inhalation for the treatment of asthma and other respiratory diseases. This route of administration appears to have a variable effect on candidal overgrowth that had been found to range from <1–7% [36,37].

Treatment with cancer chemotherapeutic agents places patients at high risk for oral infections, the majority of which are caused by *C albicans* [38]. Cancer chemotherapy also causes dry mouth, which increases the possibility of a candidal infection.

Finally, oral candidiasis can develop following a change in or suppression of the normal oral flora. This is likely to occur following the administration of antibiotics, particularly those with broad spectrum activity such as tetracycline [33]. The overgrowth is also enhanced by other environmental factors in the oral cavity, including xerostomia, smoking, and the use of dentures [35].

Chemical injuries

Chemical burns of the oral tissues are common occurrences that may be accidental (ingestion by children), or from misuse of products that are being used for self-medication. The "aspirin burn" probably represents the typical example of such a reaction that the dentist may encounter.

An increasing number of over-the-counter "do it yourself" topical agents are available for the relief of oral pain. These products may contain phenol, eugenol, or concentrated hydrogen peroxide, all of which can also burn the oral mucosa. If these remedies are used to treat dental pain that originates from the pulp or the periodontium, it is unlikely that they will provide adequate relief. The patient may then resort to prolonged or repeated applications of the material that can result in mucosal injury.

Taste aberrations

Changes in the perception of taste or "dysgeusia" are estimated to affect several million individuals [39]. Abnormal taste sensations have been attributed to a number of diverse systemic diseases [39], or the cause may be obscure or nondeterminable. The use of medications has also been implicated. When the side effect of a drug results in a taste aberration, it may be a direct effect of the medication, or an indirect effect that is mediated by, for example, a drug-induced overgrowth of *Candida* (see above) or xerostomia. A variety of abnormal taste perceptions can occur, but patients usually seek professional attention from the dentist for a metallic taste. Several categories of drugs have been associated with metallic taste and are listed in Table 1 [40]. This sensation may also become apparent after the placement or insertion of an amalgam restoration or metal prosthesis, which is then implicated as the cause.

Lichenoid drug eruptions

Lichen planus is considered to be a dermatologic condition but it frequently occurs on the oral mucosa. Dentists are likely to encounter patients with this disorder, particular if it causes any discomfort or concern. Lesions on the oral mucosa that resemble lichen planus have been linked to a number of medications that encompass a variety of pharmacologic categories. These include antibiotics, oral hypoglycemics, antihypertensives, nonsteroidal anti-inflammatory agents, and agents that contain heavy metals (eg, lithium, gold compounds) [39,41]. Lichenoid lesions have also been reported to result from direct contact with cinnamon [42] or as a manifestation of allergy to amalgam [43]. Patients with lichen planus should, therefore, have a comprehensive review of their drug history as part of their initial evaluation prior to initiating other diagnostic or treatment efforts.

Summary

The oral cavity may be the target organ for a number of diverse abnormalities that develop from side effects of medications. Because of the widespread and increasing use of prescription, over-the-counter, and herbal remedies, it is becoming increasingly likely that the dentist will encounter soft tissue or dental pathologies that represent a complication of a therapeutic agent. The more common abnormalities that may occur include gingival hyperplasia, tooth discoloration, candidiasis, chemical injuries, and altered taste perception. The dental practitioner is often the primary health care provider who can recognize, diagnose, treat, and/or prevent these conditions.

References

[1] Burnum JF. Medical practice a la mode. How medical fashions determine medical care. N Engl J Med 1987;317(19):1220–2.

[2] Marks HM. Revisiting "The origins of compulsory drug prescriptions". Am J Public Health 1995;85(1):109–15.

[3] Sandman D, Simatov E, An C. Out of touch: American men and the health care system. Commonwealth's Fund Men's and Women's Health Survey Findings. The Commonwealth Fund publication # 374. March 2000.

[4] The top 200 prescriptions for 2000 by number of U.S. prescriptions dispensed. IMS Health, Inc., Westport, CT. Available at: http://www.rxlist.com/top200.htm. Accessed August 16, 2001.

[5] Brass EP. Changing the status of drugs from prescription to over-the-counter availability. N Engl J Med 2001;345(11):810–6.

[6] Angell M, Kassirer JP. Alternative medicine: the risks of untested and unregulated remedies. N Engl J Med 1998;339(12):839–41.

[7] Bates DW, Leape L. Adverse drug reactions. In: Carruthers SG, Hoffman BB, Melmon KL, et al, editors. Melmon and Morrelli's Clinical Pharmacology: basic principles in therapeutics. 4th edition. New York: McGraw-Hill; 2000. p. 1223–56.

[8] Klaassen CD. Principles of Toxicology. In: Gilman AG, Rall TW, Nies AS, et al, editors. Goodman and Gilman's the pharmacological basis of therapeutics. 8th edition. New York: Pergamon Press; 1990. p. 49–61.

[9] Matthews TG. Medication side effects of dental interest. J Prosth Dent 1990;64(2): 219–26.

[10] Smith RG, Burtner AP. Oral side-effects of the most frequently prescribed drugs. Spec Care Dentist 1994;14(3):96–102.

[11] Wright JM. Oral manifestations of drug reactions. Dent Clin NA 1984;28(3):529–43.

[12] Ciancio SG. Medications with potential adverse oral reactions. In: Ciancio SG, editor. Biol Ther Dent 1995;11(3):15–6.

[13] Lowenstein DH. Seizures and epilepsy. In: Braunwald E, Fauci AS, Kasper DL, et al, editors. Harrison's principles of internal medicine. 15th edition. New York: McGraw-Hill; 2001. p. 2354–69.

[14] Dongari A, McDonnell HT, Langlais RP. Drug-induced gingival overgrowth. Oral Surg Oral Med Oral Pathol 1993;76(4):543–8.

[15] Seymour RA, Heasman PA. Drugs and the periodontium. J Clin Periodontol 1988;15:1–6.

[16] Triggle DJ. Mechanisms of action of calcium channel antagonists. In: Epstein M, editor. Calcium antagonists in clinical medicine. 2nd edition. Philadelphia: Hanley & Belfus, Inc; 1998. p. 1–26.

[17] Altman LK. Agency issues warning for drug widely used for heart disease. The New York Times; Sept 1, 1995. p. 1.

[18] Wynn RL. Calcium channel blocker-induced gingival hyperplasia: update. Biol Ther Dent 1995;11(2):5–7.

[19] Ellis JS, Seymour RA, Steele JG, et al. Prevalence of gingival overgrowth induced by calcium channel blockers: a community-based study. J Periodontol 1999;70(1):63–7.

[20] Fattore L, Stablein M, Bredfeldt G, et al. Gingival hyperplasia: a side effect of nifedipine and diltiazem. Spec Care Dent 1991;11(3):107–9.

[21] Calne RY, White DJ, Thiru S. Cyclosporin A in patients receiving renal allografts from cadaver .donors. Lancet 1978;2(8104–5):1323–7.

[22] Physicians' Desk Reference. 53rd edition. Montvale (NJ): Medical Economics Co; 1999. p. 2068.

[23] McGaw WT, Porter H. Cyclosporine-induced gingival overgrowth: an ultrastructural stereologic study. Oral Surg Oral Med Oral Pathol 1988;65(2):186–90.

[24] Transplant Patient Data Source. Richmond (VA): United Network for Organ Sharing. Available at: http://www.patients.unos.org/data.htm. Accessed February 16, 2000.

[25] Daly CG. Resolution of cyclosporin A (CsA)-induced gingival enlargement following reduction in CsA dosage. J Clin Periodontol 1992;19(2):143–5.

[26] Thomason JM, Seymour RA, Rice N. The prevalence and severity of cyclosporin and nifedipine-induced gingival overgrowth. J Clin Periodontol 1992;19(2):143–5.

[27] Weinstein L. Antimicrobial Agents. In: Goodman LS, Gilman A, editors. Goodman and Gilman's. The pharmacological basis of therapeutics. 5th edition. New York: Macmillan Publishing Co, Inc; 1975. p. 1183–94.

[28] Guggenheimer J. Tetracyclines and the human dentition. Compend Contin Ed Dent 1984;5(3):245–54.

[29] Ciancio SG, editor. Bleaching tetracycline-discolored teeth. Biol Ther Dent 2001;16(6):33–4.

[30] McKenna BE, Lamey PJ, Kennedy JG, et al. Minocycline-induced staining of the adult permanent dentition: a review of the literature and report of a case. Dent Update 1999; 26(4):160–2.

[31] Drugdex® System. In: Hutchison TA, Shahan DR, editors. Greenwood Village (CO): Micromedex® Health Care Series. vol. 19;2001.

[32] Tilley BC, Alarcon GS, Heyse SP, et al. Minocycline in rheumatoid arthritis: a 48 week double-blind placebo-controlled trial. Ann Intern Med 1995;122:81–9.

[33] Rossie K, Guggenheimer J. Oral candidiasis: clinical manifestations, diagnosis, and treatment. Prac Periodontol Aesth 1997;9(6):635–42.

[34] Wynn RL, Meiller TF, Crossley HL. Drug information handbook for dentistry. 6th edition. Cleveland (OH): Lexi-Comp, Inc; 2000. p. 1272–1343.

[35] Guggenheimer J, Moore PA, Rossie K, et al. Insulin dependent diabetes mellitus and oral soft tissue pathologies. II. Prevalence and characteristics of Candida and candidal lesions. Oral Surg Oral Med Oral Pathol Oral Radiol Endod 2000;89(5):570–6.

[36] Kennedy WA, Laurier C, Gautrin D, et al. Occurrence and risk factors for oral candidiasis treated with oral antifungals in seniors using inhaled steroids. J Clin Epidemiol 2000; 53(7):696–701.

[37] Lung Health Research Group. Effect of inhaled triamcinolone on the decline in pulmonary function in chronic obstructive pulmonary disease. N Engl J Med 2000;343(26): 1902–9.

[38] Mealey BL, Semba SE, Hallmon WW. Dentistry and the cancer patient: part 1. Oral manifestations and complications of chemotherapy. Compend Contin Ed Dent 1994; 15(10):1252–62.

[39] Neville BW, Damm DD, Allen C. Oral and maxillofacial pathology. Philadelphia: WB Saunders Co; 1995. p. 164–5, 247–8, 636–7.

[40] Mott AE, Grushka M, Sessle BJ. Diagnosis and management of taste disorders and burning mouth syndrome. Dent Clin NA 1993;37(1):33–71.

[41] Boyd AS, Nelder KH. Lichen planus. J Am Acad Dermatol 1991;25(4):593–619.

[42] Miller RL, Gould AR, Bernstein ML. Cinnamon-induced stomatitis venenata. Oral Surg Oral Med Oral Pathol 1992;73(6):708–16.

[43] Jainkittivong A, Langlais RP. Allergic stomatitis. Semin Dermatol 1994;13(2):91–101.

THE DENTAL
CLINICS OF
NORTH
AMERICA

Dent Clin N Am 46 (2002) 869–885

Geriatric pharmacology

Marc W. Heft, DMD, PhD[a,b,*],
Angelo J. Mariotti, DDS, PhD[c]

[a]*Claude D. Pepper Center for Research on Oral Health in Aging,
1600 Southwest Archer Road, Gainesville, FL, USA*
[b]*Department of Oral and Maxillofacial Surgery and Diagnostic Sciences,
University of Florida, Box 100416, HSC, Gainesville, FL 32610-0416, USA*
[c]*Department of Periodontics, The Ohio State University College of Dentistry,
4001 Postle Hall, 305 West 12th Avenue, Columbus, OH 43210-1241, USA*

With the demographic change that has resulted in a "graying of the population" has come a compelling interest in the health concerns of older adults. The increasing incidence and prevalence of systemic diseases, especially chronic diseases, among older adults, and the concomitant increase in medication use, have provided impetus for the subspecialty of geriatric pharmacology. Although it has long been obvious that because children are smaller than adults some reduction of drug dosage is appropriate, it was not understood until recently how elderly patients differ from younger adults. In fact, there were some widely held misconceptions about aging, as, for example, that senility or a progressive increase in blood pressure are normal concomitants of aging. Geriatric pharmacology did not emerge out of a specific incident, such as occurred with thalidomide, in which it was made clear that the fetus represents an area of special concern for the pharmacologist. Rather, the field of geriatric pharmacology has developed out of changes in demography that have been accompanied by an increasing knowledge of and sensitivity to the special physiologic, pharmacologic, pathologic, psychologic, economic, and emotional concerns of older adults.

In 1999, elderly persons 65 years of age or older numbered 34.5 million and represented 12.7% of the US population; by the year 2030, they will represent 20% and will number approximately 70 million [1]. Furthermore, not only is the total over-65 group growing faster than the population as a whole, but between the years 2000 and 2030 the group aged 85 years and older will increase from 4.3 million to 7 million [2,3].

---

* Corresponding author.
E-mail address: mwheft@nersp.nerdc.ufl.edu (M.W. Heft).

Of special interest to the dentist is that the newer cohorts of older adults are now and will be in better oral health [4]. The rate of edentulousness has declined [5–7], and the number of retained teeth among the dentate has increased [5,6,8,9]. With this trend among dentate older adults has emerged an understanding that there are similar needs for routine restorative and periodontal treatments among these individuals as exist among younger adults [6,8,10]. Accordingly, an increasing number of elderly people will need the kind of dental treatment that was formerly rare in the elderly patient, treatment that requires among other things antianxiety drugs, analgesics, local anesthetics, and anti-inflammatory drugs. It also means that the dentist will be confronted by an increasing number of ambulatory, community-dwelling elderly patients with a significant burden of systemic disease and medication use.

Normative aging studies have shown that the healthy elderly person is substantially and measurably different from younger counterparts. More recently, pharmacologists have begun to appreciate how these changes affect the pharmacokinetics and pharmacodynamics of drugs.

As people age, they are more likely to present to the dental office with a variety of diseases, especially chronic diseases, for which they take many drugs that are strong in effect and potentially toxic. Americans aged 65 years and older take a disproportionately high percentage of all drugs prescribed [11]. Furthermore, studies of ambulatory populations indicate that although 80–90% of older adults take at least one medication, most are taking two or more. The most commonly used drugs are agents affecting the cardiovascular system, analgesic and anti-inflammatory drugs, psychotherapeutic medications, and gastrointestinal preparations such as laxatives and antacids. Approximately 40% of medications are prescribed to patients to be taken "as necessary," with an average of three drugs per patient [12].

Multiple medications prescribed to individuals of any age increases the risk for adverse drug reactions, drug interactions, and other health-related problems associated with the use and misuse of medications [12,13]. The potential problems in older adults are compounded by the potential age-related physiologic changes that may place these individuals at greater risk. The misuse of medications by elderly patients is considered a major healthcare problem [14,15]. Finally, many segments of our society, not the least important of which is the healthcare provider, have become sensitized to the nonmedical problems common among the elderly (loneliness, depression, poverty, poor nutritional status) and have come to understand how these can complicate therapeutic management of elderly patients.

This article presents a view of geriatric pharmacology that deals mainly with alterations in drug responsiveness that can be attributed directly to aging, and deals only in passing with those psychosocial factors that indirectly have an impact on how elderly patients use and react to drugs.

Physiologic changes associated with aging

Studies of the aging process in community-dwelling, healthy (presumed disease-free) individuals have provided insights into the process of biologic aging. These studies have been either cross-sectional studies, in which different-aged persons are assessed at the same point in time, or longitudinal studies, in which the same individuals are assessed at different times as they "age in place." Although the former studies are easier and quicker to complete, they limit inferences to "age differences" rather than "age-related changes," because of the limitations in controlling for and measuring individual differences in biology and behavior. Results of cross-sectional and longitudinal studies have reported a gradual decline in performance from the third decade through the seventh and eighth decades in a broad range of physiologic functions, including renal function, pulmonary function, cardiac function, and nerve conduction velocity [16]. Findings from these studies have shown, however, that (1) there are broad individual intersubject differences in the rate of aging, (2) not all organ systems age at the same rate, (3) the pattern of age-related declines in organ systems can vary among individuals, (4) with increasing age, there is greater variability among individuals within an age cohort in measures of organ functioning, (5) age-associated declines are greater in more complex integrative functions (such as maximum breathing capacity) than in basic functions (such as the velocity of propagation of a nerve impulse along a nerve), and (6) the latency and capacity for achieving adaptive responses are, respectively, greater and smaller for older individuals than younger individuals. Thus, variability is a cardinal feature of the aging process. It has also been suggested that at least some of the apparent decline in functioning may reflect changes in lifestyle rather than chronologic aging per se (such as declining muscle mass associated with the adaptation of a more quiescent life-style).

Age-related changes in drug disposition that have potential importance to drug use are summarized in Table 1. These alterations affect the absorption, distribution, biotransformation, and excretion of drugs; the specific features of these changes are considered later. There also is a well-documented decline in homeostatic competence in elderly patients that accounts for the increased incidence of postural hypotension with age [17], the increasing sluggishness of thermoregulation, and the fact that the elderly are less able to compensate rapidly for the hypotensive effects, for instance, of an antihypertensive drug [18]. Elderly patients undergo physiologic changes that could be characterized as normal concomitants of the aging process, but that they also, to a greater or lesser extent, suffer changes that are disease- and medication-related. Because what we consider aging represents an interplay among the physiology of aging, disease, and the cumulative effects of behavioral and lifestyle choices (eg, sedentary living and tobacco use versus regular exercise and abstention from tobacco), the elderly population is more heterogeneous than, for instance, a population of children between birth and puberty [19].

Table 1
Summary of age-related changes that affect drug disposition in older adults

Pharmacokinetic property	Physiologic change	Possible influence on drug effect
Absorption	↑ Gastric pH	Increased absorption of drugs inactivated by stomach acid
	↓ Absorptive surface	Minor effect
	↓ Splanchnic blood flow	Minor effect
	↓ Gastrointestinal motility	Minor effect
Distribution	↓ Cardiac output	Impaired delivery of drugs to organs of elimination
	↓ Total body water	Increased concentration and effect of drugs distributed in body water
	↓ Lean body mass	Increased concentration and effect of drugs distributed in lean body mass
	↓ Plasma albumin	Increased effect of, and interaction between, drugs extensively bound to albumin
	↑ α_1-Acid glycoprotein	Minor effect
	↑ Body fat	Increased sequestration of lipophilic drugs in fat
Metabolism	↓ Hepatic mass and enzyme activity	Decrease phase I metabolism of some drugs
	↓ Hepatic blood flow	Decreased metabolism of drugs normally rapidly cleared by the liver
Excretion	↓ Renal blood flow	Decreased renal elimination of water-soluble drugs and metabolites
	↓ Glomerular filtration rate	Decreased renal excretion of water-soluble drugs and metabolites
	↓ Tubular secretion	Decreased renal elimination of drugs and metabolites actively secreted into urine

Nonphysiologic aspects of aging

Multiple disease states

Elderly people suffer from more health problems, especially chronic diseases and conditions, than younger people. The most prevalent chronic conditions among older adults are listed in Table 2. Some of these diseases are degenerative (eg, cataracts, detached retina), others are caused by

Table 2
Prevalence of selected reported chronic illnesses[a]

Condition	Prevalence by age (yr)		
	65–74	>75	All ages
Arthritis	444.7	550.4	129.9
Hypertension	372.6	373.6	121.5
Hearing impairment	273.7	380.7	90.8
Heart disease	271.8	333.6	84.1
Chronic sinusitis	176.2	167.8	139.7
Cataract formation	118.1	246.0	25.3
Deformity or orthopedic impairment	151.4	176.6	111.6
Diabetes	95.2	87.8	25.8
Visual impairment	67.4	127.6	34.7
Tinnitus	89.4	75.1	26.4

[a] Prevalence data (number of cases/1000 persons) from Adams PF, Hardy AM. Current estimates from the National Health Interview Survey, 1988. Vital and Health Statistics, Series 10, No. 173. Hyattsville (MD): US Department of Health and Human Services, Public Health Service, Centers of Disease Control, National Center for Health Statistics; 1989.

cumulative exposure to environmental contaminants (eg, cases of chronic obstructive pulmonary disease and cancer), and still others are the consequences of essentially normal processes of aging (eg, decreased bone density with increasing age). Among older adults there is an increased incidence of all varieties of heart disease (arrhythmias, myocardial infarction, valvular disease), renal disease, atherosclerosis, arthritis, diabetes, osteoporosis, a variety of gastrointestinal problems, declines in humoral- and cell-mediated immune responses (that lead to a decreased resistance to infectious diseases), and various sensory and musculoskeletal impairments. It has been estimated that more than four out of five persons aged 65 years and older have at least one chronic illness, and multiple coexisting conditions are commonplace among older adults. The leading chronic health conditions for this age group are arthritis, hypertensive disease, and heart disease [20,21].

It is not surprising that although the elderly represent less than 13% of the population, they account for 30% of hospitalizations [22] and 32% of drug use [23]. It also is noteworthy that symptoms of disease in older adults often present differently than in younger individuals. For example, infections are sometimes manifested not by fever but by tachycardia in older individuals. Furthermore, transient or episodic symptoms may be forgotten, misreported, or misinterpreted.

Numerous studies have shown that older adults, because of a higher prevalence of chronic disease, are the principal consumers of drugs [11,24]. The use of over-the-counter (OTC) with prescription medications for the treatment of chronic diseases in older adults has dual implications. These agents can provide a cure or palliative treatment of a disease in a nontoxic and economical manner. Because of the age-related changes in physiologic status and age-dependent and age-related diseases, however [25], medications can induce adverse reactions that can be a major source of morbidity or even mortality [13,26].

Adverse drug reactions

The incidence of adverse drug reactions among older adults is much greater than among younger individuals, and this increase is related for the most part to polypharmacy (multiple drug use). Important factors in the occurrence of adverse drug reactions, however, are multiple diseases (especially chronic diseases), hepatic or renal insufficiency, small body size, malnutrition, and previous drug reactions. Important adverse reactions include side effects (eg, dry mouth with tricyclic antidepressant medication), drug allergy (eg, pruritus or hives), and toxic reactions [27] (eg, digitalis toxicity). Toxic reactions are especially important in older adults and may be caused by a broad range of potential pharmacodynamic changes (age-related changes in drug sensitivity) or pharmacokinetic changes (including decreased renal function and changes in lean body mass and water content).

Adverse drug reactions can be categorized into two principal groups: unexpected and unpredictable versus predictable and preventable. An unexpected, unpredictable reaction is an unwanted consequence of drug administration that occurs at appropriate doses for prophylaxis, diagnosis, or therapy. Examples of such reactions include allergic responses, idiosyncratic reactions, or secondary pharmacologic effects. In contrast, predictable, preventable drug reactions involve an unwanted consequence of drug administration that occurs because of failure in decision making by the healthcare provider. Failure by the dentist to choose the appropriate agent can occur, as in prescribing the wrong drug for a disease or prescribing a drug with known potential adverse effects in a susceptible patient.

Because most adverse drug reactions are preventable, it is important to understand the patient's medical history, drug history, and current list of medications (OTC and prescribed), the pharmacology of each agent used, and any abnormal physiologic factors that can affect drug action. Although the incidence of adverse reactions increases among older patients, in part because of polypharmacy, actions of a single powerful agent can produce severe adverse reactions for the elderly patient. Many of the drugs commonly prescribed by dentists can produce a variety of harmful reactions in their patients. As illustrated in Table 3, a variety of drug classes used in dental practice can be of potential risk for the older patient. For example, cephalosporins commonly prescribed for the treatment of infections can produce deleterious effects. Cefoperazone, cefamandole, and cefotetan can prolong prothrombin time and partial thromboplastin time, which can impair hemostasis [28,29]. Other antibiotics, such as clindamycin, can markedly increase the incidence of such gastrointestinal problems as diarrhea and colitis in patients older than 60 years of age [30,31]. In addition to antibiotics,

Table 3
Age-related increased risk of toxicity with some commonly prescribed dental agents

Drug	Increased risk for elderly patients
Clindamycin	Diarrhea and colitis
Metronidazole	Toxic plasma concentrations (patients over 70 years of age)
Cephalosporins	Impaired clotting mechanisms and bleeding problems
NSAIDs[a]	Compromised renal or gastrointestinal function
Opioid analgesics	Increased plasma half-life, respiratory depression
Glucocorticoids	Muscle wasting and osteoporosis with chronic therapy
Benzodiazepines	Impaired memory and decrements in psychomotor performance

[a] NSAIDs, nonsteroidal anti-inflammatory drugs.

nonsteroidal anti-inflammatory drugs (NSAIDs) also can cause morbidity in the elderly population. The NSAIDs are commonly used for postoperative pain control in dental practice; however, NSAID use among older adults can be a problem, as documented by an association of NSAID intake with impaired renal function, GI toxicity, or hypertension [32–34]. Therefore, alternatives to NSAIDs can include the use of COX-2 inhibitors such as celecoxib and rofecoxib. More specifically, because NSAIDs inhibit the COX-1 and COX-2 pathways, the use of selective COX-2 inhibitors provides anti-inflammatory and analgesic properties with less GI toxicity [35].

Another dilemma encountered by older adults that complicates the dental treatment plan is medications that may cause xerostomia. Drug-induced xerostomia is a concern because (1) older adults take prescription and nonprescription medications at a higher rate than the general population, (2) there are many medications that have xerostomic potential (more than 400 medications have been implicated), and (3) the oral health sequelae of xerostomia are consequential. Xerostomia induced by sympathomimetics, diuretics, anticholinergics, tricyclic antidepressants, antihistamines, antiparkinson drugs, psychotropic agents, cardiovascular agents, and muscle relaxants can greatly impair oral health and function [36]. Potential sequelae of xerostomia include rampant dental caries, periodontal problems, difficulty in speech and swallowing, mouth soreness, impaired denture retention, greater likelihood of oral infection, and altered sense of taste [37,38].

Polypharmacy is a special attribute of drug use among older adults. One fourth of hospitalized patients over age 65 receive six or more drugs daily [39], older adults average 13 prescriptions per year [40], and approximately 90% of patients aged 75 years and older take drugs regularly, with greater than one third taking three or more drugs daily [41]. The major consequence of multiple drug use is an increased incidence of adverse drug reactions. These adverse drug reactions result from several factors, including incorrect identification of medications, multiple prescriptions from more than one health provider (because of a lack of awareness or communication among providers), and the use of medications prescribed for someone else.

Because most adverse drug reactions are preventable, dentists should take advantage of available resources to minimize the likelihood of these untoward sequelae. Consultation with other health professionals (including physicians and pharmacists) or use of a comprehensive drug reference book assists in determining the appropriate drug and dose schedule. In addition, computer-based data retrieval systems and newsletters can keep the dentist informed regarding appropriate drug selection. Finally, the dentist should always be aware of and concerned about the onset of new symptoms that do not normally arise from the anticipated course of the disease process but do follow from dental treatment.

The salient point to remember concerning adverse drug reactions in older adults is that they are largely preventable. A sound approach to avoid adverse drug reactions involves (1) understanding the physical and psychosocial changes that occur in older adults, (2) knowing the pharmacokinetics and pharmacodynamics of the medications the patient is taking and ones the dentist is planning to use or prescribe, (3) evaluating the existing prescription drug burden of an individual when considering further prescription needs, (4) prudent drug monitoring, and (5) careful record keeping.

Patient compliance

Patient compliance can be a major source of medication errors. Ample evidence exists that a substantial percentage of elderly patients make serious or potentially serious medication errors [42]. Failure to comply with drug regimens consists of omitting medications, use of medications not prescribed by the physician or dentist, and errors of dosage, sequence, and timing. Problems especially identified with the elderly that contribute to compliance errors include poor comprehension and memory, deficits in vision and hearing, financial strictures, inability to cope with the environment, self-neglect, cultural attitudes, and physical obstacles to getting medications out of the bottle (particularly the child-resistant kind) and self-administering them. Therefore, whenever possible unnecessary medications should be eliminated, and drugs with simplified dosing schedules should be selected. Prescription strategies by the dentist, including written instructions, use of drugs that require fewer doses per day (eg, doxycycline instead of tetracycline), selection of less expensive generic alternatives, and packaging of drugs in easy-open, daily dosing boxes increase the likelihood of compliance.

Psychosocial factors

Any discussion of geriatric pharmacology would be incomplete without mention of the various psychosocial and economic challenges that frequently confront the elderly. Although it is no longer true that older adults inevitably suffer a serious reduction in income, 10.5% live in poverty, and elderly single women (14% are below the poverty line) are worse off than men or couples. Furthermore, poverty rates are higher for elderly Blacks

(25%) and Hispanics (24%) than for elderly Whites (9%) [43]. The elderly may also live in increasing isolation, away from families, children, and spouses, and suffer from depression, loneliness, and sometimes senility. They also receive three times as many prescriptions for psychotropic drugs as do younger people, even though they are more vulnerable to the adverse effects of these drugs and take twice as long to recover from them than do young patients [44]. This constellation of factors places older adults at risk for many problems, including inadequate diet, poor nutrition, loss of weight, forgetfulness and inattention to medical and pharmacologic needs, and an inability or lack of desire to fill prescriptions and to take them as directed. One widely held belief about the elderly is that their nutritional status is compounded by losses in salivary secretory ability and taste acuity that are presumed to occur with aging and would naturally interfere with the enjoyment of food. Although some studies showed a decrease in parotid gland secretion and salivary amylase activity, and morphologic age-related changes in the salivary gland, most studies have not found a diminution of salivary flow in older individuals [45,46], and the decline in gustatory function is at most modest among the elderly [47]. It cannot be denied that pathologic aging may have an adverse effect on salivary function, however, and that many of the drugs and treatments to which the older person is subject can cause xerostomia of varying degrees of severity.

Pharmacologic changes associated with aging

Two basic mechanisms have been developed to explain age-related differences in drug effects [27]. The pharmacodynamic mechanism suggests that changes in drug responsiveness account for such differences [48,49]. These changes presumably involve either an alteration in the number or activity of receptors on the target cell or a change in intracellular responses to receptor activation. Documentation in support of this mechanism is modest, involving only a few drug classes. The more widely accepted pharmacokinetic mechanism suggests that age differences in drug response are related to changes in drug disposition as a result of alterations in drug absorption, distribution, metabolism, and excretion or combinations of these processes. A general review of these factors with particular regard to aging is provided in the following sections.

Pharmacokinetics of drugs

Absorption

Most medications prescribed to patients living independently are taken orally. These medications are absorbed through the gastrointestinal tract. The documented age-related alterations that might predispose older adults to potential declines in absorption are increased gastric pH, decreased absorptive surface, decreased gastric emptying, decreased splanchnic blood flow, and impaired intestinal motility [50,51]. There is little evidence, however, to support an age-related decline in absorption [49]. In fact, it is possible that decreased stomach acidity could improve absorption of drugs normally inactivated by stomach acid. An important consideration for patients of all ages is the possible interaction of medications with food. For example, the absence of food in the gastrointestinal tract improves the efficiency of absorption of some drugs, such as erythromycin. The absorption of other medications is unimpaired, however [27]. Thus, although food–drug interactions are not a problem of aging per se, they are important in older adults who have a heavier medication burden.

Distribution

The distribution of the drug to potential receptor sites occurs after absorption of the drug through the gastrointestinal tract and then into the bloodstream. Distribution is influenced by body composition (lean body mass, body water, and adipose tissue mass), plasma protein binding (particularly albumin), and blood flow to organs. The documented age-related changes that might affect drug distribution in older patients include decreased lean body mass, decreased body water, increased body fat, decreased cardiac output, and decreased albumin [51].

The change in lean body mass may reflect other factors, including a potential lifestyle change in physical activity or dietary change, rather than an aging effect per se; nevertheless, this consistent finding in older adults must be considered when evaluating the patient. The net effect is a decrease in lean body mass and total body water, and an increase in total body fat. Thus, the respective volumes of distribution for water-soluble medications and fat-soluble medications are decreased and increased, respectively [51]. Water-soluble drugs such as acetaminophen, ethanol, digoxin, and cimetidine are distributed in a smaller volume in older individuals and, therefore, have higher concentrations at the same dose [49,51]. Similarly, the more lipid-soluble drugs such as diazepam are more widely distributed (yielding a lower concentration at the receptor site) and have a longer terminal half-life in older adults [49,51].

Although decreased plasma titers of albumin are probably not a concomitant of aging, they may accompany chronic disease seen in an aging population. A decrease in plasma albumin increases the availability of highly bound drug, thereby effectively increasing the drug concentration at the receptor. A higher concentration of free drug in the plasma has been shown for salicylic acid, metronidazole [52], and phenytoin, but not for warfarin [53]. Theoretically at least, therapeutic and toxic effects should be achieved at lower blood concentrations for drugs that are extensively protein-bound [54]. This effect may be especially important with malnutrition. Furthermore, for many drugs there has been no documented age-related difference in protein binding; two examples are diazepam and penicillin G [55].

Metabolism

The metabolism of most drugs begins with the obligatory passage through the liver after absorption from the gastrointestinal tract. Hepatic metabolism depends on hepatic blood flow, the liver enzymes responsible for biotransformation of the drug, and genetic factors that influence the hepatic enzyme system [27,51]. The reported age-related declines that might be responsible for altered drug disposition include decreased liver mass and decreased hepatic blood flow [51]. It has been suggested that biologic variability, drug use, and behavioral factors (such as smoking or alcohol use), or a combination of these factors, exert a greater effect than age on hepatic metabolism.

The documented age-related effects may impair the efficiency of the phase I pathways of metabolism, namely, oxidation, reduction, and hydrolysis. The phase II pathways of glucuronidation, acetylation, and sulfation are unaffected [51]. For drugs that are rapidly cleared by the liver, the rate-limiting step in biotransformation is the hepatic blood flow. Thus, the metabolism of high-clearance drugs such a propranolol is reduced, and caution should be exercised with regard to the tricyclic antidepressant and antiarrhythmic medications. For low-clearance drugs, metabolism depends on the efficiency of the hepatic enzyme systems. Thus, some benzodiazepines (such as desmethyldiazepam) that depend on microsomal oxidation have a prolonged half-life, whereas others (such as lorazepam) that undergo conjugation are unaffected by age. It is also important to consider the route of administration when assessing the potential for hepatic metabolism. The preceding discussion presumes the oral route of administration that involves the absorption of the drug from the gastrointestinal tract and then transport through the liver by way of the hepatic portal circulation; however, the parenteral route of administration may eliminate the liver as the organ primarily influencing disposition of the drug.

Excretion

The elimination of drugs by the kidney provides the eventual pathway for removal of most medications. The documented age-related changes that might impair kidney function and excretion include decreased renal blood flow, decreased glomerular filtration rate, and decreased tubular secretion [51]. Renal function is typically evaluated by the creatinine clearance that has been reported to decline by approximately one third between the ages of 20 and 90 years in the ambulatory, community-dwelling volunteers of the Baltimore Longitudinal Study on Aging [56]. More recent data from the same study, however, have shown that for approximately one third of older subjects, renal function did not decline, and further, there were variable declines among other older subjects [57]. These latter data underscore the need to establish adequate dosing schedules for medications based on blood concentrations rather than interpretation of age-adjusted "normative" data.

Drugs that are eliminated primarily unchanged in the kidney include digoxin, gentamicin, amantadine, lithium, nadolol, and lisinopril. Dosages for drugs with a high therapeutic index, such as penicillins and cephalosporins, are usually not adjusted for older adults (in the absence of renal disease or polypharmacy). It is important to adjust dosages for medications with active metabolites, such as the benzodiazepines diazepam and flurazepam [49].

The response of elderly patients to drugs is affected not only by alterations in renal drug clearance but by the fact that altered renal function may make them more sensitive to the nephrotoxicity of such drugs as the NSAIDs and aminoglycosides. Conversely, the decreased activity of the renin-angiotensin system may blunt the effects of drugs that inhibit renin secretion, such as β-adrenergic blocking agents and the angiotensin-converting enzyme inhibitors, diminishing their therapeutic effectiveness in the treatment of hypertension [58].

The complex and potentially serious alterations in kidney function mandate that consideration be given to renal excretory capacity when prescribing drugs to the elderly. Although there is certainly a diminution in renal function that is related to age, kidney disease is, of course, not restricted to the elderly.

Pharmacodynamic changes

Studies investigating age-related changes in pharmacodynamics are difficult to pursue, and consequently scant data exist in this area. Available evidence suggests that there are no global age-related changes in drug sensitivity. Increased sensitivity to certain benzodiazepine anxiolytic medications and decreased sensitivity to β-adrenergic agonists and antagonists have been reported in older individuals.

There are several possibilities for pharmacodynamic alterations in drug reactivity with aging, including a change in the number of receptors, a change in their affinity for the drug, or a change in tissue responsiveness to drug-receptor binding. Discovering which of these possibilities accounts for a particular reaction is difficult because it requires a knowledge of receptor number, binding affinity, and quantitation of the sequential steps following the drug-receptor interaction to the final observed response. Experimental evidence exists that one or more of these changes do occur with several groups of drugs, but interpretation of the results of some of these experiments is confounded by the fact that the elderly also demonstrate decreases in homeostatic competence, speed of performance, thermoregulation, and immunocompetence.

Changes in sensitivity to β-adrenergic agonists and antagonists have been reported in several studies. Using the production of cyclic 3′-5′ adenosine monophosphate (cAMP) by lymphocytes as an indicator of responsiveness to isoproterenol in the young and old, it was found that there is a decrease in adenylate cyclase in normal subjects of ages 67 to 90 as compared with those of 18 to 27 years of age [59]. Sensitivity of young men to isoproterenol and propranolol was demonstrated to be greater than in elderly men, but it is possible that the well-documented increase in the blood concentration of norepinephrine in the elderly may create competition for receptor sites [60]. In a recent series of investigations involving rat myocardial and human lymphocytic β-adrenergic function, a decreased responsiveness of the β receptors to catecholamines was found along with decreased adenylate cyclase activity but no decline in receptor density [61].

Increased sensitivity to central nervous system depressants is a recognized fact. In tests involving nitrazepam, age-related decrements in psychomotor performance were described and linked to pharmacodynamic, not pharmacokinetic, changes [62]. Elderly patients who were given diazepam for a surgical procedure required lower doses than younger patients to reach the same level of sedation [63]. This observation has been confirmed in other studies for diazepam and temazepam [64]. Determination of the minimum alveolar concentration for isoflurane showed an 18% decrease in anesthetic requirement between young adults and older adults; similar results have been obtained with other anesthetics [65]. In contrast to the generalization that brain function in the elderly seems to be inherently more susceptible to disruption by anesthetic drugs, the greater sensitivity of older patients to etomidate seems to result from a decreased initial distribution of the anesthetic after intravenous injection [66].

In addition to pharmacodynamic changes, the genetic characteristics of an individual may also influence the behavior of drugs in the elderly. For example, the apparent volume distribution of the acetylator phenotype of isoniazid decreased significantly with age [67]. Hence, pharmacogenetics for the elderly is important because genetically determined enhancement or impairment of drug action in the body can amplify toxicity of a drug or diminish the efficacy of a drug.

Precautions for the dental practitioner

It should be clear that the elderly patient differs from the younger adult in ways that have the potential for affecting responses to drugs. Changes potentially affecting pharmacokinetics and pharmacodynamics occur during aging, but at this stage in the development of the science of geriatric pharmacology, there are remarkably few documented instances of problems with drugs that arise directly out of these changes. It is, however, well known that responses to drugs in the elderly are confounded by multiple medications, pathologic states, compliance errors, and a variety of psychologic, sociologic, and economic difficulties that beset older people. Some precautions appropriate to dentistry are listed below.

1. The elderly usually take more drugs, prescription and nonprescription, than the general adult population, and drug interactions and adverse drug reactions are more likely to result from polypharmacy. It is

important, therefore, that the dentist take a careful history of the patient's medical and pharmacologic status and update it at regular intervals during treatment.

2. Older adults are more sensitive than are young adults to the depressant effects of drugs. It may be necessary to reduce the dosages of analgesics, antianxiety drugs, sedative-hypnotics, and general anesthetics.
3. Because of the known decline in homeostatic competence, drugs that alter blood pressure, heart rate, and smooth muscle tone should be used with caution in the elderly. Conversely, immunosenescence may dictate more aggressive antibiotic therapy than normal for the prevention and treatment of infections.
4. Older adults are more susceptible to orthostatic hypotension than are younger adults. Dentists must be especially attentive when older adults are transferred from a reclining posture in the dental chair to a standing position.
5. Age-associated decline in renal function is common in otherwise healthy elderly patients, and this decline in function is compounded in patients with kidney disease. This fact should be taken into consideration when prescribing drugs whose principal route of elimination is the kidney. Conventionally, dosage intervals are increased in such circumstances, but the dose of the drug or drugs may have to be reduced.
6. The dentist should be aware of the psychosocial and economic considerations for the patient and should be sensitive to such problems as the expense of the medications and the possibility of forgetfulness and poor compliance. Special packaging, clear labeling, and simplified dose regimens may improve compliance, as may having a responsible relative or friend monitor drug therapy.

References

[1] Duncker A, Greenberg S. A profile of older Americans. Washington (DC): Administration on Aging. US Department of Health and Human Services, Public Health Service; 2000.
[2] Aging America: trends and projections: an information paper to the Special Committee on Aging, United States Senate. Washington (DC): US Government Printing Office; 1989.
[3] US Bureau of the Census. Population projections of the United States by age, sex, race and Hispanic origin: 1993 to 2050, Current Population Reports, P25–1104. Washington (DC): US Government Printing Office; 1993.
[4] Gilbert GH, Duncan RP, Crandall LA, et al. Attitudinal and behavioral characteristics of older Floridians with tooth loss. Community Dent Oral Epidemiol 1993;21:384–9.
[5] Miller AJ, et al. Oral health of US adults: The National Survey of Oral Health in US. Employed adults and seniors, 1985–1986: national findings, Publication no. (NIH) 87–2868, Bethesda (MD): US Department of Health and Human Services, Public Health Service, National Institutes of Health; 1987.
[6] US Department of Health and Human Services. National Center for Health Statistics. Third National Health and Nutrition Examination Survey, 1988–94. Public Use Data File No. 7–0627. Hyattsville (MD): Centers for Disease Control; 1997.

[7] Weintraub JA, Burt BA. Oral health status in the United States: tooth loss and edentulism. J Dent Educ 1985;49:368–78.

[8] Heft MW, Gilbert GH. Tooth loss and caries prevalence in older Floridians attending senior activity centers. Community Dent Oral Epidemiol 1991;19:228–32.

[9] Marcus SE, Drury TF, Brown LF, Zion GR. Tooth retention and tooth loss in the permanent dentition of adults: United States, 1988–94. J Dent Res 1996;75(Special issue):684–95.

[10] Gilbert GH, Heft MW. Periodontal status of older Floridians attending senior activity centers. J Clin Periodontol 1992;19:249–55.

[11] Nelson CR, Knapp DE. Medication therapy in ambulatory medical care: National Ambulatory Medical Care Survey and National Hospital Care Survey. Advance Data from Vital and Health Statistics, No. 290. Hyattsville (MD): National Center for Health Statistics; 1992.

[12] Nolan L, O'Malley K. Prescribing for the elderly: part II. Prescribing patterns: differences due to age. J Am Geriatr Soc 1988;36:245–54.

[13] Gurwitz JH, Avorn J. The ambiguous relation between aging and adverse drug reactions. Ann Intern Med 1991;114:956–66.

[14] German PS, Burton LC. Medication and the elderly. Issues of prescription and use. J Aging Health 1989;1:4–34.

[15] Morrow D, Leirer V, Sheikh J. Adherence and medication instructions. Review and recommendations. J Am Geriatr Soc 1988;36:1147–60.

[16] Shock NW. Aging of regulatory mechanisms. In: Cape RDT, Coe RM, Rossman I, editors. Fundamentals of geriatric medicine. New York: Raven Press; 1983.

[17] Caird FI, Andrews GR, Kennedy RD. Effect of posture on blood pressure in the elderly. Br Heart J 1973;35:527–30.

[18] Greenblatt DJ, Koch-Weser J. Adverse reactions to propranolol in hospitalized medical patients: a report from the Boston Collaborative Drug Surveillance Program. Am Heart J 1973;86:478–84.

[19] Vestal RE. Drug use in the elderly: a review of problems and special considerations. Drugs 1978;16:358–82.

[20] Adams PF, Hardy AM. Current estimates from the National Health Interview Survey, 1988, Vital and Health Statistics, Series 10. Hyattsville (MD): US Department of Health and Human Services, Public Health Service, Centers for Disease Control, National Center for Health Statistics; 1989.

[21] Centers for Disease Control and Prevention. Unrealized prevention opportunities: reducing the health and economic burden of chronic disease. Atlanta: National Center for Chronic Disease Prevention and Health Promotion; 1997.

[22] Graves EJ. Utilization of short-stay hospitals, United States: annual summary, vital and health statistics, 1985, Series 13, No. 91. Hyattsville (MD): US Department of Health and Human Services, Public Health Service, Centers for Disease Control, National Center for Health Statistics; 1987.

[23] Drug utilization in the U.S.–1987: eighth annual review. Publication no. PB88–146527. Springfield (VA): Food and Drug Administration, National Technical Information Service, US Department of Commerce; 1987.

[24] Ouslander JG. Drug therapy in the elderly. Ann Intern Med 1981;95:711–22.

[25] Brody JA, Schneider EL. Diseases and disorders of aging: an hypothesis. J Chronic Dis 1986;39:871–6.

[26] Porter J, Jick H. Drug-related deaths among medical inpatients. JAMA 1977;237:879–81.

[27] Lipton HL, Lee PR. Drugs and the elderly: clinical, social, and policy perspectives. Stanford (CA): Stanford University Press; 1988.

[28] Donowitz GR, Mandell GL. Beta-lactam antibiotics. Part 2. N Engl J Med 1988;318:490–500.

[29] Nichols RL, et al. Coagulopathy associated with extended-spectrum cephalosporins in patients with serious infections. Antimicrob Agents Chemother 1987;31:281–5.

[30] Gurwith MJ, Rabin HR, Love K. Diarrhea associated with clindamycin and ampicillin therapy: preliminary results of a cooperative study. J Infect Dis 1977;135:S104–10.

[31] Neu HC, et al. Incidence of diarrhea and colitis associated with clindamycin therapy. J Infect Dis 1977;135:S120–5.

[32] Adams DH, et al. Non-steroidal anti-inflammatory drugs and renal failure. Lancet 1986;1: 57–60.

[33] Berger RG. Intelligent use of NSAIDs—where do we stand? Expert Opin Pharmacother 2001;2:19–30.

[34] Gurwitz JH, Avorn J, Bohn RL, Glynn RJ, Monane M, Mogun H. Initiation of antihypertensive treatment during nonsteroidal anti-inflammatory drug therapy. JAMA 1994;272:781–6.

[35] Silverstein FE, Faich G, Goldstein JL, Simon LS, Pincus T, Whelton A, et al. Gastrointestinal toxicity with celecoxib vs nonsteroidal anti-inflammatory drugs for osteoarthritis and rheumatoid arthritis: the CLASS study: a randomized controlled trial. Celecoxib Long-term Arthritis Safety Study. JAMA 2000;284:1247–55.

[36] Sreebny LM, Schwartz SS. A reference guide to drugs and dry mouth 2nd edition. Gerodontology 1997;14:33–47.

[37] Fox PC, et al. Xerostomia: evaluation of a symptom with increasing significance. J Am Dent Assoc 1985;110:519–25.

[38] Narhi TO, Meurman JH, Ainamo A. Xerostomia and hyposalivation: causes, consequences and treatment in the elderly. Drugs Aging 1999;15:103–16.

[39] Smith CR. Use of drugs in the aged. Johns Hopkins Med J 1979;145:61–4.

[40] Lamy PP, Vestal RE. Drug prescribing for the elderly. Hosp Pract 1976;11:111–8.

[41] Law R, Chalmers C. Medicines and elderly people: a general practice survey. BMJ 1976;1:565–8.

[42] Gillum RF, Barsky AJ. Diagnosis and management of patient noncompliance. JAMA 1974;228:1563–7.

[43] Taeuber C. Diversity: the dramatic reality. In: Bass S, Kutza EA, Torres-Gil FM, editors. Diversity in aging: the issues facing the White House Conference on Aging and Beyond. Glenview (IL): Scott, Foresman; 1990.

[44] Lamy PP. Prescribing for the elderly. Littleton, MA: Pharmaceutical Sciences Group; 1980.

[45] Atkinson JC, Fox PC. Salivary gland dysfunction. Clin Geriatr Med 1992;8:499–511.

[46] Baum BJ. Salivary gland fluid secretion during aging. J Am Geriatr Soc 1989;37: 453–8.

[47] Weiffenbach JM, Bartoshuk LM. Taste and smell. Clin Geriatr Med 1992;8:543–55.

[48] Bleich HL, Boro ES, Rowe JW. Clinical research on aging: strategies and directions. N Engl J Med 1977;297:1332–6.

[49] Greenblatt DJ, Sellers EM, Shader RI. Drug therapy: drug disposition in old age. N Engl J Med 1982;306:1081–8.

[50] Bender AD. Pharmacodynamic principles of drug therapy in the aged. J Am Geriatr Soc 1974;22:296–303.

[51] Montamat SC, Cusack BJ, Vestal RE. Management of drug therapy in the elderly. N Engl J Med 1989;321:303–9.

[52] Ludwig E, et al. Age-associated pharmacokinetic changes of metronidazole. Int J Clin Pharmacol Ther Toxicol 1983;21:87–91.

[53] Verbeeck RK, Cardinal J-A, Wallace SM. Effect of age and sex on the plasma binding of acidic and basic drugs. Eur J Clin Pharmacol 1984;27:91–7.

[54] Wallace S, Whiting B. Factors affecting drug binding in plasma of elderly patients. Br J Clin Pharmacol 1976;3:327–30.

[55] Crooks J, O'Malley K, Stevenson IH. Pharmacokinetics in the elderly. Clin Pharmacokinet 1976;1:280–96.

[56] Rowe JW, et al. The effect of age on creatinine clearance in men: a cross-sectional and longitudinal study. J Gerontol 1976;31:155–63.

[57] Lindeman RD, Tobin J, Shock NW. Longitudinal studies on the rate of decline in renal function with age. J Am Geriatr Soc 1985;33:278–85.

[58] Meyer BR, Bellucci A. Renal function in the elderly. Cardiol Clin 1986;4:227–34.

[59] Dillon N, et al. Age and beta adrenoceptor-mediated function. Clin Pharmacol Ther 1980;27:769–72.

[60] Vestal RE, Wood AJJ, Shand DG. Reduced β-adrenoceptor sensitivity in the elderly. Clin Pharmacol Ther 1979;26:181–6.

[61] Scarpace PJ. Decreased β-adrenergic responsiveness during senescence. Fed Proc 1986; 45:51–4.

[62] Castleden CM, et al. Increased sensitivity to nitrazepam in old age. Br Med J 1977;1:10–2.

[63] Reidenberg MM, et al. Relationship between diazepam dose, plasma level, age, and central nervous system depression. Clin Pharmacol Ther 1978;23:371–4.

[64] Swift CG, et al. The effect of ageing on measured responses to single doses of oral temazepam. Br J Clin Pharmacol 1981;11:P413–4.

[65] Wade JG, Stevens WC. Isoflurane: an anesthetic for the eighties? Anesth Analg 1981;60: 666–82.

[66] Arden JR, Holley FO, Stanski DR. Increased sensitivity to etomidate in the elderly: initial distribution versus altered brain response. Anesthesiology 1986;65:19–27.

[67] Kergueris MF, Bourin M, Larousse C. Pharmacokinetics of isoniazid: influence of age. Eur J Clin Pharmacol 1986;30:335–40.

Dent Clin N Am 11 (2002) 887–902

THE DENTAL
CLINICS OF
NORTH
AMERICA

Subject Index to Volume 46

Volume 46

January	EVIDENCE BASED DENTISTRY, pages 1–170
April	RESTORATIVE DENTISTRY, pages 171–434
July	DENTAL INFORMATICS, pages 435–622
October	DENTAL THERAPEUTICS UPDATE, pages 623–902

Note: Page numbers of article titles are in **boldface** type

A

Abuse, ethical, 33

Acetaminophen, action of, 696
  adverse effect of, 696
  in pediatrics, 711–712

Acid etching, 277–278
  dentin following, 213, 214

Adhesive(s), dental. See *Dental adhesives*.
  for amalgam restorations, 352

Adrenoceptors, actions of, 733, 734

Adults, inhalational and enteral conscious
  sedation for, **781–802**
  older. See *Older adults*.

Aging, nonphysiologic aspects of, 872–877
  patient compliance in, 876
  pharmacologic changes associated
    with, 877–881
  physiologic changes associated with,
    871
  psychosocial factors in, 876–877

Air abrasion, 175
  advantages of, 196
  air pressure for, 202
  and high-speed drill, compared, 195,
    196–197
  benefits of, 188
  bonded restorations and, 197
  considerations for using, 197
  continuous mode with exhaust, 200
  continuous mode without exhaust, 200
  contraindications to, 202
  cutting rate in, 199–200
  diagnosis of decay for, 192–193
  directing particle stream in, 200
  dynamics of, understanding of,
    205–208

extremely conservative preparations
    produced by, 195–197
  goal of, 188
  in conservative operative dentistry,
    185–209
  instruments for, development of,
    185–186
    nozzle diameter for, 202–203
    selection of, 200
    techniques and procedures for,
      197–203
  learning to use, 186–197, 197, 203
  mechanisms of, 195
  mistakes to avoid in use of, 204
  particle type and size for, 203, 204
  patient comfort and, 201, 202–203
  patient preparation for, 198–199, 201
  science of, and anatomy of teeth, 188
  sensitivity of patient to, 201
  steps in use of, 198
  stream intensity or particle flow rate
    for, 202

Air-abrasive microdentistry system, value
  of, 195

Albuterol, in emergency, 821

Alprazolam, 795–796

Amalgam, as core material, 376
  silver, for restoration of root-surface
    caries, 388–390

Amalgam restorations, 348–354
  adhesive for, 352
  complex, amalgam preparation for,
    348–352
  complex matrices for, 352–353
  finishing of, 353, 354
  longevity of, in posterior teeth,
    308–311

Amalgam restorations (*continued*)
  preparations for, 176–178
  resin-based composite, direct, for class
    I and II cavities, 305–312
      discussion of,
        317–321

Amalgapins, 351–352

American Dental Association, standards for
  products and, 41

Analgesics, classification of, 691
  combinations of, rational use of,
    691–705
  for children, 711–713
  regimens of, 703–704

Analytic studies, 53–55

Anaphylaxis, drugs used in, 826

Anesthesia, dental electronic, 730
  general, definitions establishing
    guidelines for, 768–770
  intraosseous, 728
    systems for, 728–730
  local, 720
    advances in agents and
      techniques of, **719–732**
    adverse drug reactions to,
      747–757
      diagnosis of, 748
    allergic reactions to, 754
    anxiety associated with,
      techniques to overcome,
      759
    toxicity to, 747–750
      management of, 750
      prevention of, 749–750
      signs and symptoms of,
        747–749
    vasoconstrictor reactions to,
      750–752
      practical management of,
        752
      prevention of, 752
      signs and symptoms of,
        751–752

Anesthetics, amide, long-acting, 724–726
  ester, 721
  local, clinical pharmacology of,
    720–726
    ideal, 719
    in children, 711
    lingual infiltration of, 726–727
    periodontal ligament injections
      of, 727–728
    sulfite antioxidant reactions to,
      755
  topical, concentration of, as factor in
    efficacy, 762

  duration of application of,
    764–765
  effective, and techniques, **759–766**
  efficacy of, factors influencing,
    762
    studies of, 760–762
  formulations of, 759, 760
  site of application of, and
    duration of, 763–764

Angina/myocardial infarction, management
  of, 827–828

Antibiotics, and oral contraceptives,
  653–664
    clinical studies evaluating,
      659–661
    legal actions and opinions
      concerning, 661
    pharmacological basis of,
      657–659
  in dentistry, indications for, 635
  in odontogenic infections, **623–633**
    choice of antibiotics for,
      626–627
    culturing and, 626
    factors influencing, 623
    indications for use of, 625–627
  mechanism of action of, 624–625
  prophylactic, for endocarditis,
    prosthetic joints, and surgery,
    635–651
      for immunosuppressed patients,
        646–647
      for orthognathic surgery, 645
      for surgical removal of impacted
        third molars, 645
      in patients with prosthetic joints,
        641–644
      to prevent infective endocarditis,
        635–641

Antihistamine(s), 796
  injectable, in emergency, 820–821

Anti-inflammatory agents, nonsteroidal
  (NSAIDs), actions, side effects, and
  contraindications to, 692–693
    adverse effects of, 680
    efficacy, selection, and dosages
      of, 693–697
    for children, 712
    in chronic pain, 684

Antimicrobial agents, local delovery of, in
  periodontal therapy, **665–677**
    MEDLINE search to study,
      666

Application service providers, in dentistry,
  477–491

Argon lasers, for polymerization, 331

ART treatment technique, success rate of, 315

Articaine hydrochloride, 722–724

"Aspirin burn," 865

Asthma, acute, management of, 826

Atropine, in emergency, 822

B

Bacteremia, after dental procedures, prevalence of, 636

Barbiturate sedation, for children, 811

Barbiturates, 797–798
administration of, 798–800
recovery from, 800–801

Baseline problem, research and, 42–43

Benzodiazepines, adverse effects of, 792
dependence liability of, 792
for adult patients, 790–796
for sedation of children, 808–809
in emergency, 824–825

Biostatistical consultation, for research, **137–155**

Blue light-emitting diode, for polymerization, 332

Bonding, philosophies of, dentin adhesive systems and, 330–331

Bonding agent(s), application of, for resin composites, 342–344

Bronchospasm, management of, 826

Bupivacaine, 724–726

C

CAD/CAM procedure, **405–426**
adhesive seating for, 419–420, 423, 424
case reports of use of, 412–420
computer-aided design for, 408–409
computer-aided machining for, 409–411
development and improvements in, 406
discussion of, 420–425
for chair-side inlays and partial crowns, 412–414, 415
for chair-side partial and full crowns, 414–415, 416, 417
full crown design on screen for, 416–418, 419, 420, 421, 422
history of, 405–406
intraoral three-dimensional scanning camera for, 406–407

multitasking computer-aided design/ computer-aided machining for, 418–419, 422
scanning principle of, 407, 408
semichair-side and laboratory computer-aided design/ computer-aided machining for, 411–412

Calcium channel blockers, as cause of gingival hyperplasia, 860–861
uses of, 860

Calcium hydroxide liner, 318

Candidiasis, altered immunity and, 863–864

Carbohydrate, oral, in emergency, 821

Cardiac arrest, management of, 827

Cardiovascular disease, vasoconstrictors in, 737–739

Caries, detection of, 172
caries-detecting dye for, 193–194
lasers for, 194–195
incidence of, 247
magnification of, 172–173
nonvital, air abrasion in, 207
preparations for, conservative, **171–184**
restoration in, 173
risk of, classification of, 400, 401
root-surface, etiology of, 386–387
factors controlling, 388
incidence of, 386
materials for restoration of, 388–392
rapidly progressing, 387
slowly progressing, 387
treatment of, **385–404**
secondary, and fluoride-releasing dental materials, **247–276**
definition of, 251
development of, risk factors for, 254, 255–256
in-vitro, and fluoride-releasing dental materials, 259–262
locations of, 251, 263–264
prevention of, 254
restoration replacement in, 249
studies of, 254
treatment of, as disease, 599–600, 606
future developments in, 400–402
nonsurgical, 172
vital, air abrasion in, 206–207

Case-control studies, design of, to yield insight and identify prognostic factors, 130
in evaluation of causation, 121–123

Case simulation programs, interactive, 577

CASE STUDIES for Dentistry, 577–581
　future of, 601–602

Causation, and risk factors, in dentistry, key
　elements to determine, **117–126**
　evaluation of, case-control studies in,
　　121–123
　　key elements for, 118
　　magnitude of, 125
　　prospective cohort studies in,
　　　120–121
　　randomized controlled trials in,
　　　123–124
　　reporting of magnitude of risk
　　　factor in, 119–120
　　research studies for, 118–125
　studies of, 117–118
　　bias in, 124–125

Cavity preparation, oscillating instruments
　for, 332

Celecoxib, 680, 681, 682
　pharmacokinetics and drug
　　interactions of, 681

Cements, glass ionomer. See *Glass ionomer
　cements.*
　luting, for posts, 371

Ceramic inlays and onlays,
　contraindications to, 356–357
　indications for, 356

Ceramics, core-strengthened, 355
　for inlays and onlays, 355
　glass, 355
　strengthened, 355

Chemical injuries of mouth, 865

Children. See *Pediatric dental patients.*

Chloral hydrate sedation, for children,
　809–811

Chlorhexidine, in periodontal therapy, 667,
　668, 670–671, 672, 674

Clinical decision making, 52

Clinical dental practice, use of diagnostic
　data in, **87–115**

Clinical trials, 53–54

Cocaine, 741

Cochrane Collaboration, 1–2

Codeine, 699–701
　for children, 712–713

Cohort study(ies), 24–25
　design of, to yield insight and identify

　　prognostic factors, 130
　inception, 66

Compomers, 392

Composite inlays and onlays,
　contraindications to, 356–357
　indications for, 356

Composite resin(s), advantages of, 359
　as core material, 377
　bonding agent application for,
　　342–344
　fluoride-releasing, 591, 615
　for root-surface restorations, 390
　materials used for, 344
　matrix systems for, 343–344
　placement of, 344–347
　posterior, formation of contact area
　　for, 347–348
　posterior restorations using, 342
　rebonding of, 348

Composite resin restorations, direct, for
　class I and II cavities, 303–305
　new developments in, 328–330
　preparations for, 178–179, 180

Composites, indirect composite materials
　and, 356
　shade guide for, 316

Computer(s), clinical decision making
　using, **521–538**
　dental patient and, 522–523
　for clinical decision making, 529–530
　for diagnostics, 525–527, 529
　for patient history and dental record,
　　523–524
　for treatment planning and
　　pretreatment, 527–529
　handheld, applications of, 545–548
　　dental applications of, 548–551
　　description of, 539–540
　　features of, 540–545
　　in dentistry, **539–551**
　　softwear for, 546, 548–551
　　　Dental Lexi-Drugs, 549
　　　Dentalog, 549
　　　DocAlert, 548
　　　ePocrates QID, 548
　　　ePocrates qRx, 548
　　　Five-minute Clinical
　　　　Consult, 549
　　　Palm Corporate Dental
　　　　Application, 550
　　　STAT growth charts,
　　　　550–551
　in dentistry, 477–478, 565,
　　575–576
　recommendations for, 530–532

Computer systems, office, application
  service providers, 481–482
      benefits and drawbacks of,
        482–486
      examples of, 486–488
      functions of vendor of, 489
      security and, 489
      hardware failures in, 480–481
      network failures in, 480–481
      operator error and, 479–480
      power failures and, 480
      software failures and, 480
      traditional, 478–481
      type of Internet connection for,
        488

Concordance, diagnostic tests and, 108–109

Confidence-interval estimates, 140–141

Confidence intervals, 57

Convergence, diagnostic tests and, 108–109

Copper-band matrices, 353

Core-strangthened ceramics, 355

Correlation coefficient(s), intraclass,
  reliability of measurements and, 95
  reliability of measurements and, 95

Corticosteroids, and candidiasis, 864
  in emergency, 823

COX-1, 680

COX-2, 680

COX-2 inhibitors, **679–690**
  adverse effects of, 685–687
  cardiovascular effects of, 686–687
  currently under review by FDA, 687
  gastrointestinal effects of, 685–686
  renal effects of, 687
  selective, acute orofacial pain
      management with, 683–684
      analgesic efficacy and anti-
        inflammatory effect of, 681–
        683
      chronic orofacial pain manage-
        ment with, 684–685

Criteria for causality, 58–59

Cross-sectional surveys, 53

Crown segment, 215

Cyclooxygenase, in pain, 680

Cyclooxygenase-2 inhibitors. See *COX-2
  inhibitors.*

Cyclosporine, as cause of gingival
  hyperplasia, 861–862

D

Data bases, electronic, for literature
  searches, 47–49

Data integration, fundamental informatics
  principles and, 606–610
  meaning of, to practicing dentist,
    605–615
  optimizing value of information in,
    614–615
  transforming principles into practice,
    610–614

Data management, for statistical research,
  151–152

Decay, diagnosis of, 193

Decision analysis, diagnostic, 89–92

Decision making, clinical, 52

Dental adhesives, advantages and
  disadvantages of, 283
  "all-in-one," 290–293
  clinical trials of, 293–296
  cytotoxicity of, 221
  laboratory tests of, 296, 297
  new philosophies on, 290
  types of, 283

Dental anxiety scale, 773

Dental caries. See *Caries.*

Dental education, and continuing dental
  education, interactive multimedia
    patient simulations in, **575–587**
  basic science made clinically relevant,
    581–582
  clinical problem solving in, 582
  continuing, and dental education,
      interactive multimedia patient
      simulations in, **575–587**
      background of, 589–590
      education courses and listings, on
        Web, 591
      emerging Web technologies,
        600–601
      on World Wide Web, **589–604**
        instructional quality of,
          592–595
        quality course review and,
          596–600
      Web-based, location of, 590–592
  creation of standardized patients for,
    583–584
  goal of, 576
  hard-to-find patients for, 582–583
  teaching of self-evaluation in, 584
  transfer problem in, 576–577

Dental materials, cytotoxicity of, 221–222

Dental postoperative pain, in children, 710
    management of, medications and
        dosage for, 714
        protocol for, 715
        recommendations for,
          713–715

Dental postoperative pin, in children,
    management of, **707–717**

Dental practice, clinical, use of diagnostic
    data in, **87–115**

Dental practitioners, statistical needs of,
    138, 142–143
    statistical training for, 143–144
    treating older patients, precautions
        for, 881–882

Dental procedures, infective endocarditis
    and, studies of, 637–638
    prevalence of bacteremia after, 636
    surgical, prevention of infection
        following, 644–645

Dental research. See *Research.*

Dental researcher(s), biostatistician and,
    145–146
    statistical needs of, 144–145

Dentin, abnormal forms of, sealing of,
    problems associated with, 224–225
    as porous barrier, 213
    collagen banding in, 282–287
    contaminated with bacteria,
        permeability of, 233–235, 236
    effects of growth factors on, 236–238
    following acid etching, 213, 214
    fractured mineralized, 213, 214
    hybridization of, 288, 291, 295
    hydraulic conductance of, 217, 218
    initial seal, restoration of, 220–221
    middle, dentin tubules in, 278, 281
    peripheral seal, restoration of, 220
    permeability of, effects of dentin
        thickness on, 215–216
        effects on restorative dentistry,
          211–245
        intertubular, versus tubular
          permeability of, 225–229,
          230
        regional differences in, 216–218
    postoperative sensitivity of, 217–218
    sealing of, with resins, problems
        associated with, 222–224
    thickness of, effects on permeability,
        215–216
    tubular structure of, 282

Dentin adhesive systems, and bonding
    philosophies, 330–331

Dentin bonding, as function of dentin
    structure, **277–301**
    "wet-bonding" technique and, 287–288

Dentin bonding systems, categories of, 278

Dentin substrate, ideal, 278–290

Dentist, practicing, meaning of data
    integration to, **605–615**

Dentistry, clinical practice of, decision
    making in, 11
        surgical component of, 11
    evidence-based. See *Evidence-based*
        dentistry.
    product testing in, 2

Descriptive studies, 52–53

Diabetic emergencies, management of, 828

Diagnosis(es), validity of, and reference
    standard, 98–99

Diagnostic data, principles of decision
    analysis and, 89–90
    test characteristics and, 99–109
    use and interpretation of, in diagnostic
        decision analysis, 89–90

Diagnostic decision analysis, 89–92
    threshold approach for,
        90–92
    use and interpretation of diagnostic
        data in, 89–90

Diagnostic process, 88–89

Diagnostic test(s), concordance and,
    108–109
    convergence and, 108–109
    evidence-based dentistry in, 160
    gold standard and new, contingency
        comparison between, 109
    likelihood ratios and monograms for,
        109–113
    parallel testing with, 108
    sensitivities, specificities, and
        likelihood ratios of, 102
    series testing with, 107–108

Diazepam, 793
    for children, 808–809

DICOM standard, advantages of, 566–567
    as accepted standard, 566
    committee, 568
    conformance statement of, 568–569
    description of, 566
    in dentistry, American Dental
        Association and, 569–570
        practical demonstrations of,
          570–571
    use and implication of, **565–573**

in perspective, 567
latest version of, specialties supported
by, 567–568
parts of, 568
streamlined, interoperability within,
571
groups participating in,
572–573
validation tests of,
571–572

Digital imaging and communication in
medicine. See *DICOM standard.*

Dimension reduction procedure, 146

Disease, classification of, 88–89
determinants of, 52
distribution of, 52
principles of, 88

Doxycycline, effects on ethinyl estradiol and
norethindrone, 660
in periodontal therapy, 668, 669,
670–671

Drill, high-speed, and air abrasion,
compared, 195, 196–197

Drug(s), alterations in responsiveness to, in
aging, 870, 872
and taste aberrations, 865
dental, toxicity of, age-related risk of,
875
emergency, **815–830**
categories of, 816
essential, 817–822
supplementary, 817, 822–825
interactions of, related to pain
management, 694–695
with vasoconstrictors, 740–744
pharmacokinetics of, in older adults,
877–881
taken by older adults, 870

Drug eruptions, lichenoid, 865

Drug reactions, adverse, among older
adults, 874–876
to local anesthesia, **747–757**
diagnosis of, 748
classification of, 858, 859

Drug therapy, oral manifestations
of, **857–868**
and etiology of, 859

Dye, caries-detecting, for detection of
caries, 193–194

E

Emergency kit, dental office, contents of,
775–777

Emergency(ies), drugs in, **815–830**
medical, dentist in, 815–816
specific, drug use in,
825–829

EMLA, for topical anesthesia, 762–763

Endocarditis, infective, antibiotic
prophylaxis to prevent, 635–636
dental procedures requiring,
638–640
efficacy of, 641
risk and cost benefit of,
640–641
cause of, questions concerning,
636–644
dental procedures and, studies of,
637–638
patients at risk for, 638, 639
prosthetic joints, and surgery,
antibiotic prophylaxis for,
635–651

Endodontically treated tooth, restoration
of, **367–384**

Entacapone, 744

Ephedrine, in emergency, 823

Epidemiologic studies, 52

Epidemiology, definition of, 52

Epinephrine, 733, 735, 741
in emergency, 818–820

Ethical abuse, 33

Ethical concerns, clarifying relationships in,
34

Ethical situation, 34

Ethics, common principles of, 30–31
definition of, 32, 33
discursive approach to, 31–33
general approaches to, 30–35
insensitivity to, 33
issues of, approach to, 31
of experimenting in dental practice,
29–44
of research, literature on, 40–43
organizations concerned with, 30
test of, 33–35
therapeutic alliance and, 32

Ethinyl estradiol, action of colonic bacteria
on, 658
and norethindrone, effects of
doxycycline on, 660
effects of rifampin on, 655, 656

Etidocaine, 724–726

Etoricoxib, 687

Evidence-based dentistry, **1–164**
   accounting for patients entered in trial, 3
   application of, to patients, **157–164**
   application of prognostic information in, 161–162
   application of therapeutic improvements in, 162–163
   basic approach in, 42–43
   beneficiaries of, 8
   blind comparison with reference standard in, 6
   blinding of patients, clinicians, and study personnal in, 3–4
   clinical outcomes of, consideration of, 4–5
   definition of, 1
   design architecture for, **51–59**
   diagnostic tests in, 160
   follow-up studies in, 5
   groups in, equal treatment of, 4
      similarity of, 4
   model of, steps in, 157, 158
   outcome criteria in, objective and unbiased, 5
   patient input and, 159
   randomized assignment to treatment in, 2–3
   reported outcomes and, predictive value of, 163
   research on sample of patients and, 158–159
   results of, benefit of, in caring for patients, 5
   specific applications of, 159–163
   statistical analysis in, terminology and, 6
   to determine therapy, 2–5
   to evaluate need for diagnostic test, 6–7
   value of testing and, 6–7
   what is it?, **1–9**
   what it is not, 7

Exclusion criteria, 55

Experimenting, in dental practice, ethics of, **29–44**

Experiment(s), categories of, 36
   definition of, 35
   in dental practice, 35–37
   in practice. See *Practice experiments.*
   scientific investigation as, 35–36

Extension-for-prevention approach, 196

F

Fissure(s), assessment and management of, 173, 174

definition of, 172

Flumazenil, in dental office emergency kit, 777
   in emergency, 825

Fluoride, amount of, in dental materials, 258
   availability from glass ionomers, 271
   release of, methods of, 257–258

Fluoride-releasing composite resins, 591, 615

Fluoride-releasing materials, 589, 614–617
   caries-preventive mechanisms of, 271
   fluoride recharge in, 393, 394
   fluoride release from, 393
   plaque and, 268–270
   recharging of, 270
   remote effect of, 262–268
   secondary caries and, **247–276**
      in-vitro, 259–262

Fluoride(s), compounds, common, 833
   dietary supplements of, 832–834
   gels and foams, 836
   in restorative materials, 834–835
   OTC dentifrices, 838–839
   practitioner's guide to, **831–846**
   prescription, 832–835
   professionally applied, 835–838
   prophylaxis pastes, 836–837
   self-applied, 834
   toxicity to, 839–840
   varnishes, 837–838

Food and Drug Administration, standards for products and, 41

G

Geriatric pharmacology, **869–885**

Gingival hyperplasia, as complication of drug therapy, 859

Glass ceramics, 355

Glass ionomer(s), as core material, 377
   fluoride availability from, 258–259, 268
   resin-modified, 267–268, 391–392
      as core material, 377

Glass ionomer cements, 257
   for posterior restorations, discussion of, 321–326
      failure rate of, 312–314
      longevity of, 313

Glucagon, in emergency, 822

Groove, definition of, 172

Growth factors, effects of, on dentin, 236–238

H

Handheld computing. See *Computer(s), handheld.*

Health care research, designs for, experimental, 62
    observational, 62

Health Insurance Portability and Accountability, **553–563**
    and dentistry, 555–556
    areas covered by, 553–554
    Department of Health and Human Services and, 553
    electronic transaction standards and, 556–557
    health care issues addressed by, 553
    national employer identifier and, 562
    national provider identifier and, 561
    privacy rule of, 557–559
    security and, 559–561
    summary table, 554

Histogram, bell-shaped curves and, 138–140

Hydrocodone, 701

Hydroxyzine, 797

Hypotension, management of, 828

I

Imidazopyridines, 796

Immunity, altered, and candidiasis, 863–864

Immunosuppressed patients, antibiotic prophylaxis for, 646–647

Implant surgery, antibiotic prophylaxis in, 646

Implant therapy, single-tooth, search strategies for, 48

Inception cohort study, 66

Inclusion criteria, 55

Infection(s), following surgical dental procedures, prevention of, 644–645
    odontogenic, antibiotic therapy in, **623–633**
        as polymicrobial, 624
        diagnosis and management of, myths concerning, 627–631
        step-by-step approach for, 631–632
    of in-dwelling devices, antibiotic prophylaxis in, 647–648

reduced resistance to, antibiotic prophylaxis in, 647

Informatics principles, fundamental, data integration and, 606–610

Information management processes, 611, 612

Information problem, for continual learner, 79–80
    solution to, 80–81

Informed consent, 34–35

Inlays, and onlays, ceramic, contraindications to, 356–357
        indications for, 356
    composite, contraindications to, 356–357
        indications for, 356
    luting technique for, 361–362
    placement of, preparation for, 358–359

Institute of Medicine, report of, patient simulations and, 585

Instruments, oscillating, for cavity preparation, 332

Internet, advanced filtering and, 451, 452
    Boolean keyword search and, 441, 442
    catalogs and, 440, 441
    current problems associated with, 458–459
    genetic algorithms and, 460–461
    InfoFinder agent and, 460
    information and, need for, 436–437
        retrieval of, 437
            advanced concepts for, 442–459
            basic concepts for, 438–441
        versus knowledge, 437–438
    information economics and, 459
    information retrieval on, **435–462**
    intelligent agents and, 460
    keyword search and, 440–441
    knowledge management and, 437–438
    meta search engines and, 449–451
    natural-language queries and, 451, 453
    newsgroup search and, 454
    outlook for, 459–461
    picture search and, 454, 456
    ranking and matching criteria on, 445–447
    ranking by relevance on, 447
    search engine list, 446–447
    search for personal conversation and, 457
    search methods and, 440–441
    search with special purpose search engine, 443–445
    searchbots and, 454, 455

Internet advanced (*continued*)
    searching by example on, 448
    semantic search engine and, 459–460
    structure of, 435
    traditional search engines and,
        438–439, 473
    type of connection for office computer
        systems, 488
    WebWatcher project and, 460

Internet Grateful Med, 47–48

Intervention studies, 53–54

J

Joints, prosthetic, antibiotic prophylaxis in,
    641–642
            guidelines for, 642–643
            overview of, 644
            regimens for, 643–644
        endocarditis, and surgery, anti-
            biotic prophylaxis for,
            635–651
        infections around, dental-induced
            bacteremia in, 642
            microbiology of, 642

Journals, peer-reviewed, for conducting
    literature searches, 46–47

K

Kappa scores, reliability of measurements
    and, 97

L

Lasers, argon, for polymerization, 331
    for caries detection, 194–195

Levonordefrin, 733, 735

Lichenoid drug eruptions, 865

Lidocaine hydrochloride, 721–722

Light polymerization units, 331–332

Liner, calcium hydroxide, 318

Literature, about prognosis, designs of
    studies to yield, 129–130
        evaluation of, 128
            clinical situation illustrat-
            ing, 128–129
        conducting search of, **45–49**
            electronic data bases for, 47–49
            peer-reviewed journal sources
            for, 46–47
            sources for, 45
            traditional reference sources for, 46
    on ethics of research, 40–43

recent focus of, 80
    systematic reviews of, overview and
        meta-analysis of, **79–86**
    user's guide to, **127–136**

Lonesome Doc Document Ordering service,
    48, 49

Longitudinal data analysis, and research,
    146–147

Lorazepam, 795

Luting materials, 360–361

M

Macrodentistry, 185–186

Matrix systems, for resin composites, 343–
    344

Max pin, 349–351

Means, comparison of, 141–142

Measurement(s), and tests, reliability of, 95,
    96
    reliability of, and correlation
        coefficients, 95
        and intraclass correlation
        coefficients, 95
        Kappa scores and, 97
        variability of examination
        equipment and environment
        influencing, 93
        variability of examiners
        influencing, 93–94
        variation in system measured
        influencing, 92–93
    validity of, and reference standard,
        97–98

Measures of association, 55–57

MEDLINE, for search of literature, 47–49
    for systemic reviews of literature,
        79–80, 82
    search terms for use on, 16–17

Memex, 435

Meperidine, 701–702

Mepivacaine hydrochloride, 722

Methemoglobinemia, 753

Metronidazole, in periodontal therapy, 667

Microdentistry, 185–186
    air abrasion in. See *Air abrasion.*
    basic principle of, 188
    caries-detecting dye in, 193–194

Microdentistry system, air-abrasive, value
    of, 195

Midazolam, 795

Minikin pins, 350

Minocycline, as cause of tooth
discoloration, 862–863
in periodontal therapy, 668, 670–671,
672, 674

Molars, endodontically-treated, post
placement in, 368–369
mandibular, Rainey Ridge of, 189
subocclusal oblique transverse
ridge of, 189–192
third, impacted, surgical removal of,
antibiotic prophylaxis for, 645

Morphine, 699–701
in emergency, 823–824

Multimedia patient simulations, interactive,
in continuing dental education and
dental education, **575–587**

N

Naloxone, in emergency, 824

Nanoleakage, 229–233

Nifedipine, as cause of gingival hyperplasia,
861

Nitroglycerin, in emergency, 820

Nitrous oxide, for conscious sedation, 781,
782
health hazards associated with,
787–788
prevention of, 788
in emergency, 824

Nitrous oxide inhalation sedation, for
children, 806–807

Nitrous oxide/oxygen inhalational sedation,
administration of, 784–785
physical properties, pharmacokinetics,
and pharmacodynamics of,
782–783
recovery from, 785–786
safety precautions for, 786–787

Nonopioids, 692, 697, 698

Norethindrone, and ethinyl estradiol, effects
of doxycycline on, 660
effects of rifampin on, 655, 656

O

Observational comparison studies, in
research, 65–68

Observational studies, 54–55
selection bias in, 66–67

selection of subjects based on recall, 67
to evaluate harmful exposures, 67–68

Odontogenic infections. See *Infection(s),
odontogenic.*

Older adults, adverse drug reactions among,
874–876
alterations in responsiveness to drugs
in, 870, 872
dental practitioners treating,
precautions for, 881–882
drug absorption in, 877–878
drug distribution in, 878
drug excretion in, 879–880
drug metabolism in, 879
drugs taken by, 870
multiple disease states in, 872–874
numbers of, 869
pharmacodynamic changes in,
880–881
polypharmacy in, 875

Onlays, modifications of, 359–360

Operative dentistry, conservative, air
abrasion in, **185–209**

Opioids, actions and effects of, 698
as specific receptors, 692
for sedation of children, 807
specific considerations for use of,
699–704
therapeutic use of, 698–699

Oral contraceptives, antibiotics and,
653–664
clinical studies evaluating,
659–661
legal actions and options
concerning, 661
pharmacological basis of,
657–659
interactions with penicillin and
tetracycline, 655–657
interactions with rifampin, 655
pharmacology of, 654
side effects of, 654
types of, 654

Orthodontic referrals, via TeleDent
Southwest, **507–520**
background of, 507–509
capturing clinical data, clinical
examination for, 510
images of models and
radiographs for, 510
obtaining advice in,
511–513
comments on, 515–516
effect on dentists, 518
effect on patient care, 516–517, 518

Orthodontic referrals (*continued*)
    method of, 509–510
    results and discussion of, 513–514
        cases referred, 514–515
        process of referral, 514
        use of equipment, 514

Orthognathic surgery, antibiotic
    prophylaxis in, 645

Oxycodone, 701

Oxygen, in emergency, 817–818

P

P-values, 141

Pain, acute orofacial, selective COX-2
        inhibitors in, 683–684
    children and, 710
    control of, for ambulatory dental
        patients, 679–680
    definition of, 709–710
    management of, drug interactions
        related to, 694–695
        in children, changing philosophy
            of, 708
    postoperative dental. See *Dental
        postoperative pain.*

Parecoxib, 687

Patient simulations, and accreditation
        standards, 585–587
    in curriculum, 581
    interactive, computer-based, 576–577
        early in dental education, 582
    report of Institute of Medicine and,
        585

Patient(s), caring for, benefits of
        evidence-based dentistry in, 5
    input of, evidence-based dentistry and,
        159
    interests of, as first concern in
        experimentation, 37–38
    questions of, to reflect wishes and
        priorities, 13–14

Pediatric dental patients, pain in, 710
    postoperative pain in, management of,
        707–717
    sedation for, **803–814**
        precautions in use of, 811–812
        regimens for, 805

PEDNET (Professional Ethics in Dentistry
    Network), 30

Penicillin, interactions with oral
    contraceptives, 655–657

Pentazocine, 702

Periodontal disease, effect of antibiotic and
    scaling and root planing therapy on, 56

Periodontal therapy, using local delivery of
        antimicrobial agents, **665–677**
    MEDLINE search to study, 666

Pharmacology, geriatric, **869–885**

Phenytoin, as cause of gingival hyperplasia,
    860

Phosphoric acid, for acid etching, 277–278

Pilot data, definition of, 149
    loss of attachment study illustrating,
        sample size estimator for, 150
    sources of, 149–151

Plaque, fluoride-releasing materials, 268–270

Plasma arc curing units, for polymerization,
    331–332

Polymerization, argon lasers for, 331
    blue light-emitting diode, 332
    plasma arc curing units for, 331–332
    "softstart," 331

Polypharmacy, in older adults, 875

Post(s), antirotation of, 375
    canal preparations for, 370
    cement placement for, 371
    core materials for, 376–377
    crown bevel and, 376
    design of, 369–370
    diameter of, 370
    length of, 370
    luting cements for, 371
    metallic, active, 372
        passive parallel, 372
        passive tapered, 372
        prefabricated, 372
    non metallic, carbon fiber, 373
        tooth colored, 373–375
    placement of, indications for, 368–369
    restorations retained by, retention and
        resistance of, 375–376
    surface preparation for, 370
    types of, 371–375
    vertical remaining tooth structure and,
        376

Power analysis, primary steps in carrying
    out, 150

Practice experiments, 36–37
    ethics of, 37–40
    expectation of success of, 38–39
    heroic, 40
    patient's interests and, 37–38
    standard of care and, 38
    systemic approach to, 39
    visible, 40

Practice system, information systems, 612, 613
  integrated, 612, 613, 614
  interfaced, 611, 612

Pregnancy, vasoconstrictors in, 739–740

Prilocaine hydrochloride, 722

Procaine, 721

Product testing, in dentistry, 2

Promethazine, 797

Propoxycaine, 721

Propoxyphene, 702

Prospective cohort studies, in evaluation of causation, 120–121

Q

Question(s), **11–19**
  background, 15
  conversion of patient's problem into, 16
  description of patient and, 15
  evidence to answer, 12–13
  foreground, 15
  framing of, 16
  how they arise, 11–12
  of patient, to reflect wishes and priorities, 13–14
  of searcher, finding answer for, 14–15
  search terms and, 16–17
  titles and abstracts in literature and, 17–18
  types of, 15–16

R

Randomized controlled trials, 24, 25–26
  in evaluation of causation, 123–124
  in research, 63–65

Receiver operating characteristic analysis, test characteristics and, 105–106

Reference standard, validity of diagnosis and, 98–99
  validity of measurements and, 97–98

Research, accounting for all subjects in, 74–75
  administration and execution of, 152–153
  baseline problem and, 42–43
  bias in, 124–125
    can lead to inappropriate treatment selection, **61–78**
  bias in methods of, 70–76
  biostatistical consultation for, **137–155**
  blind participants in, 70–71
    calibration and training of examiners in, 73–74
  case reports and case studies in, 68
  clinical, 62
  data used appropriately in, 75–76
  ethics of, literature on, 40–43
  factors complicating, 146–147
  generalizability of, 42
  health care, designs for, experimental, 62
    observational, 62
  hierarchy of design of, and bias control, 62–70
  historical control groups in, 68–70
  internal versus external validity of, 41–42
  longitudinal data analysis and, 146–147
  observational comparison studies in, 65–68
  published findings of, credibility of, 41
  randomized controlled trials in, 63–65
  role of statistical consultant in, 145
  same treatment of all subjects in, 71–73
  sample size and power analysis in, 148–149

Research studies, assessment of validity of, 57–58
  confidence intervals and, 57
  findings of, criteria for causality in, 58–59
  in evaluation of causation, 118–125
  measures of association and, 55–57
  samples of subjects in, 55
  types of, 51–55

Researchers, dental, biostatistician and, 145–146
  statistical needs of, 144–145

Resin composite(s). See *Composite resin(s)*.

Resin-modified glass ionomer restorative materials, 267–268, 377, 391–392

Resin restoration, preventive, 179, 180

Resins, sealing of dentin with, problems associated with, 222–224

Restoration(s), amalgam. See *Amalgam restorations*.
  bonded, air abrasion and, 197
  composite, direct, longevity of, in posterior teeth, 303–304, 306–307
  composite resin, direct, for class I and II cavities, 305–315
    preparations for, 178–179, 180
  definitive, of endodontically treated tooth, 377–378

Restoration(s), amalgam (*continued*)
  direct, materials for, 341–354
  failure of, reasons for, 249, 250–251
  in caries, 173
  indirect, material selection for,
    354–355
  longevity of, 249, 250–251
  posterior, direct, clinical results of,
    and new developments,
    303–339
      clinical trials in, design of,
        326–327, 328
      factors influencing longevity
        of, 326–327
      in class I and II cavities,
        303–315
      new developments in,
        327–332
    glass ionomer cements,
      discussion of, 321–326
      failure rate of, 312–314
      longevity of, 313
    using resin composites, 342
  replacement of, in secondary caries,
    249
  resin-based composite, direct class I
    and II cavities, 303–305
    direct for class I and II cavities,
      discussion of, 315–317
    new developments in,
      328–330
  single-tooth, complex, **341–365**
  tunnel, 180–181
    failure rate of, 314–315
  types of, 248–249

Restoration system, fill-ceramic,
  chair-side computer-aided design/
  computer-aided machining.
  See *CAD/CAM*
  procedure.

Restorative dentistry, effects of dentin
  permeability on, **211–245**

Restorative materials, adhesive, 197

Retrospective studies, types of, 66

Rifampin, effects on ethinyl estradiol and
  norethindrone, 655, 656
  interactions with oral contraceptives,
    655–657

Risk factors, and causation, in dentistry,
  key elements to determine, **117–126**
  magnitude of, 125
    reporting of, 125

Rofecoxib, 680, 681–683
  pharmacokinetics and drug
    interactions of, 681

Root canal therapy, single-tooth, search
  strategies for, 49

Root-caries. See *Caries, root-surface.*

S

Salivary glands, dysfunction of, causes of,
  847

Scientification investigation, as experiments,
  35–36

Search terms, for use on MEDLINE, 16–17

Sedation, conscious, definition of, 768–769
  for dentistry, **767–780**
    general office preparedness for,
      776–779
    patient preparation for, 773–775
    patient selection and preparation
      for, 770–775
    physical assessment for, 770–772
    psychologic assessment for,
      772–773
    training requirements for,
      775–776
  deep, definition of, 769–770
  enteral, with single agent, 789–797
  for pediatric dental patients, **803–814**
  inhalational and enteral conscious, for
    adult dental patient, **781–802**
  safe, definitions establishing guidelines
    for, 768–770

Sedation/anesthesia, definitions in, 804

Seizures, management of, 828–829

Self-etching primers, 278, 286

Shade guide, for composite materials, 316

Siloranes, 330

Silver amalgam, for restoration of
  root-surface caries, 388–390

Sjögren's syndrome, 847, 852

Smear plug, 278, 286

Soft tissue abnormalities, due to drug
  therapy, 859–862

Statistical consultant, role in dental
  research, 145

Statistical hypotheses and methods, 146

Study(ies), analytical, 24
  bias of clinician and, 27
  biologic response and clinical response
    demonstrated by, 26–27
  cohort, 24–25
  comparative, 24–25
  designs of, to yield insight and identify

prognostic factors, 129–130
measurements of, determination of, 24
outcome assessment and, 24
prospective, 24
randomized controlled trials, 24, 25–26
results of, expression of, 26
    leading to selection or avoidance
        of therapy, 135
    precision of estimates of
        likelihood and, 134
    size of likelihood of outcome
        event and, 132–134
    statistical significance and, 26
    use for reassuring or counseling
        patients, 135
    value to practitioners caring for
        patients, 134
retrospective, 24, 25
setting for gathering in, referral filter
    bias and, 159
structure of, and applicability to
    patients, 24
subjects in, eligibility decisions for, 23
    screening for, 23
    study parameter and, 23
validity of, assessment of, primary
    guides of, 131–132

Study samples, 55

Success, definition of, as controversial, 27

Sulfite intolerance, vasoconstrictors and,
    744–745

Syncope, in dentistry, management of,
    825–826

Systematic reviews of literature, features
    illustrating, 81–83
    overview and meta-analysis of, **79–86**
    questions to consider in, 83–85

T

Taste aberrations, drugs and, 865

TeleDent Southwest, orthodontic referrals
    via. See *Orthodontic referrals, via
    TeleDent Southwest.*

Test characteristics, and test thresholds,
    criteria for selection of, 103–104
    definitions and calculations for,
        100–101
    diagnostic data and, 99–109
    effects of prevalence on, 106–109
    posttest likelihood of, 108
    predictive values in, 106
    pretest likelihood and, 106
    receiver operating characteristic
        analysis and, 105–106

Test thresholds, criteria for selection of, test
    characteristics and, 103–104

Tetracycline, as cause of tooth
    discoloration, 862
    in periodontal therapy, 668, 669,
        670–671, 672, 674
    interactions with oral contraceptives,
        655–657

Therapeutic alliance, ethics and, 32

Therapy, determination of, dental education
    and, 21
        evaluation of reports for, 23
        factors influencing, 21–22
        risk information and, 22
        sources of information for, 22–23

Therapy anecdote, experience, of evidence?,
    21–28

Tolapone, 744

Toluidine blue test, as example of diagnostic
    test, 106–107

Tooth(Teeth), anatomy of, science of air
    abrasion and, 188
    anterior, endodontically-treated, post
        placement in, 368–369
    discoloration of, minocycline as cause
        of, 862–863
        tetracycline as cause of, 862
    full coverage, indications for, 362
    posterior, longevity of direct
        composite restorations in,
        303–304, 306–307
    premolar, endodontically-treated, post
        placement in, 369
    unsound, new systems to diagnose, 199

Tramadol, 696–697
    for children, 712

Triazolam, 793–794

Tunnel restorations, 180–181
    failure rate of, 314–315

U

United Kingdom National Health Service,
    507

V

Valdecoxib, 680, 683

Vasoconstrictors, drug interactions with,
    740–744
    for enhancement of local anesthesia,
        735–736
    for increased safety of anesthetics, 737

Vasoconstrictors (*continued*)
    for intraoperative hemostasis, 736
    in cardiovascular disease, 737–739
    in pregnancy, 739–740
    indications for, 735–737
        and precautions in use of,
            733–746
    mechanism of action of, 733–735
    precautions in use of, 737–745
    sulfite intolerance and, 744–745

Virtual reality articular, adjustment of,
        preliminary and matching procedures
        for, 495–496
    conception of, 495
    DentCAM, 496–497
        evaluation of, 497–498
        modules of, 498–500
    development of, in cooperation with
        Fraunhofer institute, 500–502
    educational settings of, 502–504
    in dentistry, **493–506**
    need for, 493–495
    outlook for, 504–505

W

Website(s), categories of information
    checklist, 465–466
    companies and resources to help put
        online, 467–469
    dental practice, **463–475**
        background of, 463
    design of, guide to, 463–467
    designing and maintaining own, 470
    future of, in dentistry, 474
    promotion of, 472–474
    uses of, for dental practices, 470–472

World Wide Web, continuing dental
        education on, **589–604**
    search results, 590

X

Xerostomia, clinical trials for, interventions
        assessed in, 849
    management of, discussion on,
        851–853
        literature on, flaws in, 850–851
        methods of, 848
    radiotherapy-induced, 851
    treatment of, **847–856**

Z

Zolpidem, 796

Changing Your Address?

Make sure your subscription changes too! When you notify us of your new address, you can help make our job easier by including an exact copy of your Clinics label number with your old address (see illustration below.) This number identifies you to our computer system and will speed the processing of your address change. Please be sure this label number accompanies your old address and your corrected address—you can send an old Clinics label with your number on it or just copy it exactly and send it to the address listed below.

We appreciate your help in our attempt to give you continuous coverage. Thank you.

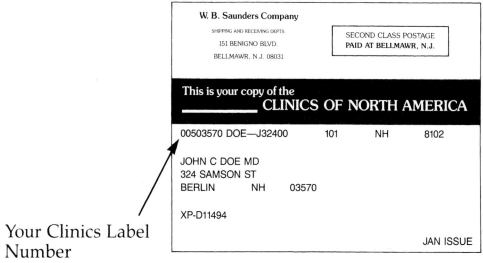

W. B. Saunders Company

SHIPPING AND RECEIVING DEPTS.

151 BENIGNO BLVD.

BELLMAWR, N.J. 08031

SECOND CLASS POSTAGE
PAID AT BELLMAWR, N.J.

This is your copy of the
_____ **CLINICS OF NORTH AMERICA**

00503570 DOE—J32400   101   NH   8102

JOHN C DOE MD
324 SAMSON ST
BERLIN   NH   03570

XP-D11494

JAN ISSUE

Your Clinics Label Number

Copy it exactly or send your label along with your address to:
W.B. Saunders Company, Customer Service
Orlando, FL 32887-4800
Call Toll Free 1-800-654-2452

Please allow four to six weeks for delivery of new subscriptions and for processing address changes.

United States Postal Service
Statement of Ownership, Management, and Circulation

1. Publication Title	2. Publication Number								3. Filing Date
Dental Clinics of North America	0	0	1	1	-	8	5	3	2	9/15/02

4. Issue Frequency	5. Number of Issues Published Annually	6. Annual Subscription Price
Jan, Apr, Jul, Oct	4	$135.00

7. Complete Mailing Address of Known Office of Publication (*Not printer*) (*Street, city, county, state, and ZIP+4*)

Elsevier Science
6277 Sea Harbor Drive, Orlando, FL 32887-4800, Orange County

Contact Person

Amy Snyder

Telephone

215-238-8319

8. Complete Mailing Address of Headquarters or General Business Office of Publisher (*Not printer*)

Elsevier Science, The Curtis Center, Independence Square West, Philadelphia, PA 19106-3399

9. Full Names and Complete Mailing Addresses of Publisher, Editor, and Managing Editor (*Do not leave blank*)

Publisher (*Name and complete mailing address*)

Glen Campbell, Elsevier Science, The Curtis Center, Independence Square West, Philadelphia, PA 19106-3399

Editor (*Name and complete mailing address*)

John Vassallo, Elsevier Science, The Curtis Center, Independence Square West, Philadelphia, PA 19106-3399

Managing Editor (*Name and complete mailing address*)

Heather Cullen, Elsevier Science, The Curtis Center, Independence Square West, Philadelphia, PA 19106-3399

10. Owner (*Do not leave blank. If the publication is owned by a corporation, give the name and address of the corporation immediately followed by the names and addresses of all stockholders owning or holding 1 percent or more of the total amount of stock. If not owned by a corporation, give the names and addresses of the individual owners. If owned by a partnership or other unincorporated firm, give its name and address as well as those of each individual owner. If the publication is published by a nonprofit organization, give its name and address.*)

Full Name	Complete Mailing Address
Wholly owned subsidiary of	4520 East-West Highway
Reed/Elsevier, US holdings	Bethesda, MD 20814

11. Known Bondholders, Mortgagees, and Other Security Holders Owning or Holding 1 Percent or More of Total Amount of Bonds, Mortgages, or Other Securities. If none, check box ▶ None

Full Name	Complete Mailing Address
N/A	

12. Tax Status (*For completion by nonprofit organizations authorized to mail at nonprofit rates*) (*Check one*)
The purpose, function, and nonprofit status of this organization and the exempt status for federal income tax purposes:
 Has Not Changed During Preceding 12 Months
 Has Changed During Preceding 12 Months (*Publisher must submit explanation of change with this statement*)

(*See Instructions on Reverse*)

PS Form 3526, October 1999

13. Publication Title	14. Issue Date for Circulation Data Below
Dental Clinics of North America	April 2002

15. Extent and Nature of Circulation			Average No. Copies Each Issue During Preceding 12 Months	No. Copies of Single Issue Published Nearest to Filing Date
a.	Total Number of Copies (*Net press run*)		3725	2800
b. Paid and/or Requested Circulation	(1)	Paid/Requested Outside-County Mail Subscriptions Stated on Form 3541. (*Include advertiser's proof and exchange copies*)	2042	1835
	(2)	Paid In-County Subscriptions Stated on Form 3541 (*Include advertiser's proof and exchange copies*)		
	(3)	Sales Through Dealers and Carriers, Street Vendors, Counter Sales, and Other Non-USPS Paid Distribution	407	368
	(4)	Other Classes Mailed Through the USPS		
c.	Total Paid and/or Requested Circulation [*Sum of 15b. (1), (2), (3), and (4)*] ▶		2449	2203
d. Free Distribution by Mail (*Samples, complimentary, and other free*)	(1)	Outside-County as Stated on Form 3541	78	82
	(2)	In-County as Stated on Form 3541		
	(3)	Other Classes Mailed Through the USPS		
e.	Free Distribution Outside the Mail (*Carriers or other means*)			
f.	Total Free Distribution (*Sum of 15d. and 15e.*) ▶		78	82
g.	Total Distribution (*Sum of 15c. and 15f.*) ▶		2527	2285
h.	Copies not Distributed		748	515
i.	Total (*Sum of 15g. and h.*) ▶		3275	2800
j.	Percent Paid and/or Requested Circulation (*15c. divided by 15g. times 100*)		97%	96%

16. Publication of Statement of Ownership

Publication required. Will be printed in the **October 2002** issue of this publication.   Publication not required

17. Signature and Title of Editor, Publisher, Business Manager, or Owner   Date

Jean M. Fanucci

John M. Fanucci, Director of Subscription Services   9/15/02

I certify that all information furnished on this form is true and complete. I understand that anyone who furnishes false or misleading information on this form or who omits material or information requested on the form may be subject to criminal sanctions (including fines and imprisonment) and/or civil sanctions (including civil penalties).

Instructions to Publishers

1. Complete and file one copy of this form with your postmaster annually on or before October 1. Keep a copy of the completed form for your records.
2. In cases where the stockholder or security holder is a trustee, include in items 10 and 11 the name of the person or corporation for whom the trustee is acting. Also include the names and addresses of individuals who are stockholders who own or hold 1 percent or more of the total amount of bonds, mortgages, or other securities of the publishing corporation. In item 11, if none, check the box. Use blank sheets if more space is required.
3. Be sure to furnish all circulation information called for in item 15. Free circulation must be shown in items 15d, e, and f.
4. Item 15h., Copies not Distributed, must include (1) newsstand copies originally stated on Form 3541, and returned to the publisher, (2) estimated returns from news agents, and (3), copies for office use, leftovers, spoiled, and all other copies not distributed.
5. If the publication had Periodicals authorization as a general or requester publication, this Statement of Ownership, Management, and Circulation must be published; it must be printed in any issue in October or, if the publication is not published during October, the first issue printed after October.
6. In item 16, indicate the date of the issue in which this Statement of Ownership will be published.
7. Item 17 must be signed.

Failure to file or publish a statement of ownership may lead to suspension of Periodicals authorization.